Combination Therapies

Biological Response Modifiers in the
Treatment of Cancer and
Infectious Diseases

Combination Therapies

Biological Response Modifiers in the Treatment of Cancer and Infectious Diseases

Edited by
Allan L. Goldstein

The George Washington University School of Medicine
Washington, D.C.

and
Enrico Garaci

University of Rome
"Tor Vergata"
Rome, Italy

Sponsored by The Institute for Advanced Studies in Immunology and Aging

Springer Science+Business Media, LLC

Library of Congress Cataloging-in-Publication Data

Combination therapies : biological response modifiers in the treatment
  of cancer and infectious diseases / edited by Allan L. Goldstein and
  Enrico Garaci ; sponsored by the Institute for Advanced Studies in
  Immunology and Aging.
        p.   cm.
    Proceedings of the First International Symposium on Combination
  Therapies, held March 14-15, 1991, in Washington, D.C.
    Includes bibliographical references and index.
    ISBN 978-1-4613-6472-6   ISBN 978-1-4615-3340-5 (eBook)
    DOI 10.1007/978-1-4615-3340-5
    1. Biological response modifiers--Congresses. 2. Cancer-
  -Treatment--Congresses. 3. Communicable diseases--Treatment-
  -Congresses. 4. Chemotherapy, Combination--Congresses.
  I. Goldstein, Allan L. II. Garaci, E. (Enrico) III. Institute for
  Advanced Studies in Immunology & Aging. IV. International Symposium
  on Combination Therapies (1st : 1991 : Washington, D.C.)
    [DNLM: 1. Biological Response Modifiers--congresses. 2. Combined
  Modality ·Therapy--congresses. 3. Communicable Diseases--therapy-
  -congresses. 4. Drug Therapy, Combination--congresses.
  5. Immunotherapy--congresses. 6. Neoplasms--therapy--congresses.
  WB 330 C731 1991]
  RC271.B53C66 1992
  615'.704--dc20
  DNLM/DLC
  for Library of Congress   91-45507
                                                                CIP

Proceedings of the First International Symposium on Combination Therapies:
New and Emerging Uses for Biological Response Modifiers in the Treatment
of Cancer and Infectious Diseases, held March 14–15, 1991, in Washington, D.C.

ISBN 978-1-4613-6472-6

PREFACE

Over the past decade many of the key lymphokines, hormones and growth factors that help regulate the immune system have been defined. These molecules, termed biological response modifiers (BRMs), have been sequenced, synthesized and produced in large enough quantities to test in animals and humans resulting in the development of new approaches to the treatment of human disease, in particular, cancers and infectious diseases. Advances in this area have also led to rethinking therapies against a range of autoimmune disorders and other diseases associated with immune and endocrine imbalances. BRMs currently are being applied clinically as both primary and adjunctive therapy to enhance the effectiveness of traditional treatments by maximizing their activities and to protect critical tissues against intolerable chemotherapeutic and radiation damage.

Present constraints against the use of BRMs revolve around the nature of these substances in vivo, where many of their actions and the majority of their interactions and synergies remain to be elucidated. For example, as these molecules are thought to exert their effects locally, the systemic administration of lymphokines, cytokines and growth factors at doses adequate to produce a wanted anti-tumor effect in many instances is intolerably toxic. Efforts to overcome this formidable problem have led scientists to begin to explore the transfer of genes known to encode for these molecules into cells which otherwise inadequately elicit or produce anti-tumor or anti-infective responses.

The decade of the 1990's offers prospects for the integration of immune augmentation and hematopoietic and gene regulation that will have broad implications for both basic scientists and clinical investigators. The majority of BRMs appear to be central to normal cellular functions which, when dysregulated by the effects of an infectious agent or the unknown events leading to the formation of neoplasia, themselves exacerbate the disease process. The cautious use of BRMs in human disease conditions and the newly emerging data suggesting that BRMs may synergize are expanding knowledge of their use and, at the same time, opening windows on the underlying mechanisms utilized by neoplasia and infectious agents to evade destruction by the immune system. The growing ability to intervene in these dysfunctions with one or more BRMs in combination with the other BRMs or conventional therapies is rapidly expanding the body of knowledge concerning the ways in which the immune system is regulated.

To advance the understanding of the role of BRMs in these schemes, the first International Symposium on Combination Therapies was held on March 14 and 15, 1991, at The George Washington University in Washington, D.C., sponsored by the Institute for Advanced Studies in Immunology and Aging in collaboration with the George Washington University School of Medicine and the University of Rome "Tor Vergata." The symposium brought together outstanding international researchers with a variety of diverse interests in the field of BRMs. The program included reports of experimental and clinical work in cancer and infectious diseases, as well as basic research elucidating the ever-widening range of BRMs. The book is divided into 5 sections.

The first section of the book details several of the preliminary results of novel clinical approaches by Drs. Garaci, Gale and Fefer using BRMs in combination with either chemotherapy or bone marrow cells in the treatment of far advanced cancers and as a means to reduce relapses following bone marrow transplantation. This section also includes an important chapter by Weinstein on new concepts for designing and analyzing experiments utilizing combination therapies.

The second section of the book reports on clinical progress in the use of BRMs alone and in combination with conventional therapies in the treatment of renal cell carcinoma, malignant melanoma, breast cancer, lung cancer, multiple myeloma, colorectal carcinoma, head and neck cancer and a number of other advanced cancers. This section would be of particular interest to clinicians who are interested in the toxicities, pharmacokinetics and possible applications of single and/or combined BRM therapies in the treatment of refractory malignancies after intensive chemotherapy.

The third section of the book deals with the use of BRMs as therapy for viral infections. Therapy of cancers and chronic viral infections share many problems which are being elucidated by advanced technology and the rapidly expanding knowledge of immune mechanisms. As well as proving valuable against a range of cancers, BRMs are being studied as primary and adjunctive therapy and for prevention of viral and fungal infections.

One example of this growing knowledge is seen in the chapter by Cassone that describes the BRM-like properties of two protein constituents of Candida albicans, one of which causes T cell proliferation, while the other appears to be responsible for the opposite effect. The production of cytokines in Candida infection, once thought to be caused by monocytes, was described as due to the stimulatory antigen moiety of the pathogen.

Novel studies reported in this section include the report by Lopez Berenstein of the use of liposomal constructs for the treatment of systemic fungal infections and that of Hsia documenting the potential use of aspirin as a BRM by virtue of its action in inhibiting prostaglandin production by the macrophage resulting in upregulation of T-cells. The synergism between many anti-HIV drugs and the targeting of several of the viruses' life cycle stages will allow lower doses of any one drug, which should result in lower toxicity and better outcomes than those obtained by single drugs directed against one site.

The use of the thiol immunomodulator, DTC and the cyanoaziridine compound, Imexon, was described by Hersh as being able to prevent the development of disease in MAIDS (murine retrovirus-induced immunodeficiency and to reverse infection when administered later. The substances were shown to be synergistic with AZT in clinical trials of patients with symptomatic HIV infection and caused improvement across a wide range of symptoms. The treated patients were reported to have had a significant reduction of opportunistic infections.

Several interesting chapters in this session featured the use of various thymic hormones. One by Ershler describes the use of thymosin alpha 1 as an adjuvant which has been shown to enable elderly persons to respond to influenza vaccine. Vaccines cannot "take" in many older persons because of their decreased ability to produce various T cell cytokines and thus, antibodies. A Phase II study using thymosin alpha 1 in patients with chronic, active hepatitis B infection was described by Mutchnick. Seventy-five percent of patients treated with thymosin alpha 1 as opposed to 25 percent of controls achieved complete remission for as long as 2 years of follow-up. This compares very favorably with α interferon where less than a 40% response rate is seen. In addition, there was no toxicity or significant side effects of thymosin treatment.

The fourth section of the book analyzes what is known about the mechanism of action of BRMs. Several interesting papers discussed new approaches based upon the modulation of immune responses. For example, differences in response rates to standard chemotherapeutic and radiation regimens are well known, with a percentage of patients achieving and remaining in remission, while others relapse. Harris detailed the differences in tumorcidal function by macrophages and monocytes; when the cells of patients with ovarian and non-small cell lung cancers and those with endometritis and non-malignant lung disease are stimulated by a battery of growth factors and lymphokines, those with cancers were found to have significantly less activity. The apparently abnormal tumorcidal activities of cells from cancer patients could be overcome by a mouse monoclonal antibody directed against the CD3 epitope, by co-cultivation with allogenic lymphocytes and by the addition of indomethacin, a prostaglandin antagonist.

In his chapter Schreiber explores the possible relationship of the expression of Fcγ receptors on cells of the monocyte/macrophage lineage with several human autoimmune disorders, as well as with the response to therapy and relapse of cancer patients. A number of Fcγ receptor genes have now been cloned, and as their mechanisms of action are defined, these may be candidates for gene transfers to enhance the activities of this important domain of IgG.

The chapters in the fifth section of the book are more experimental and discussed future directions using animal models to better define effective combination therapies with BRMs. In this session Favalli provided the rationale for further human therapeutic approaches using thymic hormones, IL-2 and α interferon in combination with chemotherapy. Several interesting chapters in this section outline additional uses of BRMs in the treatment of cancer and in infectious diseases. Wiltrout presented an overview of cytokine based combination modality approaches in the treatment of murine renal cancer. Novel pre-clinical approaches with triazine compounds were also discussed in this section.

The conclusion of the symposium left participants with much to consider. Old approaches to vaccines as only preventives and to the reduction of microbial and cancer burdens with drugs with dose-limiting toxicities clearly are beginning to yield to advanced BRM therapies to enhance the body's own immune and anti-tumor defenses. The use of the many known BRMs as primary therapy and as adjuncts to current regimes is being approached with caution, however, and the participants emphasized that, as exciting as many of these are in theory, to date gains are modest, with small incremental improvements to be expected as knowledge and experience accumulates. However, all agreed that this is the area of study and experimentation from which enormous improvements in the treatment of important diseases -- cancers, infections and autoimmune conditions -- are most likely to come in the near future.

This volume should provide a good overview of current and projected clinical applications of BRMs that are currently being explored in this very new and exciting area of biomedicine. The volume should be of great interest to all scientists and clinicians currently working in this area as well as for those interested in catching up with the most recent developments in this very rapidly moving and exciting new field.

A.L. Goldstein
E. Garaci

CONTENTS

PART IV - MECHANISM OF ACTION AND SYNERGY BETWEEN DRUGS, BIOLOGICAL RESPONSE MODIFIERS, AND/OR VACCINES IN COMBINATION THERAPIES

PART V - PROSPECTS AND FUTURE DIRECTIONS USING ANIMAL MODELS TO DEFINE EFFECTIVE COMBINATION THERAPIES WITH BIOLOGICAL RESPONSE MODIFIERS

COMBINATION THERAPY WITH THYMIC HORMONES AND CYTOKINES AFTER CHEMOTHERAPY IN CANCER TREATMENT

Enrico Garaci and Cartesio Favalli

Department of Experimental Medicine and
Biochemical Sciences, University of Rome
"Tor Vergata" , 00173 Rome, Italy

INTRODUCTION

Although there is general agreement on the central role of immune anti-tumoral defences and on the possibility of using immunopotentiating substances in tumor therapy, the clinical use of these substances has not produced the expected results. Thus an amount of skepticism has arisen about the therapeutical potentiality of the immunostimulating substances and about the importance of the immune system itself towards neoplasia [1,2,3]

Among the immunomodulators at our disposal, the substances of physiologic origin are certainly the most interesting and include the interleukins (ILs)[4,5,6] the interferons (IFNs) [7,8],the thymic hormones (THs) [9,10], the tumor necrosis factors (TNFs) [11], the colony stimulating factors (CSFs) etc. These cytokines are physiologically involved in the regulation of the ontogenesis and of the activation of different immune cells and are characterized by a certain selectivity of action. Because of their powerful effects on the immune response and their availability in considerable quantities by the DNA recombinant technique and by chemical synthesis, they are under intense experimental and clinic investigations [12,13,14,15,16,17]. Although results have been encouraging, when applied alone, these substances display only restricted efficacy. This is to be attributed to numerous and, as yet, not well defined factors, including the possibility of tumor cell resistance to cytokines [18]. This phenomenon has, in fact, been demonstrated by several authors who described a resistance of tumor cells to cytokines treatment. This resistance could be attributable either to non-responsiveness of host killer cells to cytokines stimulating action, or to tumor cells resistance to the direct toxic effects of cytokines. However, it seems that a single cytokine is not able to arrest tumoral progression [19]. Consequently many research groups are trying the route of combination therapies with more cytokines, with or without chemotherapy [20,21,26].

Our research group has been studying the combination among immunomodulators and in particular among THs combined with IFN and interleukin 2 for several years [22,23,24,25,26,27]. In this chapter we report part of

Combination Therapies, Edited by A.L. Goldstein and
E. Garaci, Plenum Press, New York, 1992

the results of our studies by using Thymosin α1 (Tα1) in combination with IFN in the control of tumor growth in experimental animal models. Moreover, here we report the characteristics and the preliminary results of two pilot clinical studies in inoperable, stage III & IV, non small cell lung carcinoma (NSCLC) and in metastatic melanoma patients.

EFFECTS OF COMBINATION BETWEEN THYMIC HORMONES AND INTERFERON IN EXPERIMENTAL ANIMAL MODELS

The first evidence for a synergistic effect between THs and IFNs on the immune response dates back to a few years ago, when we demonstrated that Tα1, a well identified and extensively studied synthetic thymic hormone [28], and murine α-ß IFN are able to induce the stimulation of natural killer (NK) activity in animals immunodepressed by means of cyclophosphamide (CY). These experiments demonstrated that, as one expected, a single injection of IFN αß (3 x 10^4 IU/mouse, i.p.) significantly stimulated NK activity in normal animals, while the same treatment could not stimulate such an activity in animals inoculated 4 days before with CY. On the other hand, when IFN was administered after a pre-treatment with Tα1, no further increase in NK activity was observed in normal mice, while a significant stimulation in CY-suppressed mice was observed [22]. More recently we have demonstrated that a combined treatment with Tα1 and IFN αß, can powerfully stimulate NK activity in B-16 melanoma tumor-bearing, immunodepressed animals. In this study we observed that during the growth of experimental tumors, animals develop a state of non-responsiveness to the treatment with IFN alone, which is correlated to the growth of tumor burdens, and which can be restored by pretreatment with THs[23].

Since it has been demonstrated that cytotoxic killer cells play an important role in host defence against tumors, we examined the possible correlation between cytotoxic activities and the effect on tumor growth. The results of these studies have shown that a certain slowing-down in B16 Melanoma or Lewis Lung carcinoma (3LL) tumor growth could be obtained when IFN treatment was, in any one case, preceeded by Tα1 injections and combination treatment was started in an early phase after tumor implantation. Utilizing regimen of combination treatments with Tα1 and IFN, according to the above mentioned

Table 1. Hypotheses on the synergy between chemotherapy and immunotherapy

----

1) increased immunosensitivity of the tumor cells which have been partially damaged by chemotherapy treatment;
2) increased chemosensitivity of the tumor cells which were not irreversibly damaged by immune response;
3) increase of the immunogenicity of tumor cells;
4) positive modulation by the drug of the host immune response by eliminating for example part of T suppressor cells;
5) release of chemotactic factors for phagocytic and cytotoxic cells by tumor cells damaged by chemotherapeutic treatment

----

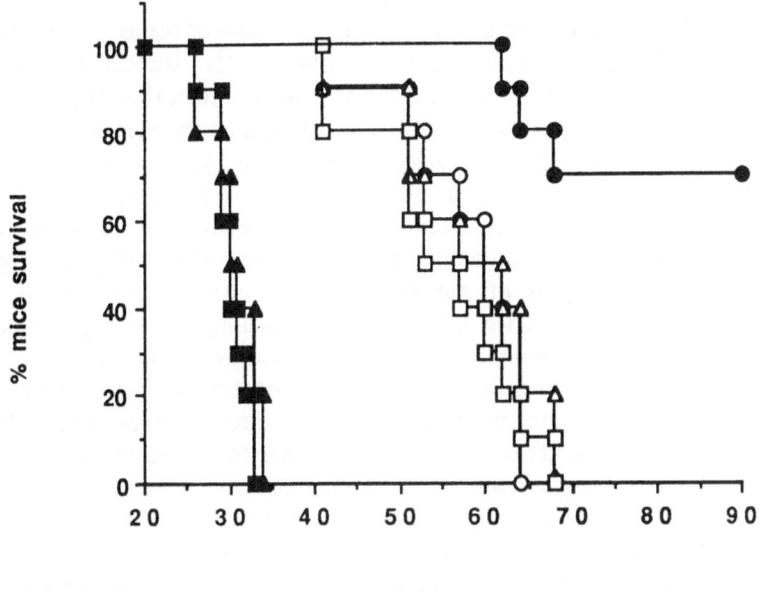

Fig.1 Effect of combined chemoimmunotherapy treatment on the survival of 3LL-bearing mice. Mice were injected s.c. with 3LL tumor cells on day 0. ■ untreated mice, ▲ mice treated with Tα1 on days 1-4 plus IFN on day 4, ○ CY on day 8, △ CY on day 8 and Tα1 on days 10-13, □ CY on day 8 and IFN on day 13, ● CY on day 8 and Tα1 on days 10-13 plus IFN on day 13.

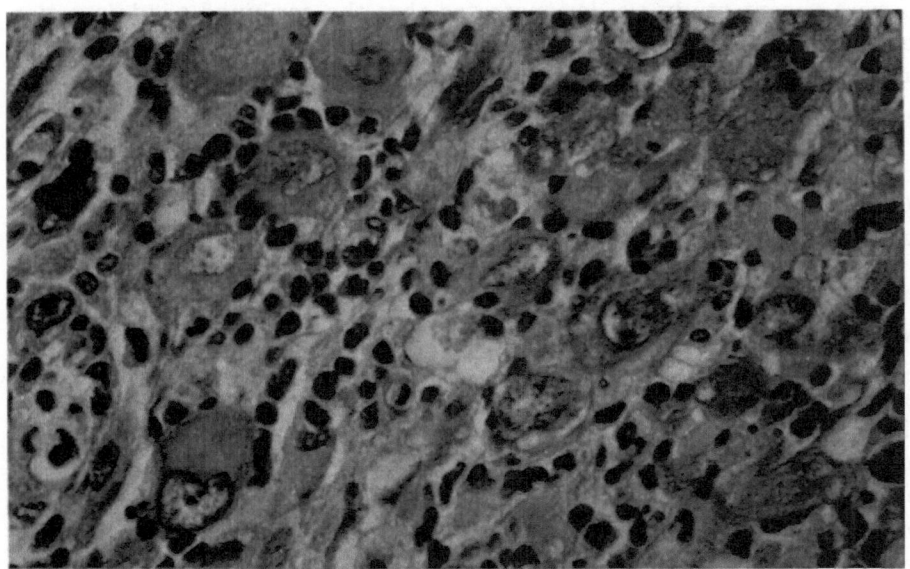

Fig.2 Histological analysis of the effect of combined chemoimmunotherapy treatment (CY on day 8 after 3LL tumor inoculation, plus Tα1 on days 10-13 and IFN on day 13). A tumor cell completely surrounded by lymphoid cells is shown.

criteria, we were able, indeed, to also obtain an increase of animal survival time but, in no case has long-term survival been obtained [25]. During the past few years it has been evident that immunotherapy and chemotherapy could act synergistically. Even if the mechanisms involved in this synergic effect are still unknown, several hypoteses can be formulated (Table 1).

We have thus attempted to establish if Tα1 and IFN combination treatment could prove more effective if administered with chemotherapy. The results of this study demonstrated that the combination treatment with Tα1 (200 μg/Kg) for four days, followed by a single injection of murine IFN αß (3 x 10^4 IU/mouse), starting two days after CY treatment (200 mg/Kg, single injection) caused the disappearance of tumors in a high percentage of mice bearing Lewis lung carcinoma (3LL). The chemoimmunotherapy protocol was effective even on the long-term survival. In fact we have observed a high percentage (75%) of living, tumor-free mice even after 60 days after tumor inoculation. Results were significantly different when compared to those obtained in mice treated with the single agents at the same doses and time of administration in conjunction with chemotherapy (Tα1 = 35% of survival; IFN = 10% of survival) or to chemotherapy itself (10% of survival)[26] (Fig.1). In order to explain the mechanism of the antitumoral action, immunological studies were carried out. The results of these experiments have shown that the same regimen utilized in controlling the tumor growth was able to strongly stimulate the cytotoxicity against NK-sensitive YAC-1 target cells and cytotoxicity against NK-resistant autologus 3LL tumor cells, in 3LL tumor bearing mice, whereas treatments with each agent singularly did not or only slightly modified the cytotoxic activity towards both YAC-1 and 3LL target cells. The killer cells stimulated by chemoimmunotherapy combination treatment bear the phenotypic characteristics of asialo GM1 positive cells. A histological study has shown a high number of infiltrating lymphoid cells in tumors obtained from mice treated with combination chemoimmunotherapy [26] (Fig.2).

In a more recent study we demonstrated that the combined administration with Tα1, plus IL-2, after CY treatment, was much more effective than either BRMs alone and induced a complete tumor regression in 100% of mice studied. Combination immunotherapy alone without CY caused only a slight slowing of the rate of tumor growth. The combined chemoimmunotherapy with CY and Tα1 plus IL-2 also increased the cytotoxicity of spleen cells and markedly enhanced long-term survival in all treated animals. The results of these experiments are reported in details by Favalli et al. in another chapter of this book.

EFFECTS OF COMBINATION BETWEEN THYMIC HORMONES AND INTERFERON IN CANCER PATIENTS

The results of the experiments on the effect of combination therapy with chemotherapeutic agents and Tα1 plus IFN in tumor bearing mice, proved to be very encouraging and indicated that such treatment regimens could be easily transferred to clinical practice since additional side effects caused by immunotherapy were not expected in humans. We have thus decided to extend our studies on combination chemoimmunotherapy to humans. For ethical reasons and in order to compare the results obtained with a combination chemoimmunotherapy treatment to those obtained with chemotherapy alone, we selected two neoplastic diseases, quite common and quite refractary to chemotherapy alone treatment. These neoplastic diseases are also characterized by the fact that no other treatment other than chemotherapy can be reasonably proposed to the patients. Moreover, standard chemotherapy regimens were not altered, but the combination immunotherapy treatment was inserted between the courses of chemotherapy itself. These clinical studies are in progress at the moment, and here we report their characteristics and some preliminary results. In particular we are performing two pilot clinical studies in inoperable, stage III & IV, non small cell lung carcinoma (NSCLC) and in metastatic melanoma patients. The main objectives of these studies are: 1) the evaluation of systemic effects of combination therapy with Tα1 plus IFN in association with chemotherapy on the immune response in NSCLC and metastatic melanoma patients; 2) the evaluation of the possibility that immunotherapy with Tα1 plus IFN could potentiate the effect of chemotherapy in NSCLC and metastatic melanoma patients. The characteristics of the patients selected for the studies are reported in table 2. We are able at the moment to report the results obtained in the first evaluated twelve melanoma patients, while the evaluation of NSCLC patients is still in progress. Treatment schedule for NSCLC patients consists of cisplatin 20 mg/mq i.v. on days 1 to 5 , etoposide 100 mg/mq i.v. on days 1 to 5, Tα1 1mg s.c. on days 8 to 11 and 15 to 18, natural α-IFN 3M U.I. i.m. on days 11 and 18. Courses are repeated every 28 days for six months or until disease progression. Treatment schedule for metastatic melanoma patients

Table 2.   Characteristics of the patients enrolled for the clinical studies on the effectof the combination between thymic hormones plus interferon and chemotherapy.

PATIENTS
NUMBER
            NSCLC: 60 of both sex at the end of the study
            Melanoma: 30 of both sex at the end of the study

DIAGNOSIS
            histologically confirmed inoperable nor eligible
            for radiation therapy, eligible for chemotherapy,
            stage III & IV NSCLC.
            Mestastatic melanoma with measurable cutaneous,
            nodals or viscerals metastases, unresectable nor
            eligible for radiation therapy.

PERFORMANCE
SCORE   0-2 Eastern Cooperative Oncology Group (ECOG)
            or >70 Karnofsky index;
            life expectancy > 3 months.

PRIOR
TREATMENT   none of patients received other treatment than
            surgery or radiation therapy.

----

consists of dacarbazine (DTIC) 200 mg/mq i.v. on days 1 through 4, Tα1 1mg s.c. on days 8 through 11 and 15 through 18, natural α-interferon 3M U.I. i.m. on days 11 and 18. Also with these patients courses are repeated every 28 days for six times or until disease progression. Five of the evaluated melanoma patients observed until now, received, as thymic hormone, the synthetic pentapeptide thymopentin instead of Tα1, at the dose of 50 mg s.c., according to the same regimen described above. Each patient underwent a thorough medical and immunological evaluation before therapy, and after at least 3 cycles of treatment. Immunological monitoring consists of flow cytometry analysis of peripheral blood lymphocyte subsets and testing cytotoxic activity against NK-sensitive and, in some cases, NK-resistant target cell lines. The toxicity is established according to WHO grading criteria. A response is considered to be complete (CR) if all measurable tumors disappear and to be partial (PR) if the sum of the products of the longest perpendicular diameters of all lesions decreases by at least 50% and if no tumor has any increase and no new tumors appear. Less than 50% decrease or no appreciable modification of the lesions is considered as a no change (NC). The management of the NSCLC patients is performed in collaboration with Dr. M. Lopez (Regina Elena Istitute for Cancer Research, Rome), Dr. M. D'Aprile and Dr. F. Angelini (S.M. Goretti Hospital, Latina), and Dr. G. Bonsignore (Respiratory Phisiopathology Institute of C.N.R., Palermo). The management of the melanoma patients is performed in collaboration with Dr. E. Terzoli and Dr. F. Izzo (Regina Elena Istitute for Cancer Research, Rome).

No major side effects attributable to the immunotherapy have been observed up until now in patients affected by both the neoplastic diseases, and treated with the new chemoimmunotherapy regimens. Toxicity, as expected, has been evident in the same percentage of patients and with the same features as in patients treated with chemotherapy alone. About 20% of the patients presented a light and transient fever enhancement with myalgias, attributable to IFN treatment. No side effects or toxicity attributable to thymic hormones were observed. The immunological monitoring of the melanoma patients has shown a high variability of NK activity during the therapeutic regimen. The variability seems to be correlated to the phase of the course of treatment. The trend of these variabilities is shown in figure 3, in which the mean values of cytotoxicity detected in different phases of the first, the third and the sixth course of chemoimmunotherapy, in twelve melanoma patients are reported. Moreover, it is possible to distinguish the trend of the variability between patients who could have been considered as responder (CR+PR) to the therapy and those who could have been considered as non-responder(NC or Progression), according to the clinical evaluation criteria. The mean values were then separately cumulated for these two groups of patients. Results reported in figure 3 show a cyclic variation in the cytotoxicity, with a dramatic decline after chemotherapy and an evident boosting on day 12, i.e. after immunotherapic treatment, which occurs repeatedly during each cycle. Patients classified as non-responder seem not to be stimulated by immunotherapy whilst undergoing treatment, demonstrating a relationship between immunological response to thymic hormone plus IFN and the progression of the neoplastic disease. Similar results were obtained in NSCLC enrolled until now, in which the treatment with Tα1 plus IFN, after chemotherapy, stimulated NK response. Moreover both in Melanoma and NSCLC patients, immunotherapy treatment induced the stimulation of cytotoxic response against Daudi, NK resistant target cells, in about 20% of cases. None of patients that received only chemotherapy, or normal donors we have observed, have shown cytotoxic activity against the same target, demonstrating that combination therapy with Tα 1 and IFN is able to specifically induce, even if in a limited number of cases, this effect.

The study of CD4+ and CD8+ subpopulations, by flow cytometry, demonstrated that in patients treated with combination immunotherapy there was an increase either in percentage or in absolute number of CD4+ subpopulation, an absolute increase of CD8+ cell population, and an icrease of CD4+/CD8+ ratio.

Regarding to the clinical results, we have completed the evaluation, at at least 6 months, of the first twelve melanoma patients, while the evaluation of NSCLC is still in progress. Results obtained in melanoma patients are reported in table 3. Among the patients, treated with chemotherapy plus combination immunotherapy, evaluated up until now for response to the therapy according to the WHO criteria, the percentage of objective responses (complete responses and partial responses) is higher and remissions long lasting as compared with groups of patients previously treated by us or with results reported by other authors with similar chemotherapy or chemotherapy plus IFN alone regimens [29,30]. The results are thus promising both in terms of tolerance and efficacy of treatment. Also in NSCLC patients, the clinical results, even if preliminary,

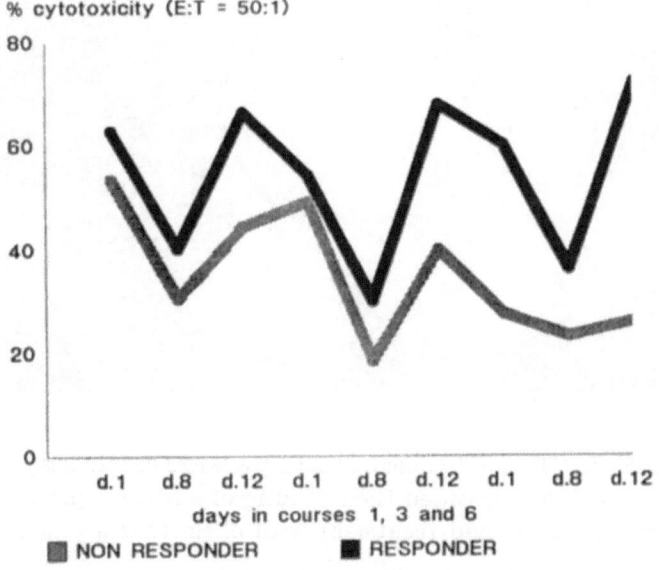

Fig.3 Natural killer activity of peripheral blood lymphocytes collected from melanoma patients treated with DTIC plus Tα1 and IFN combined chemoimmunotherapy. Results represent the cumulative mean values obtained in responder (CR+PR) or non responder (NC+Progr.) patients at days 1, 8 and 12 of the first, the third and the sixth course respectively.

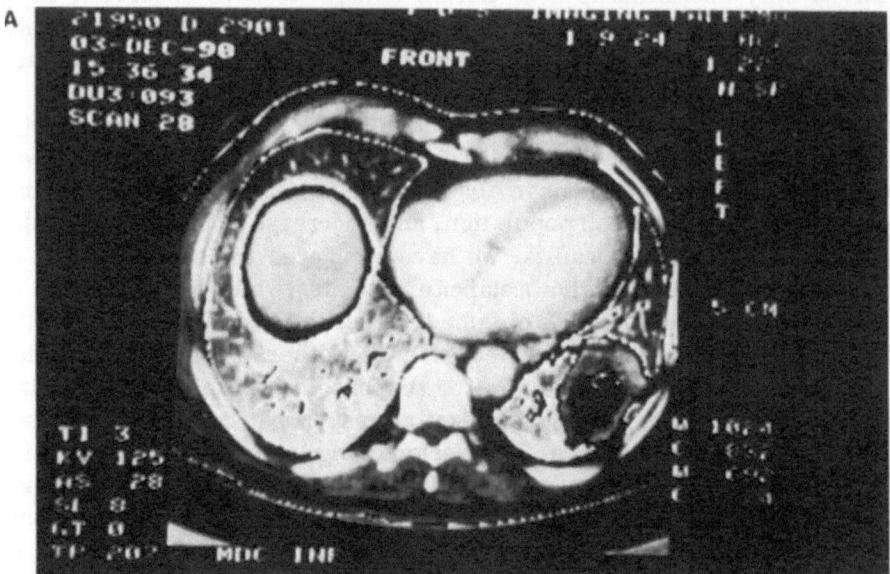

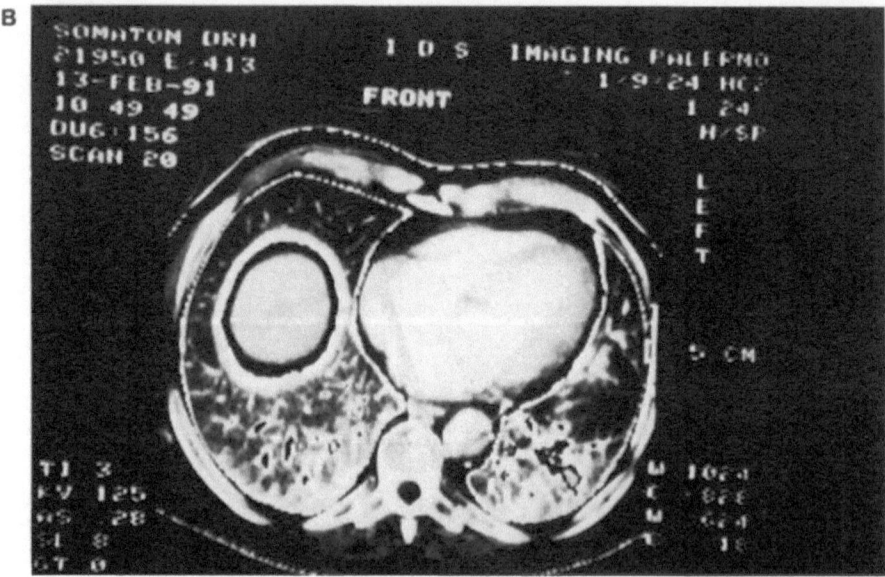

Fig. 4 A. Thoracic CT section demonstrating a large carcinoma, which has almost completely invaded the left lung of a NSCLC patient, before starting the combined treatment with chemotherapy and Tα1 plus IFN.

B. Thoracic CT section of the same patient reported in fig. 4A, after two courses of chemoimmunotherapy. The tumor mass is no more detecteble. A very small residual lesion, presumably consisting of fibrous tissue, can be observed.

Table 3. Clinical features of 12 evaluated melanoma patients.

Pat. No.	Age/ Sex	Prior Therapy	Site of Metastatic Disease	Response	Duration
°1	64/F	Surgery	Lymph nodes (sub-mandibular)	Progr.	
°2	69/F	Surgery	Lymph nodes (groin) subcutaneous (thigh)	PR	> 6
°3	74/M	Surgery	Lung	CR	> 6
°4	75/M	Surgery	Lymph nodes (axilla mandibular, neck) subcutaneous	PR	1
°5	44/F	Surgery	Lung, l. nodes, pelvic mass, subcutaneous	Progr.	
°6	47/F	Surgery	Lymph nodes (groin)	CR	6
°7	42/F	Surgery	Lymph nodes (groin)	Progr.	
*8	41/F	Surgery	Lymph nodes (axilla)	CR	> 28
*9	32/M	Surgery	Lymph nodes (axilla)	Progr.	
*10	64/M	Surgery	Lymph nodes (groin)	CR	12
*11	70/F	Surgery	Liver	Progr.	
*12	32/M	Surgery	Lymph nodes (groin)	Progr.	

° Thymosin α1
* Thymopentin

----

seem be very encouraging, since a number of responses have been observed. In some cases the response was very impressive and dramatic as shown in figures 4A and 4B.

CONCLUSIONS

Our results, obtained in experimental animal models, have demonstrated how very effective the combined treatment protocols with CY followed by thymosin α1 plus IFN or IL-2 in the control of neoplastic growth are. In fact, we submitted evidence that combined chemoimmunotherapy treatment is able to induce tumor regression without the appearance of any toxic or side effect, even if it is started when the tumor burden is developed and easily detectable. Moreover our results allow us to explain, at least in part, the mechanism by wich the combined treatments with thymosin α1 and IFN, or IL-2, exert this powerful antitumorous action in animals treated with CY. In fact, the results obtained on the stimulation of cytotoxic activity of the splenic cells against 3LL tumor cells as target cells, would seem to indicate that such stimulation might play an important role in the antitumorous mechanism of combined chemoimmunotherapy. The loss of the antitumor response following <u>in vivo</u> depletion of immune cells by irradiation or antibody treatment, clearly indicates an involvement of cells belonging to both NK and T compartments in the phenomena observed after chemoimmunotherapy treatment.

On the basis of these results, we extended our studies to humans. The immunological results are confirming that, as in experimental animal models, the combined treatment with Tα1 plus IFN strongly stimulates cytotoxic activities in NSCLC or melanoma patients treated with chemotherapy. These studies are also demonstrating that TH combined with IFN strikingly potentiate the antitumorous action of chemotherapy. The results are promising both in terms of tolerance and efficacy of treatment. However, in order to point out the importance of these results in a more definite way, we must wait for the end of our clinical trials, when a more elevated number of patients will have been enrolled and a longer observation time will have past.

Acknowledgements

This work was supported in part by Ministero dell'Università e della Ricerca Scientifica e Tecnologica (MURST).

REFERENCES

1. M. J. Mastrangelo, D. Berd, and H.C. Maguire, Current condition and prognosis of tumor immunotherapy: a second opinion. Cancer Treat. Rep. 68: 207 (1984).
2. G. Mathe', M. Kamel, M. Dezfulian, O. Halle-Pannenko, G. Bourut, An experimental screening for "systemic adjuvants of immunity" applicable in cancer immunotherapy. Cancer Res. 33:1987 (1973).
3. E. Mihich. Relationship between chemotherapy and immunotherapy: a brief overview, in: "Rationale of Biologcal response modifiers in cancer treatment," E. Tsubura, I. Urushizaki, T. Aoki, eds., p.105, Excerpta Medica, Amsterdam (1985).
4. M.T. Lotze, L.W. Frana, S.O. Sharrow, R.J. Robb, and S.A. Rosenberg, In vivo administration of purified human interleukin-2. I. Half life and immunological effects of Jurkat cell-line derived interleukin-2. J. Immunol. 134: 157 (1985).
5. M.T. Lotze, Y.L. Marory, S.E. Ettinghausen, A.A. Rayner, S.O. Sharrow, C.A.Y. Seipp, M.C. Custer, and S.A. Rosenberg, In vivo administration of purified human interleukin-2. II. Half life immunologic effects and expansion of peripheral lymphoid cells in vivo with recombinant IL-2. J. Immunol. 135: 2865, (1985).
6. S.A Rosenberg, E.A. Grimm, M. Mcgrogan, M. Doyle, E. Kawasaki, and D.F. Mark, Biochemical activity of recombinant human interleukin 2 produced in Escherichia Coli. Science 223: 1412 (1984).
7. P.A. Bunn, C.D. Ihde, and K.A. Foon, The role of recombinant interferon alfa-2a. Cancer 57: 1689 (1986).
8. H.S. Jaffe, R.B. Herberman, Rationale for recombinant human

interferon-gamma adjuvant immunotherapy for cancer. J.Natl. Cancer Inst. 80: 616 (1988).

9. A.L. Goldstein, and R.S. Schulof, Thymosins in the treatment of cancer, in: "Immunity to cancer," A.E. Rei and M.S. Mitchell, eds, p. 469, Acad.Press Inc., Orlando (1984).

10. J.A. Hooper, M.C. McDaniel, G.B. Thurman, G.H. Cohen, R.S. Schulof, and A.L. Goldstein. Purification and properties of bovine thymosin. Ann. N.Y. Acad. Sci.,249: 125 (1975).

11. F. Dammacco, A. Vacca, S. Benvestito, G. Pantaleo, Tumor necrosis factor: biologic and immunochemical properties and potential therapeutic applications, in: "Recent advances in autoimmunity and tumor immunology", F. Dammacco, ed., p.157, Edi-Ermes, Milano (1988).

12. M.H. Cohen, P.B. Chretien, D.C. Ihde, et al. Thymosin fraction V and intensive combination chemotherapy prolonging the survival of patients with small-cell lung cancer. J. Am. Med. Assoc. 241: 1813 (1979).

13. A.F. Figlin, J.B. De Kernion, J. Maldzys, et al. Treatment of renal cell carcinoma with (human leukocyte) interferon and vinblastine in combination: a phase I-II trial: Cancer Treat. Rep. 69: 263 (1985).

14. S.D. Fossa, and S.T. De Garis, Further experience with recombinant interferon alfa-2a with vinblastine in metastatic renal cell carcinoma: a progress report. Int. J. Cancer Supplement 1: 36 (1987).

15. J.A. Neidhard, Interferon therapy for the treatment of renal cancer. Cancer 57: 1696 (1986).

16. R.J. Quesada, Biologc Response Modifiers in the therapy of metastatic renal cell carcinoma. Seminars in Oncology 15: 396 (1988).

17. R.S. Schulof, M.S. LLoyd, P.A. Cleary, S.R. Palaszynski, Mai D.A., J.W. Cox, O. Alabaster, and A.L. Goldstein, A randomized trial to evaluate the immunorestorative properties of synthetic thymosin alpha 1 in patients with lung cancer. J. Biol. Response Mod. 4: 147 (1985).

18. J.J. Killion, and I.J. Fidler, Evasion of host responses in metastasis: implications of cellular resistance to cytokines. Current Opinion in Immunology 2: 693 (1990).

19. J.W. Hadden, New strategies of immunotherapy, in: "Advances in immunomodulation," B. Bizzini and E. Bonmassar, eds., p. 327, Pythagora Press, Roma (1988).

20. C. Favalli, A. Mastino, and E. Garaci, Experimental models of chemoimmunotherapy of tumors, in: "Immunoregulation and lymphoproliferative disorders: basic and clinical aspects", F. Dammacco, ed., p.187, Edi-Ermes, Milano (1989).

21. S. Silagi, R. Dutkowski, and A. Schaefer, Eradication of mouse melanoma by combined treatment with recombinant human interleukin 2 and recombinant murine interferon-gamma, Int. J. Cancer 41: 315 (1988).

22. C. Favalli, T. Jezzi, A. Mastino, C. Rinaldi-Garaci, C. Riccardi, and E. Garaci, Modulation of natural killer activity by thymosin alpha 1 and interferon. Cancer Immunol. Immunother. 20: 189 (1985).

23. C. Favalli, A. Mastino, T. Jezzi, S. Grelli, A.L. Goldstein, and E. Garaci, Synergic effect of thymosin alpha 1 and alpha-beta interferon on NK activity in tumor-bearing mice. Int. J. Immunopharm. 11: 443 (1989).

24. E. Garaci, A. Mastino, T. Jezzi, and C. Favalli, Thymic hormones and cytokines: a synergystic combination with high therapeutic potentialities. In: "Recent advances in autoimmunity and tumor immunology," F. Dammacco, ed., p.211, Edi-Ermes, Milano (1988).

25.E. Garaci, A. Mastino, and C. Favalli, Enhanced immune response and antitumor immunity with combinations of biological response modifiers. Bull. N.Y. Acad. Med. 65: 111 (1989).

26. E. Garaci, A. Mastino, F. Pica, and C. Favalli, Combination treatment using Thymosin α 1 and interferon after cyclophosphamide is able to cure Lewis lung carcinoma in mice. Cancer Immunol. Immunother. , 32: 154 (1990).

27. A. Mastino, C. Favalli, S. Grelli, F. Innocenti, and E. Garaci, Thymosin α 1 potentiates interleukin 2-induced cytotoxic activity in mice, Cell. Immunol., 133: 196 (1991).

28. A.L. Goldstein, T.L. Low, M. Adoo, J. Mc Clure, G.B. Thurman, G. Rossio, C.Y. Lay, D. Chang, S.S. Wang, C. Harwey, A.H. Ramel, and J. Meienhofer, Thymosin alpha 1: isolation and sequence analysis of an immunologically active thymic polypeptide. Proc. Natl. Acad. Sci. 74: 725 (1977).

29. D.A. Vorobiof, G. Falkson, C.W. Voges, DTIC versus DTIC and recombinant interferon alpha 2b (2IFNα2b) in the treatment of patients with advanced melanoma, Proc.Am.Soc.Clin.Oncol., 8: 2 (1989).

30. S.S. Legha, Current therapy for malignant melanomas, Sem. Oncol., 16 (suppl. 1): 34 (1989).

IMMUNE THERAPY OF HUMAN CANCERS*

Robert Peter Gale and Anna Butturini

Department of Medicine, Division of Hematology-Oncology, UCLA
School of Medicine, University of California, Los Angeles, California
90024-1678 and Department of Pediatrics, Division of Hematology and
Oncology, University of Parma, Parma 43100, Italy

ABSTRACT

There is considerable controversy whether the immune system is important in controlling
human cancers. We review data regarding leukemia control in recipients of bone marrow
transplants. These data indicate that several distinct immune-mediated anti-leukemia
mechanisms operate. We consider how these mechanisms might be used to treat human
cancers.

Considerable data in animal models suggest a role for the immune system in controlling
cancer (for review see[1,2]). However, most experimental models differ substantially from
human cancers. Experimental tumors are often immunogenic because of tumor-related or
-specific antigens such as histocompatibility antigens or virus or chemical induced antigens.
In contrast, there is little evidence of tumor-specific antigens in human cancers. Growth
characteristics and other biologic features of experimental tumors also differ considerably
from those of most human cancers. For example, retroviruses cause most leukemias in
animals; this seems not so in humans.

Convincing evidence of a role of the immune system in most human cancers is lacking.
It is also not certain that tumors in humans evoke an immune response. For example,
persons with immune deficiency disorders are not at increased risk to develop age-related
cancers. More often, they develop B-cell related leukemia or lymphoma from uncontrolled
Epstein-Barr virus (EBV) proliferation or multifocal polyclonal cancers, like Kaposi
sarcoma, from uncontrolled growth factor production by HIV-1 infected cells.[3] Additional
examples are transplant recipients and persons with autoimmune disorders receiving immune
suppressive drugs.[4,5] These persons are not at increased risk to develop age-related cancers
but rather skin cancers, Kaposi sarcoma and lymphomas preferentially involving the central

---

* Address correspondence and reprint requests to: Robert Peter Gale, MD, PhD, Department
of Medicine, Division of Hematology-Oncology, UCLA School of Medicine, Los Angeles,
CA 90024-1678, USA. TEL: 213-825-9677 (x803) FAX: 213-206-5511

Combination Therapies, Edited by A.L. Goldstein and
E. Garaci, Plenum Press, New York, 1992

nervous system. Furthermore, over the past 50 years extensive trials of immune therapy in human cancers showed no convincing benefit (for reviews see[2]). Although some recent immune therapy trials seem promising,[6,7] it is uncertain whether the benefit observed results from immune mechanisms.

Because bone marrow transplants can be envisioned as an extreme approach to immune therapy, we studied whether anti-cancer immune mechanisms operate in this setting. Transplants were developed as a way to give high-dose chemotherapy and/or radiation pretransplant. In many instances, especially leukemias, transplants are associated with fewer relapses compared to chemotherapy.[8,9] However, it soon became apparent that intensive pretransplant therapy could not completely explain the increased anti-leukemia efficacy of transplants. For example, persons with and without graft-versus-host disease (GvHD) had different probabilities of leukemia recurrence despite receiving similar pretransplant chemotherapy and/or radiation.[10] Also, diverse posttransplant immune suppression, such as with methotrexate or cyclosporine, resulted in different leukemia relapse rates.[10,11]

Additional data support the notion of immune-mediated anti-leukemia effects. Several years ago we and others reported an increased probability of relapse in recipients of transplants from genetically-identical twins.[12,13] Although some of this effect might result from absence of GvHD, relapse risk was increased even when compared to recipients of HLA-identical sibling transplants without GvHD.[14] Most recently, we reported increased relapses in some recipients of T-cell depleted transplants even after adjusting for GvHD.[15] Here we review these data indicating different likelihoods of leukemia eradication in persons receiving comparable pretransplant high-dose chemotherapy and radiation. These data are the most convincing evidence that the immune system operates in human cancers. Whether these immune-mediated effects operate when donor and recipient are genetically-identical, whether they are active in cancers other than leukemia, and whether they can be used in non-transplant settings requires further study.

Relative risks of leukemia relapse among over 2000 recipients of HLA-identical sibling transplants reported to the International Bone Marrow Transplant Registry (IBMTR) are reviewed in Table 1.[16] The data indicate that acute and chronic GvHD significantly decrease relapse risk in acute lymphoblastic leukemia (ALL), acute myelogenous leukemia (AML) and chronic myelogenous leukemia (CML). Data in Table 1 also indicate that T-cell depletion increases the likelihood of relapse, especially in CML. This increased risk is only partially explained by the corresponding decrease in GvHD associated with T-cell depletion. Results of transplants between genetically-identical twins are also reviewed in Table 1. These data indicate an increased relative risk of relapse even after adjusting for GvHD.

In additional analyses in recipients of HLA-identical sibling transplants, the IBMTR reported that alternate forms of posttransplant immune suppression were associated with different risks of leukemia relapse in persons with ALL.[17,18]. This correlation remained after adjusting for GvHD. Risk of relapse was greatest with cyclosporine, intermediate with cyclosporine and minimal doses of methotrexate, and least with relatively higher doses of methotrexate. Whether it results from a direct anti-leukemia effect of methotrexate or from inhibition of an immune-mediated anti-leukemia effect by cyclosporine is uncertain.

The data reviewed suggest that multiple immune-mediated anti-leukemia mechanisms operate in transplants. One is an anti-leukemia effect of GvHD. A similar effect is well documented in experimental models (reviewed in[19]). This effect is most likely directed against disparate non-HLA histocompatibility antigens on leukemia cells; qualitative or quantitative abnormalities in HLA-antigens may sometimes be involved.[20-23] Most data

Table 1. Relative Risk of Relapse after Transplants[1,2]

	ALL		AML		CML	
	RR	P	RR	P	RR	P
HLA-Identical						
No GvHD	1.00	—	1.00	—	1.00	—
Acute GvHD only	0.36	0.004	0.78	0.26	1.15	0.75
Chronic GvHD only	0.44	0.16	0.48	0.12	0.28	0.16
Both	0.38	0.02	0.34	0.0003	0.24	0.03
HLA-Identical, T-depleted						
No GvHD	1.48	0.33	1.57	0.33	6.91	0.0001
Acute and Chronic GvHD	0.98	0.97	0.80	0.60	4.45	0.003
Twins	0.99	0.99	2.58	0.008	2.95	0.08

[1] Adapted from reference 16.
[2] ALL, acute lymphoblastic leukemia; AML, acute myelogenous leukemia; CML, chronic myelogenous leukemia. ALL and AML in 1st remission; CML in chronic phase. GvHD, graft-versus-host disease.

suggest this GvHD-related anti-leukemia effect is mediated by T-cells.[2,19] There are no convincing data that this effect is leukemia-specific.

These data also suggest a second distinct GvHD-independent immune-mediated anti-leukemia effect operating only in the context of genetically-non-identical transplants. We term this allogeneic graft-versus-leukemia (GvL). Although it is likely that this effect is also mediated by T-cells, convincing data are lacking. Although the target antigen(s) of this effect is unknown, there are no convincing data that it is leukemia-specific. Attempts to modulate GvL without increasing GvHD in humans with leukemia, such as by transfusing additional T-cells or decreasing posttransplant immune suppression, were unsuccessful.[24,25] However, some recent data suggest a benefit of these approaches in some subjects with CML.[26]

A third T-cell mediated anti-leukemia effect may operate after transplants. This is illustrated by the markedly increased relative risk of relapse after T-cell depleted transplants in CML independent of GvHD. It is not certain whether this effect is distinct from the aforementioned allogeneic GvL effect.

In summary, these data indicate that several potent, immune-mediated anti-leukemia mechanisms operate after bone marrow transplants. Some recent preliminary data suggest similar effects may operate in transplants for lymphomas[27] and neuroblastoma.[28] These concepts are not yet tested in transplants for more common tumors such as breast or lung cancers.

Understanding the mechanism(s) by which these anti-leukemia mechanisms operate is essential if one wishes to use these effects in non-transplant settings. It makes sense to perform these studies before initiating large clinical trials.

ACKNOWLEDGEMENT

Supported in part by grant CA 23175 from the NCI, NIH, USPHS, DHHS and by the Center for Advanced Studies in Leukemia. RPG is the Wald Foundation Scholar in Biomedical Communication and President of the Center for Advanced Studies in Leukemia. We thank Emanuel Maidenberg for technical assistance and Katharine Fry for typing the manuscript.

REFERENCES

1. A. Fefer and A. L. Goldstein, "The Potential Role of T Cells in Cancer Therapy," Raven Press, New York (1982).
2. R. L. Truitt, R. P. Gale, and M. M. Bortin, "Cellular Immunotherapy of Cancer," Alan R. Liss, New York (1987).
3. A. H. Filipovich, D. Zerbe, B. D. Spector, and J. H. Kersey, Lymphomas in persons with naturally occurring immunodeficiency disorders, *in*: "Pathogenesis of Leukemia and Lymphomas: Environmental Influences," I. Magrath, G. T. O'Connor, and B. Ramot, eds., Raven Press, New York (1984).
4. I. Penn, The occurrence of cancer in immune deficiencies, *Curr. Problems Cancer* 6:1 (1982).
5. M. A. Epstein, Infection and tumor induction, *Nature* 321:653 (1986).
6. S. A. Rosenberg, M. T. Lotze, L. M. Muul, A. E. Chang, F. P. Avis, S. Leitman, W. M. Linehan, C. N. Robertson, R. E. Lee, and J. T. Rubin, A progress report on the treatment of 157 patients with advanced cancer using lymphokine-activated killer cells and interleukin-2 or high-dose interleukin-2 alone, *N. Engl. J. Med.* 316:889 (1987).
7. R. I. Fisher, C. A. Coltman, J. H. Doroshow, A. A. Rayner, M. J. Hawkins, J. W. Mier, P. Wiernik, J. D. McMannis, G. R. Weiss, and K. A. Margolin, Metastatic renal cancer treated with interleukin-2 and lymphokine-activated killer cells: A phase II clinical trial, *Ann. Intern. Med.* 108:518 (1988).
8. R. P. Gale and A. Butturini, Chemotherapy versus transplantation in acute leukemia, *Br. J. Haematol.* 72:1 (1989).
9. E. D. Thomas and R. A. Clift, Indications for marrow transplantation in chronic myelogenous leukemia, *Blood* 73:861 (1989).
10. K. M. Sullivan, P. L. Weiden, R. Storb, R. P. Witherspoon, A. Fefer, L. Fisher, C. D. Buckner, C. Anasetti, F. R. Appelbaum, and C. Badger, Influence of acute and chronic graft-versus-host disease on relapse and survival after bone marrow transplantation for HLA-identical siblings as treatment of acute and chronic leukemia, *Blood* 73:1720 (1989).
11. L. Backman, O. Ringden, J. Tollemar, and B. Lonnqvist, An increased risk of relapse in cyclosporin-treated patients: long term follow up of a randomized trial, *Bone Marrow Transplant.* 3:463 (1988).
12. R. P. Gale and R. Champlin, How do transplants cure leukemia? *Lancet* 2:28 (1984).
13. A. Fefer, K. M. Sullivan, P. Weiden, C. D. Buckner, G. Schoch, R. Storb, and E. D. Thomas, Graft versus leukemia effect in man: the relapse rate of acute leukemia is lower after allogeneic than after syngeneic marrow transplantation, *Prog. Clin. Biol. Res.* 244:401 (1987).
14. R. P. Gale, M. M. Horowitz, and M. M. Bortin, Identical twin transplants for leukemia, *Blood* 76(Suppl. 1):540a (1990).
15. A. M. Marmont, M. M. Horowitz, R. P. Gale, R. C. Ash, D. W. van Bekkum, R. E. Champlin, K. A. Dicke, J. M. Goldman, R. A. Good, R. H. Herzig, R. Hong, T.

Masaoka, R. J. O'Reilly, H. G. Prentice, A. A. Rimm, O. Ringdén, B. Speck, R. S. Weiner, and M. M. Bortin, T-cell depletion of HLA-identical transplants in leukemia, *Blood* (in press).

16. M. M. Horowitz, R. P. Gale, P. M. J. M. Goldman, J. Kersey, H.-J. Kolb, A. A. Rimm, O. Ringdén, C. Rozman, and B. Speck, Graft-versus-leukemia reaction after bone marrow transplantation, *Blood* 75:555 (1990).

17. International Bone Marrow Transplant Registry (IBMTR), Effect of methotrexate on relapse after bone marrow transplantation for acute lymphoblastic leukemia, *Lancet* 1:535 (1989).

18. A. J. Barrett, M. M. Horowitz, R. P. Gale, J. C. Biggs, K. G. Blume, B. M. Camitta, K. A. Dicke, E. Gluckman, R. A. Good, R. H. Herzig, M. B. Lee, A. L. Marmont, T. Masaoka, N. K. C. Ramsay, A. A. Rimm, B. Speck, F. E. Zwaan, and M. M. Bortin, Marrow transplantation for acute lymphoblastic leukemia: Factors affecting relapse and surviva, *Blood* 74:862 (1989).

19. J. P. Okunewick and R. P. Meredith, "Graft-versus-Leukemia in Man and Animal Models," CRC Press, Boca Raton, Florida (1981).

20. C. Perreault, F. Deary, S. Brochu, M. Gyger, R. Belanger, and D. Roy, Minor histocompatibility antigens, *Blood* 76:1269 (1990).

21. P. Marrack and J. Kappler, T cells can distinguish between allogeneic major histocompatibility complex products on different cell types, *Nature* 322:840 (1988).

22. W. R. Heath, M. E. Hurd, F. R. Carbone, and L. A. Sherman, Peptide-dependent recognition of H-2kb by alloreactive cytotoxic T lymphocytes, *Nature* 341:749 (1989).

23. G. T. Nepom, The effects of variations in human immune-response genes, *N. Engl. J. Med.* 321:751 (1989).

24. K. M. Sullivan, H. J. Deeg, J. Sanders, et al. Hyperacute graft-v-host disease in patients not given immunosuppression after allogeneic bone marrow transplantation, *Blood* 67:1172 (1986).

25. K. M. Sullivan, R. Storb, C. D. Buckner, A. Fefer, L. Fisher, P. L. Weiden, R. P. Witherspoon, F. R. Appelbaum, M. Banaji, and J. Hansen, Graft-versus-host disease as adoptive immunotherapy in patients with advanced hematological neoplasms, *N. Engl. J. Med.* 320:828 (1989).

26. H. J. Kolb, J. Mittermuller, C. Clemm, E. Holler, G. Ledderose, G. Brehm, M. Heim, and W. Willmans, Donor leukocyte transfusions for treatment of recurrent chronic myelogenous leukemia in marrow transplant patients, *Blood* 76:2462 (1990).

27. R. J. Jones, R. F. Ambinder, S. Piantadosi, and G. W. Santos, Evidence of a graft-versus-lymphoma effect associated with allogeneic bone marrow transplantation, *Blood*, 77:649, (1991).

28. M. C. Favrot, D. Floret, S. Negrier, P. Cochat, E. Bouffet, D.C. Zhou, C. R. Franks, T. Bijman, M. Burnat-Mentigny, and I. Philip, Systemic interleukin-2 therapy in children with progressive neuroblastoma after high dose chemotherapy and bone marrow transplantation, *Bone Marrow Transplant.* 4:449 (1989).

USE OF IL-2 AND LYMPHOCYTES FOLLOWING BONE

MARROW TRANSPLANTATION

A. Fefer, C. Higuchi, M. Benyunes, C. Beach, C. Lindgren, C.D. Buckner,
and J.A. Thompson

University of Washington
and
Fred Hutchinson Cancer Research Center
Seattle, Washington 98195

High-dose chemoradiotherapy and bone marrow transplantation (BMT) can cure
some patients with acute leukemia or lymphoma refractory to conventional therapy [1]. The
success of BMT is limited largely by a high relapse rate [1]. Attempts to use additional
chemotherapy or radiation to decrease the relapse rate have been hampered by the cross-
resistance of the tumor to the various agents and by their shared cumulative side effects. The
systemic administration of IL-2 with or without reinfusion of *ex vivo*-generated LAK cells
[2] represents one possible consolidative treatment modality which, if used after BMT, might
exert an anti-tumor effect against the minimal residual disease which is assumed to persist
after BMT, and thereby prevent or delay recurrence of the malignancy.

This paper will present the rationale for this approach, provide some very preliminary
data obtained in recipients of autologous marrow and identify some of the issues relevant to
performing similar studies in recipients of allogeneic marrow. Results of any therapy trials
to reduce relapses will not be available for at least two years.

The magnitude of the problem is suggested in Table 1, which presents the actuarial
five year estimates for relapse and disease-free survival as a function of the type and stage of
malignancy for which an allogeneic HLA matched sibling marrow transplant is performed
[1].

Table 1. Results of Allogeneic BMT

	Actuarial 5-Year Estimates (%)	
Disease	Relapse	Disease-Free Survival
AML, first remission	20-30	45-60
CML, chronic phase	20-25	50-80
Advanced leukemia or lymphoma	40-80	15-35

Combination Therapies, Edited by A.L. Goldstein and
E. Garaci, Plenum Press, New York, 1992

The survival of patients with even the best prognosis, i.e., those who undergo a transplant for AML in first complete remission, or for CML in the chronic phase is limited by a 20-30% probability of relapse. Patients who undergo BMT transplantation for advanced leukemia or lymphoma. i.e., beyond the first complete remisssion, have a significantly lower probability of disease-free survival, largely due to a 40-80% probability of relapse.

Autologous BMT for such advanced leukemia or lymphoma is associated with an even higher relapse rate. For example, in a series of 101 lymphoma patients who underwent autilogous BMT in Seattle, the group exhibited an 84% probability of relapse, with a median time to relapse of only about 2-4 months after BMT [3].

The rationale for using IL-2 ± LAK cells as consolidative therapy after BMT for patients who are at high risk for relapse can be summarized as follows:

(a) Human leukemia and lymphoma cells can be lysed in vitro by LAK cells [4, 5]; (b) the therapy may be non-cross-resistant with chemotherapy [6]; (c) in phase I/II trials, treatment with IL-2 ± LAK has induced partial or, rarely, complete remissions in some patients with hematologic malignancies [7, 8, 9]; (d) a state of minimal residual disease is readily attained by the conditioning regimens used for transplantation--a setting in which immunotherapy should theoretically be more effective; (e) in autologous marrow recipients, IL-2/LAK should theoretically be able to eradicate whatever clonogenic malignant cells might be present and reinfused with the stored marrow and thus should obviate the need for purging the marrow of tumor cells; and (f) in allogeneic marrow recipients, IL-2/LAK might induce or amplify a graft-versus-leukemia effect exerted by the foreign donor cells from the marrow [10]. Indeed, although strong circumstantial evidence for a GVL effect appears to exist only in recipients of allogeneic marrow [10]--especially those who exhibit GVHD--one cannot rule out the possibility that a GVL effect also exists in recipients of autologous marrow and can be amplified by IL-2 and/or cells.

If IL-2 ± LAK cell therapy were to be used after BMT, it would have to be administered late enough for the patient to have established a graft and to have recovered from the major BMT-related toxicities, but early enough before the malignancy would be likely to recur. Moreover, IL-2-responsive LAK precursor cells would have to be present in the circulation at that time.

Our studies thus far have focused on recipients of autologous rather than allogeneic marrow, so as to avoid the unknown effects of IL-2 in the more complex setting presented by immunologic barriers between the marrow donor and recipient. The resultant sequence of studies planned is shown in Table 2.

Table 2. Sequence of Studies Planned

1. Study reconstitution of LAKp after ABMT
2. Perform Phase I trial of IL-2 after ABMT
3. Perform a trial of IL-2 + LAK cells after ABMT to decrease relapse of lymphoma
4. Initiate similar studies after allogeneic BMT

To determine whether IL-2-responsive LAK precursor cells were present in the circulation early after autologous BMT, peripheral blood mononuclear cells were obtained from 21 patients with acute leukemia or lymphoma 17 to 83 days after BMT. The cells were

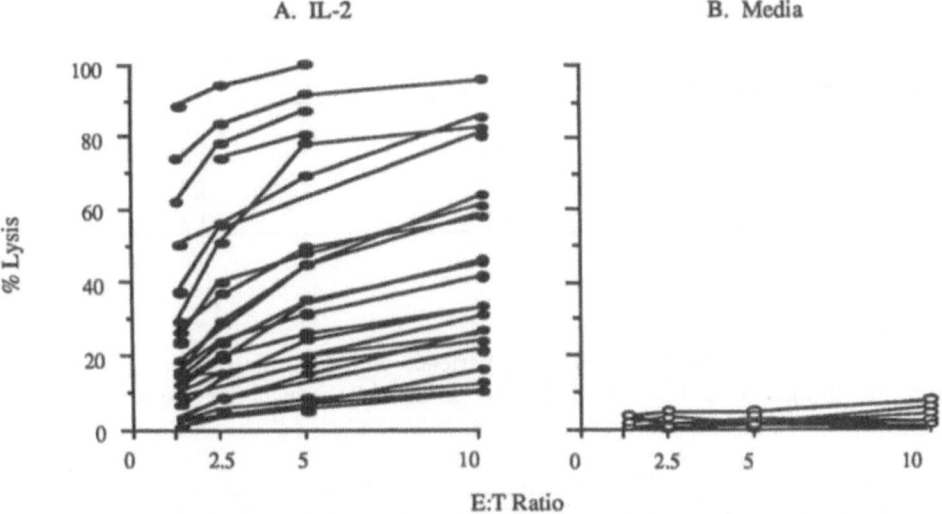

A. IL-2　　　　　　　　　　　　　　B. Media

PBMC obtained from 21 patients with refractory hematological malignancies who were at various intervals within 3-12 weeks after ABMT were cultured for 4 or 5 days with (A) IL2 (1000 U/ml), or (B) culture media without IL2 supplementation. Cells were assessed for cytolytic reactivity against Daudi.

Figure 1. LAK precursor activity is detectable after ABMT.

cultured with IL-2 at 1,000 to 2,000 U/ml for 4 to 5 days, and tested for their ability to lyse the LAK-sensitive target Daudi at different effector:target ratios [11].

The results are shown in Figure 1.

Each curve represents the lysis by cells from a single patient obtained at a single point in time after they have been incubated with IL-2, or in media alone. Despite the heterogeneity of the patients studied--in terms of diagnosis, conditioning regimen and marrow manipulation--LAK precursor activity was detectable in the circulation of virtually every patient tested at every point in time tested. Positive and negative selection experiments on the FACS revealed that, as in cells from non-BMT patients, most of the LAK activity was mediated by CD3$^-$ CD56$^+$ cells with a minor subset of cells which stained dimly for CD8 and coexpressed CD56 [11, 12].

The possibility was considered that early after BMT patients might be too susceptible to IL-2 toxicity--especially in terms of the viability of the marrow graft and the capillary leak syndrome--and/or might not be able to respond immunologically to IL-2 administration. Therefore, a Phase Ib clinical trial with IL-2 alone was carried out after autologous BMT to identify the maximum tolerated dose of IL-2 and to assess immunologic responses to it, if any [13]. The design is shown in Table 3. Patients were sequentially assigned to escalating IL-2 (recombinant IL-2 kindly provided by Hoffman-LaRoche) "induction" doses of 0.3-4.5 x 10^6 U/m^2/day on day 1-5. After a rest period, all patients received a low-dose "maintenance" infusion of IL-2 at 0.3 x 10^6 U/m^2/day on day 12-21. Patients received induction IL-2 in the hospital and maintenance IL-2 as outpatients in the clinic.

Table 3. Design of Phase Ib Trial of IL-2 After Autologous BMT

Group	No. Pts.	"Induction" dose ($\times 10^6$ U/m^2/d) (d 1-5)	"Maintenance" dose ($\times 10^6$ U/m^2/d) (d 12-21)
I	4	0.3	0.3
II	4	1.0	0.3
III	6	3.0	0.3
IV	2	4.5	0.3

The trial design was based on our experience with non-transplant cancer patients and on the design of a trial of IL-2 plus LAK cells which we expected to use subsequently.

Sixteen patients, aged 15 to 59 (median, 34), with AML, HD, NHL or myeloma, who had been conditioned for BMT with chemotherapy, with or without TBI, recieved IL-2 by continuous intavenous infusion as early as 14 to 91 days (median, 33) after BMT.

Dose-related toxicities consisted largely of fever, nausea, diarrhea, skin rash and mild fluid retention. Dose limiting toxicities were hypotension and thrombocytopenia. All toxicities reversed quickly after stopping IL-2. The maximal tolerated induction dose was identified as 3×10^6 U/m^2/day.

Hematologic and immunologic tests were performed on days 0, 7, 12 and 23, i.e., before IL-2 was begun just after completing the induction course, and at the beginning and end of the IL-2 maintenance phase. Since early after BMT the marrow graft is often tenuous, the possibility of myelosuppression by IL-2 and/or LAK cells with resultant neutropenia and infection was considered. However, neutropenia was <u>not</u> observed. Indeed, Figure 2 shows that the neutrophil counts tended to <u>rise</u> in all groups during IL-2 treatment, probably due to induction of GM-CSF secretion.

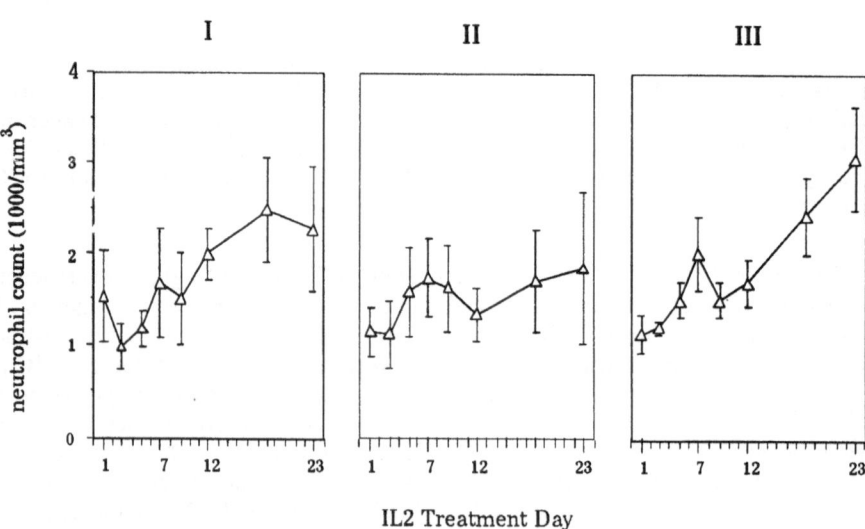

Figure 2. IL-2 Therapy Raises the Neutrophil Counts

Figure 3 shows that, as in non-BMT cancer patients, IL-2 induced a transient lymphopenia followed by a rebound lymphocytosis 24 hours after completion of the IL-2 "induction" course. Although the increases represented largely cells expressing CD3 and CD8, the highest dose of IL-2 also increased the percentage of circulating lymphocytes expressing the CD56 surface marker associated with LAK activity, as shown in Figure 4.

Peripheral blood lymphocytes were also tested serially for LAK precursor (LAKp) and LAK effector (LAKe) activities. LAKp are defined as cells which, when cultured in IL-2, acquire LAK activity, i.e., lyse Daudi; LAKe are cells which have direct LAK activity without requiring exposure to IL-2 *in vitro*.

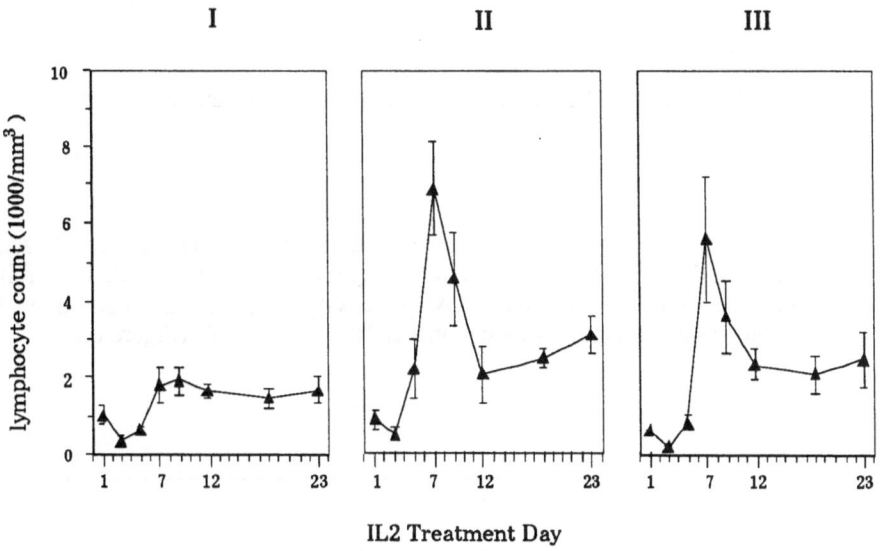

Figure 3. Effect of IL-2 Therapy on the Lymphocyte Count

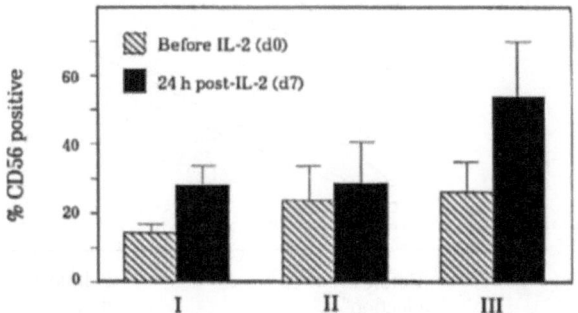

Figure 4 . IL-2 "Induction" Therapy Increases the Percentage of CD56$^+$ Cells

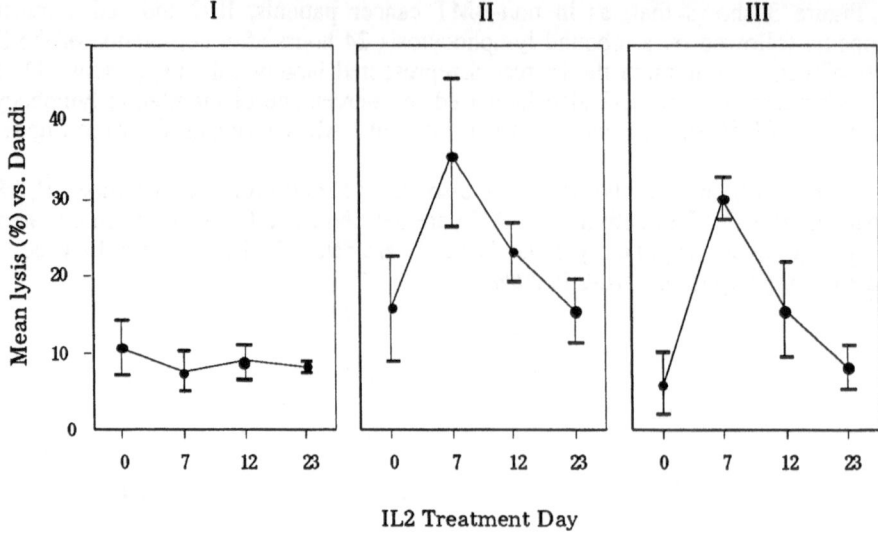

Figure 5 . IL-2 Therapy Augments LAK Effector Activity

Figure 5 shows that most patients tested had low levels of spontaneous LAKe activity on day 0, i.e., before IL-2 therapy, and those receiving the higher doses of IL-2 exhibited a substantial increase in LAKe activity. LAKp activity was also augmented by IL-2 "induction" therapy, as represented by lytic units per 10^7 effector cells (Figure 6).

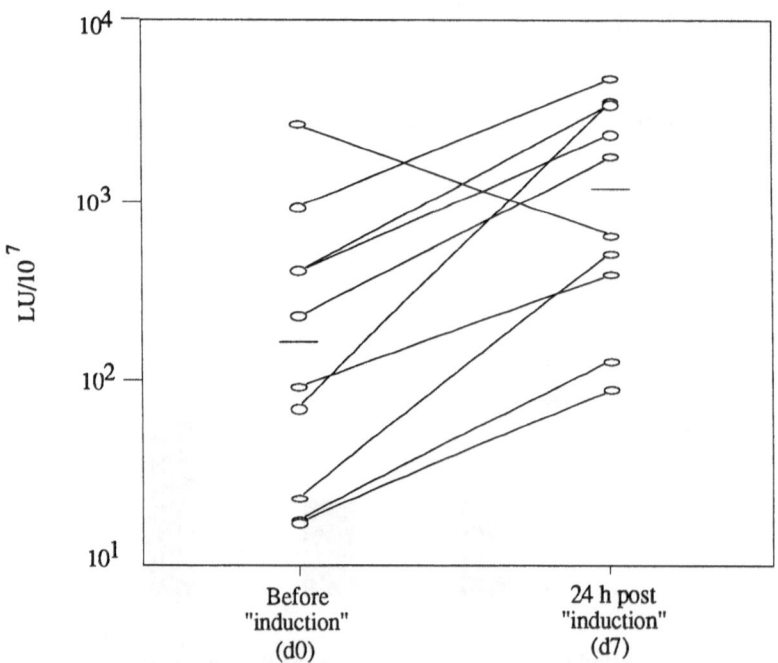

FIGURE 6. IL-2 "Induction" Therapy Increases LAK Precursor Activity

Thus, in the course of this phase I trial we identified a safe IL-2 regimen which patients will tolerate early after ABMT and to which they will respond immunologically. The toxicities and immunologic changes were consistent with those reported by 2 other groups with different regimens and sources of IL-2 [14, 15].

Based on those results, a trial of IL-2 plus LAK cells after autologous BMT was recently initiated in an attempt to reduce the relapse rate of lymphoma and AML in patients who are at high risk for relapse [16]. The design of the protocol is shown in Table 4.

Table 4. Design of IL-2/LAK Protocol

IL-2 (3×10^6 U/m^2/d)	D 1-5
PHERESIS	D 7-9
LAK INFUSION	D 12-14
IL-2 (3×10^5 U/m^2/d)	D 12-21

IL-2 at the maximal tolerated dose of 3×10^6 U/m^2/day was administered by continuous intravenous infusion on day 1-5. The patients underwent leukapheresis daily on days 7, 8 and 9. The cells were incubated with IL-2, 1000 U/ml for 5 days, and the resultant LAK cells were infused daily on days 12 through 14. A low maintenance dose of IL-2 at 3×10^5 U/m^2/day on days 12-21 was administered. The low dose was based on the assumption that less IL-2 may be required to maintain than to induce LAK activity.

To date, six patients have been treated 27-83 days after BMT. Thrombocytopenia and hypotension remain the major but reversible toxicities, as predicted by the phase I trial. Impressive lymphocytosis was observed and they have received a total of 6.9-14.1 x 10^{10} LAK cells. Obviously, more patients will have to be accrued on this trial, and ultimately a randomized prospectively controlled trial of IL-2 + LAK versus neither will be performed to definitively determine effect on relapse rates, if any.

Similar studies are warranted in patients who have undergone allogeneic BMT in an effort to induce or amplify a GVL effect exerted by cells from the foreign donor marrow infused. There is cogent circumstantial clinical evidence for the existence of a GVL effect in vivo after allogeneic BMT in humans. It can be summarized as follows [10]: a) the incidence of leukemic relapse is lower after allogeneic than after syngeneic BMT, b) the incidence of leukemic relapse is lower in allogeneic marrow recipients who develop acute and/or chronic GVHD than in allogeneic marrow recipients who do not develop GVHD, c) the incidence of leukemic relapse is lower in recipients of allogeneic marrow without GVHD than it is in recipients of syngeneic marrow, and d) the incidence of leukemic relapse is higher in recipients of T-cell depleted allogeneic marrow than in recipients of unmodified allogeneic marrow. Effector cells which mediate the GVL effect in animals and humans may include [10]: a) cytotoxic T-lymphocytes (CTL) specific for minor histocompatibility antigens present on both normal host tissue and leukemic cells and/or against antigens expressed only or preferentially on malignant cells, b) lymphocytes which mediate their antitumor effects via secondary lymphokine secretion, and/or c) cytolytic T- or non-T-cells that mediate their anti-tumor effect through an MHC-unrestricted mechanism, such as LAK. IL-2 can stimulate the proliferation and function of all the above-mentioned effector cells.

Data from some murine models, though sparse and variable, suggest that IL-2 with or without LAK cells can induce or amplify a GVL effect and cure tumor-bearing mice [17]. The principal potential complication of IL-2/LAK therapy after allogeneic BMT is the induction or exacerbation of severe GVHD. In murine models, most notably those by Sykes and Sachs [18, 19], IL-2 can induce, exacerbate, or even protect against GVHD, depending on the model and the timing. What any given regimen of IL-2 (± LAK) will do in human recipients of allogeneic marrow cannot be predicted. We have just initiated a phase Ib trial of IL-2 in recipients of HLA-matched sibling marrow who have no evidence of GVHD off immunosuppressive [16]. The results will determine the design of a trial of IL-2 plus LAK cells to decrease relapse rates after allogeneic BMT. Some results should be generated within the next two years.

In conclusion, there is a substantial experimental rationale for attempts to use lymphokines and lymphocytes after BMT to decrease the relapse rate of hematologic malignancies. The area is in its infancy but is receiving increasing investigative attention internationally. In the course of the next several years, should encouraging results be obtained with IL-2 alone or with IL-2 plus LAK cells in autologous or allogeneic BMT, emphasis will be placed on improving the therapeutic index by exploring ways to decrease the toxicity and increase the efficacy of the therapy. This will require a better understanding of the mechanism which mediates the toxicity and the anti-tumor effects. Should exogenously generated cells turn out to contribute significantly to the end results of therapy, then approaches will have to be developed to better identify the effector cells responsible and to study ways to preferentially augment their generation and function. It must be emphasized that the LAK cells being infused in these and similar studies are heterogeneous in nature and represent only a fraction of the cells being infused. It is conceivable that other cells that are in the bags being infused may be beneficial or even essential. Indeed, the ultimate hope is to identify, expand and use tumor-specific T lymphocytes rather than the non-T, non-MHC-restricted cells, as an adjunct to BMT [17].

This research was supported by grants CA 18029-16, 5 P01 CA47748-02, 2 T32 CA09515-6 from the National Institutes of Health and CCA-8510 from the U.S.-Spain Joint Committee.

Acknowledgements: The authors thank M.J. Schreifels and H. Todd for their expert technical assistance, J. Factor for secretarial help and Hoffmann-LaRoche, Inc. for providing the IL-2.

REFERENCES

1. Fefer, A. and K. Sullivan. Bone marrow transplantation for hematologic malignancies. *Medical Oncology: Basic Principles and Clinical Management of Cancer,* Calabresi and Schein, eds. Elmsford, NY: Pergamon Press, Inc., in press.

2. Rosenberg, S.A., M.T. Lotze, J.C. Yang, et al. Experience with the use of high-dose interleukin-2 in the treatment of 652 cancer patients. *Ann. Surgery.* **210**:474, 1989.

3. Petersen, F., F. Appelbaum, R. Hill, et al. Autologous marrow transplantation for malignant lymphoma: A report of 101 cases from Seattle. *J Clin Oncol.* **8**:638, 1990.

4. Oshimi, K., Y. Oshimi, M. Akutsu, et al. Cytotoxicity of Interleukin 2-activated lymphocytes for leukemia and lymphoma cells. *Blood.* **68**:938, 1986.

5. Adler, A., P. Chervenick, T. Whiteside, et al. Interleukin-2 induction of lymphokine-activated killer (LAK) activity in the peripheral blood and bone marrow of acute leukemia patients. I. Feasibility of LAK generation in adult patients with active disease and in remission. *Blood.* **71**:709, 1988.

6. Allavena, P., G. Damia, T. Colombo, et al. Lymphokine-activated killer (LAK) and monocyte-mediated cytotoxicity on tumor cell lines resistant to antitumor agents. *Cellular Immunology.* **120**:250, 1989.

7. West, W.H., K.W. Tauer, J.R. Yannelli, et al. Constant-infusion recombinant interleukin-2 in adoptive immunotherapy of advanced cancer. *N Eng J Med.* **316**:898, 1987.

8. Rosenberg, S.A., M.T. Lotze, L.M. Muul, et al. A progress report on the treatment of 157 patients with advanced cancer using lymphokine-activated killer cells and interleukin-2 or high-dose interleukin-2 alone. *N Eng J Med.* **316**:889, 1987.

9. Foa, R., G. Meloni, S. Tosti, et al. Treatment of residual disease in acute leukemia patients with recombinant interleukin 2 (IL2): Clinical and biological findings. *Bone Marrow Transplantation.* **6**:98, 1990.

10. Fefer, A., R.L. Truitt and K.M. Sullivan. Adoptive cellular therapy: Graft-vs-tumor responses after bone marrow transplantation. *Biologic Therapy of Cancer: Principles and Practice* DeVita, Hellman and Rosenberg ed. Philadelphia: JB Lippincott Co., in press.

11. Higuchi, C.M., J.A. Thompson, T. Cox, et al. Lymphokine-activated killer function following autologous bone marrow transplantation for refractory hematological malignancies. *Cancer Res.* **49**:5509, 1989.

12. Ortaldo, J.R., A. Mason and R. Overton. Lymphokine-activated killer cells. *J Exp Med.* **164**:1193, 1986.

13. Higuchi, C.M., J.A. Thompson, F.B. Petersen, et al. Toxicity and immunomodulatory effects of Interleukin 2 after autologous bone marrow transplantation for hematologic malignancies. *Blood,* in press.

14. Gottlieb, D.J., M.K. Brenner, H.E. Heslop, et al. A phase I clinical trial of recombinant interleukin 2 following high dose chemo-radiotherapy for haematological malignancy: Applicability to the elimination of minimal residual disease. *Br J Cancer.* **60**:610, 1989.

15. Blaise, D., D. Olive, A.M. Stoppa, et al. Hematologic and immunologic effects of the systemic administration of recombinant Interleukin-2 after autologous bone marrow transplantation. *Blood.* **76**:1092, 1990.

16. Benyunes, M., C. Higuchi, F. Peterson, et al. Clinical trials of Interleukin-2 +/- lymphokine-activated killer cells after BMT for hematologic malignancies. Abstr #253. *Proceedings of ASCO.* 1991.

17. Fefer, A., J. Thompson, C. Higuchi, et al. The future of cellular immunotherapy of cancer. *Apheresis in Cellular Immunotherapy and Stem Cell Collection* Brubaker and Kasprison ed. Bethesda, MD: American Association of Blood Banks, in press.

18. Sykes, M., M.L. Romick and D.H. Sachs. Interleukin 2 prevents graft-versus-host disease while preserving the graft-versus-leukemia effect of allogeneic T cells. *Proc Natl Acad Sci USA*. **87**:5633, 1990.

19. Sykes, M., M.L. Romick, K.A. Hoyles and D.H. Sachs. *In vivo* administration of interleukin 2 plus T cell-depleted syngeneic marrow prevents graft-versus-host disease mortality and permits alloengraftment. *J Exp Med*. **171**:645, 1990.

COMBO: NEW CONCEPTS AND METHODS FOR DESIGNING AND ANALYZING EXPERIMENTS ON COMBINATION THERAPY

John N. Weinstein* and Barry Bunow*

* National Cancer Inst., NIH, Bethesda, MD 20892
** Civilized Software, Inc., Bethesda, MD 20814

INTRODUCTION

Prompted by data from our own experiments on therapy of AIDS, we have taken a fresh look at the problem of analyzing potentiation, synergy, antagonism, enhancement of therapeutic index, and other types of drug interactions (1-3). Initial stages of that inquiry revealed the need for new concepts and new analytical methods that include:

1. Flexible choice of interaction models (clearly, no single type of model can fit all types of interactions).

2. Appropriately robust statistical methods to estimate p-values and confidence intervals (a sound statistical basis is critical in this field, if one is to be confident that there actually is an interaction).

3. Flexibility with respect to experimental design (e.g., checkerboard, constant-ratio, etc.).

4. Statistical techniques for reducing the size of experiments by reducing the number of replicates needed.

These requirements motivated development of a computer program package, COMBO, that operates in the MLAB computing environment on personal computers (Civilized Software, Inc., Bethesda, MD). COMBO provides a variety of models, e.g. "robust potentiation", "robust antagonism", "pure potentiation", and "eff-tox" (the latter for instances in which both efficacy and toxicity are observed simultaneously). COMBO can also be used for experiments on single drugs. Graphical displays, multiple statistical diagnostics, and identifiers of aberrant data are included. Confidence intervals and p-values are obtained by both parametric and non-parametric (Monte Carlo) techniques.

In the context of AIDS, we have used the COMBO paradigm and program package to design and/or analyze experiments on combinations that include AZT, ddC, ddI, ddA, dipyridamole, interferons, tumor necrosis factor, suramin, CD4-pseudomonas exotoxin, and protease inhibitors, *inter alia*. In the context of cancer, we have used it for combinations including doxorubicin, suramin, tumor necrosis factor, dipyridamole, interferons, and dideoxynucleosides. Initial

Combination Therapies, Edited by A.L. Goldstein and
E. Garaci, Plenum Press, New York, 1992

applications of the new principles and the COMBO program package can be found in references (1-3). Here, we summarize major features of this approach, illustrated using two examples from therapy of HIV infection *in vitro*. These formulations were developed on the basis of *in vitro* data, but we have applied them to *in vivo* studies as well.

DRUG INTERACTION MODELS

The interaction models used in COMBO are derived from enzyme kinetics-based "pseudo-molecular" formulations for drug interaction. Each of these represents an elaboration of the logistic dose-response curve that frequently characterizes the behavior of single drug assay systems. As indicated in Figure 1a, the single-drug logistic curve is characterized by four parameters: the zero-dose response (A), the high-dose response (D), the mid-point dose (e.g., the IC50), and the mid-point slope (B).

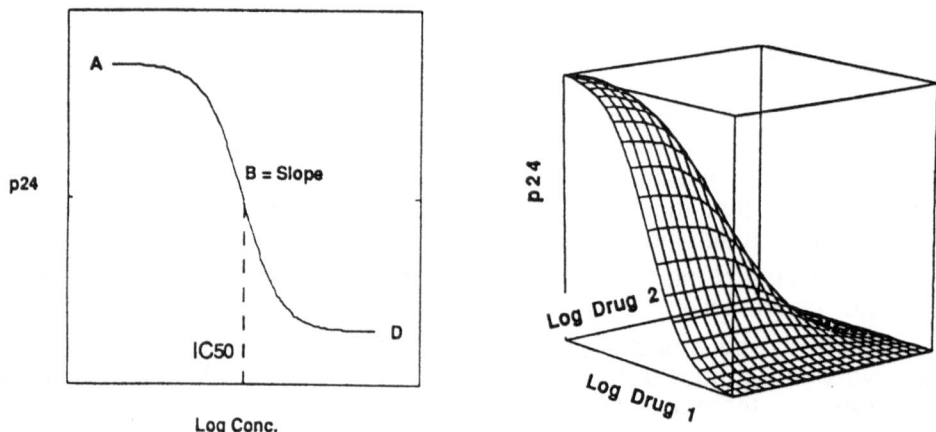

Fig. 1. (Left-hand panel) Logistic dose-response curve for a single drug, showing zero dose response (A), high dose response (D), mid-effect dose (IC50), and mid-effect slope (B). (Right-hand panel) Generalization of the logistic to two-drug combination. From ref. (2).

With two drugs, the idea is to project the logistic curve into an extra dimension (Figure 1b) to accommodate the second drug. Assuming no interaction, there are two new parameters, the IC50 and mid-point slope for drug 2. Non-additive interaction enters through one or more additional parameters, and we refer to this as a "robust potentiation" model. Most effort in the literature has been devoted to the issues of synergy and antagonism *per se* (2-14). However, flexibility in the choice of models and interaction types is also important. For example, if an assay measures both efficacy and toxicity simultaneously, and if the two overlap, then a different class of models is required. To handle this situation, we have developed "eff-tox" (efficacy-toxicity) models. If the dose-response curve of a biological response modifier is "biphasic" (i.e., non-monotonic), as is often the case, models incorporating this behavior can be invoked. Issues with respect to choice of models and with respect to confusions in the terminology of drug interaction have been discussed previously (3).

OVERVIEW OF COMBO

Briefly, the COMBO algorithms use iteratively reweighted nonlinear least squares techniques for data fitting (although robust regression is also an option provided). If desired, the weights are computed by a Gaussian kernel technique based on estimated responses. Statistical diagnostics available (2) include the weighted sum of squares, normal theory standard error estimates, variance-covariance matrix, parameter dependency values, RMS-weighted deviation errors, mean fractional deviation per data point, residuals, and weighted residuals. Various graphical outputs are generated for summary of data fits, residuals, and statistics.

COMBO offers the following features: 1. checkerboard, constant-ratio, and other experimental designs are supported; 2. overlapping efficacy and toxicity can be analyzed simultaneously; 3. all data points can generally be included (i.e., without removing those near 0 and 100% effect); 4. global parameters are computed for potentiation, synergy, antagonism, and (if appropriate) therapeutic index; 5. a flexible choice of data models can be invoked; 6. a flexible choice of error structures is provided (including Gaussian kernel error estimation --which permits the data set to specify its own error structure); 7. both parametric and distribution-free confidence intervals are calculated for model parameters, the latter obtained by Monte Carlo techniques related (but not identical) to the Bootstrap method of Efron (15,16); 8. statistical criteria for rejection of outliers can be calculated; 9. experimental designs with fewer replicates are facilitated (2). This last is perhaps the most important feature, given the requirement for large numbers of data points in experiments on combinations. The most significant disadvantage of the COMBO "tool box" is that the Monte Carlo methods and outlier selection algorithms are computer-intensive.

THE "ROBUST POTENTIATION" MODEL

Using a combination of ideas arising from the theory of multiple inhibitors in enzyme kinetics, the isobologram representation of Berenbaum (17), and the median effect analysis of Chou and Talalay (12), we obtained the following effect equation (3) for a pair of drugs, one or both of them intrinsically active:

$$1 = (1/z-1)^{-1/B_1}(c_1/IC_{50_1})(1+(c_2/PC_{50_2})^{BP_2})$$
$$+(1/z-1)^{-1/B_2}(c_2/IC_{50_2})(1+(c_1/PC_{50_1})^{BP_1}) \tag{1}$$

where $z = (a-y)/(a-d)$ is the normalized effect. y, in this case the measured p24 level in natural units, defines a surface over c_1 and c_2; c_1 and c_2 are the concentrations of the two drugs; IC_{50_1} and IC_{50_2} are the 50%-effect concentrations; B_1 and B_2 are the 50%-effect slopes for the two drugs acting individually; PC_{50_1} and BP_1 are the 50%-effect concentration and slope for the potentiation of drug 2 by drug 1; PC_{50_2} and BP_2 are the 50%-effect concentration and slope for the potentiation of drug 1 by drug 2; a is p24 in the absence of drug; d is p24 at indefinitely high drug levels. PC_{50_i} is defined as the concentration of drug i required to increase the apparent potency of the other drug (i.e., decrease its apparent IC_{50}) by a factor of 2 (beyond what would be expected on the basis of the intrinsic activity of drug i). The lower the value of

PC50$_i$, the stronger the potentiation; additivity corresponds to PC50$_1$ and PC50$_2$ approaching infinity. Note that this equation reduces to the expected explicit expression for z if B$_1$ = B$_2$.

Thus, the key parameters of interaction, PC50$_i$, are analogous to the IC50's in that a value approaching infinity indicates no effect, and a value approaching 0 indicates strong effect. The parameter $P \equiv IC50_i/PC50_i$ gives a useful dimensionless characterization of the strength of potentiation. $P_i = 0$ indicates additivity; $P_i > 0$ indicates potentiation. An alternative form of eqn. 1 (not shown) represents antagonism (with $P_i < 0$).

In the absence of interaction, equation (1) simplifies to that of Syracuse and Greco (13), who were the first to recognize the need for an implicit interaction equation when slope parameters for the two drugs are unequal. This was an important observation. Their equations and ours differ, however, when interaction is present. One aspect of this difference is that the equation in ref. (13) contains only one interaction parameter, α. Equation (1) above is a more general form containing 4 interaction parameters, although it can be simplified in the obvious way to include 0, 1, 2, or 3 interaction parameters as required (and/or justified) by the data. This flexibility allows for analysis of more complex interactions and better fitting of a wide range of experimental data. It also emphasizes the relationship between "synergy" and "mutual potentiation." To date the most useful models have included interaction parameters PC50$_1$ and BP$_1$ or PC50$_2$ and BP$_2$, but not both sets simultaneously. It is often important to include the slope parameter.

To illustrate application of the "robust potentiation" model, we consider an experiment by Ashorn, et al. (1) in which reverse transcriptase inhibitors were combined with a chimeric CD4-pseudomonas exotoxin conjugate (CD4-PE40) to eliminate HIV from human T-cell cultures. See ref. (1) for details of the experiments and analysis.

Figure 2 shows a two-drug dose-response surface representing a fit of the robust potentiation model to data on CD4-PE40 in combination with dideoxyinosine (ddI). For most of the data points, the fit appears to be quite good. Note that the slopes for the two drugs are very different. Table 1 summarizes the parameter estimates obtained for combinations of CD4-PE40 with ddI and azidothymidine (AZT). Fits were done in two ways: (i) with CD4-PE40 considered as the potentiating agent, and (ii) with the reverse transcriptase inhibitor taken as the potentiating agent. Table 1 shows that CD4-PE40 potentiated each RT inhibitor (p<0.01) and that each RT inhibitor potentiated CD4-PE40 (p<0.01). The PC50 values were at least several times smaller than the corresponding IC50 values, indicating strong potentiation. The four values of P corresponding to the four table entries are 6.53, 3.15, 7.44, and 6.56, respectively. This mutual potentiation corresponds to "synergy" (1).

Figure 3 shows "stadium" plots which illustrate graphically the potentiation of CD4-PE40 by ddI and AZT. The lefthand panels show three-dimensional dose-response surfaces for the indicated pairs of drugs, based on the best fits to the experimental data. The righthand panels show the appearance that the surfaces would have had if the agents had been simply additive (i.e., if PC50 had been infinite). The lefthand panels show a pronounced inward bowing characteristic of potentiation, whereas the righthand panels necessarily show straight tie-lines between points of equal effect on the individual drug axes. For all panels, the tie-lines are three-dimensional projections of the contours appearing in the classical isobologram (17).

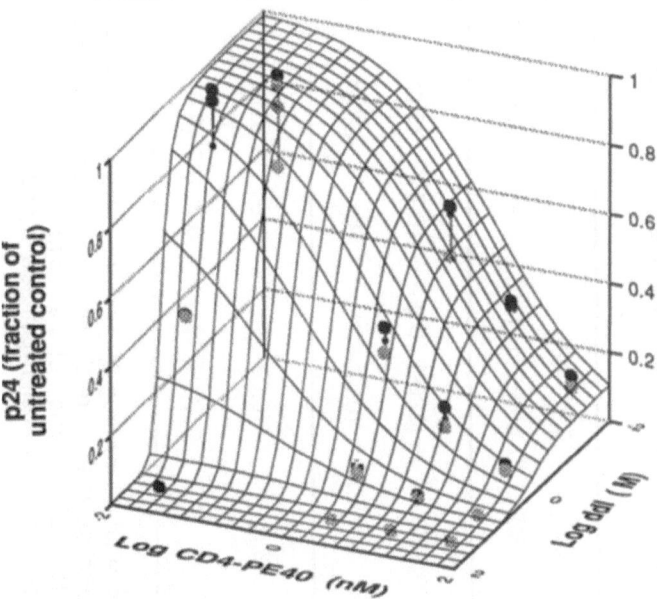

Fig. 2. Net plot of the dose-response surface for CD4-PE40 and ddI, showing quality of fit to data. Large filled circles represent data points above (black) or below (gray) the fitting surface. Small black filled circles represent corresponding calculated points on the surface. Straight connecting lines indicate the residuals. The two horizontal axes are log drug concentrations, and the vertical axis is the response (here, HIV p24 antigen). Note logistic curves on the individual drug axes. Because log concentrations were used for the axes in order to spread out the data points, this surface appears to be bowed outward (cf Fig. 1B). If plotted with absolute concentrations (cf. Fig. 3), the surface would appear inwardly bowed, indicating synergy.

THE "EFF-TOX" MODEL

To illustrate application of the "eff-tox" model (which takes account of simultaneous, overlapping antiviral efficacy and cell toxicity), we consider an experiment on the anti-HIV activity and cytotoxicity of AZT for CEM-SS T-lymphoblastoid cells in the presence and absence of dipyridamole (DPM) (2,3). See ref. (3) for details on the methods and analysis. The fitted curves in Fig. 4 were calculated using the following equations:

$$X = ((c_1/IC50_1)(1+(c_2/PC50_2)^{BPe_2})^{Be_1}) \qquad (2a)$$

$$num = av+X \qquad (2b)$$

$$den = 1+X(1+(c_1/IC50t_1)/(1+(c_2/PC50t_2)^{BPt_2})^{Bt_1}) \qquad (2c)$$

Table 1. Prameter values obtained for analysis of synergy between CD4-PE40 and dideoxynucleoside drugs using the "robust potentiation" model.

Drug 1	Drug 2	$IC50_1$ (nM)	$IC50_2$ (nM)	B_1	B_2	BP_1	BP_2	$PC50_1$ (nM)	$PC50_2$ (nM)	95% conf. limits on $PC50_2$ (nM)	F*	p-value for additivity**
CD4-PE40 ←ddl		3.9	4,900	0.67	5.4	-	1.8	-	750	(320-1,100)	10.7	<0.01
CD4-PE40 →ddl		2.9	4,800	0.59	2.7	0.54	-	0.92	-	(0.08-8.8)	8.1	<0.01
CD4-PE40 ←AZT		6.2	29	0.74	2.6	-	1.7	-	3.9	(0.03-10)	9.6	<0.01
CD4-PE40 →AZT		5.9	29	0.69	2.5	0.50	-	0.90	-	(~0-9.6)	9.3	<0.01

See text for definitions and calculations. ← indicates calculation for potentiation of drug 1 by drug 2; → indicates the reverse. Confidence limits were calculated for all parameters, but only those for the potentiation parameter are shown. Calculations were done using all 34 points except for one obvious outlier in the no-drug quadruplicate for AZT. Inclusion of that point made only minor differences in parameter estimates. *Pseudo F-statistic relative to best additive model fit; **Two-tail; hypothesis of additivity rejected at 1% level. Modified from ref. [Ashorn, 1990 #107]

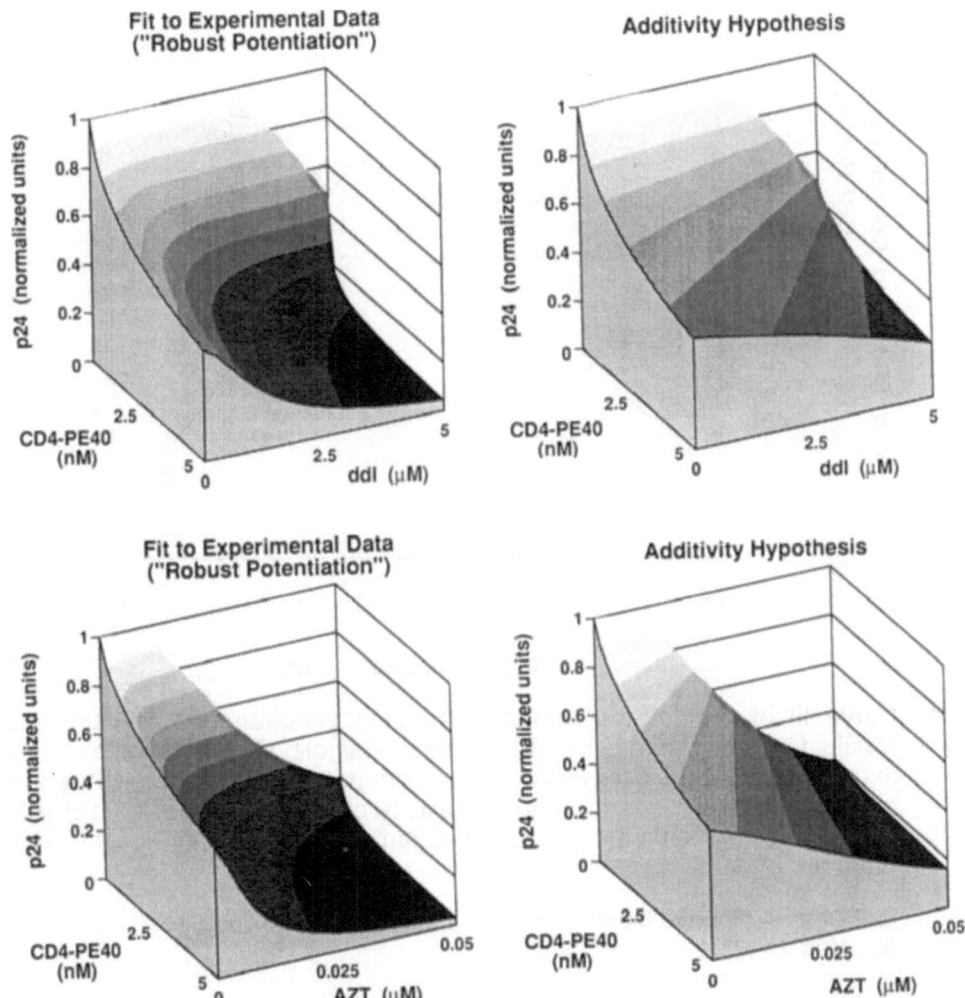

Fig. 3. "Stadium" plots showing synergistic interaction of CD4-PE40 with ddI *(upper panels)* and AZT *(lower panels)* in primary T-cell cultures. The dose-response surfaces were constructed from the parameter estimates in Table 1. *Left:* Best fits of the experimental data using the "robust potentiation" model. Inward bowing indicates synergy. *Right:* Surfaces (with straight tie-lines) that would have been obtained in the absence of synergy. From ref. (1).

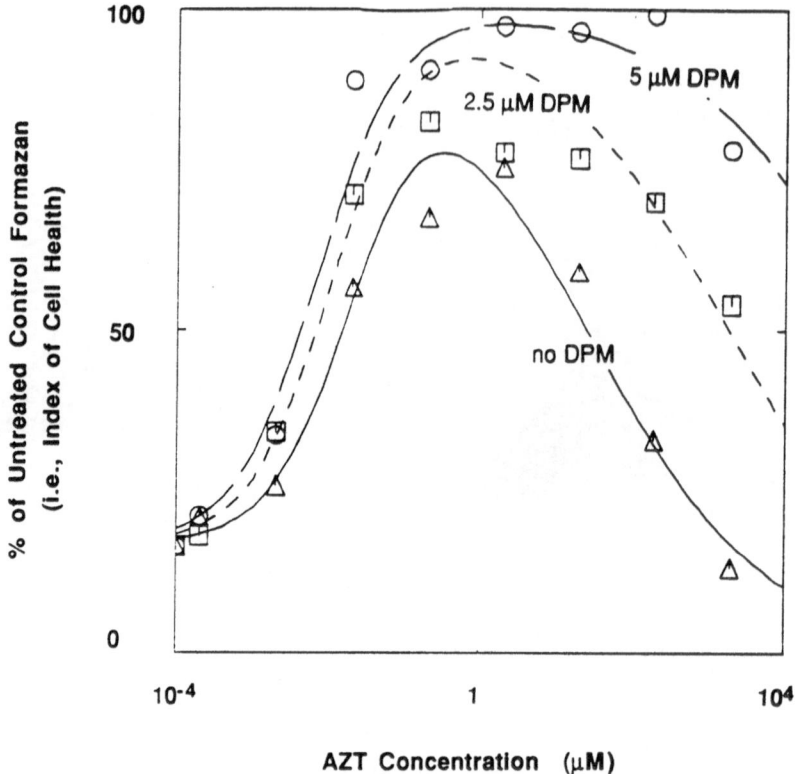

Fig.4. Curve fit of the "eff-tox" model describing simultaneous efficacy and toxicity for the drug combination AZT-dipyridamole. The figure shows that in cultured CEM-SS cells dipyridamole both potentiates the anti-HIV effect of AZT and decreases the cellular toxicity of AZT. The assay (18) was based on colorimetric analysis of formazan dye produced by healthy cells. From ref. (2, 3).

Q: Does AZT have intrinsic antiviral activity? Cytotoxic effect?
A: Yes ($p < 0.01$)   Yes ($p < 0.01$)

Q: What is the therapeutic index of AZT alone?
A: The best estimate is a 3,300-fold difference between IC50e and IC50t. There is a 95% chance that the "true" value lies between 800- and 8,300-fold.

Q: Does DPM potentiate the antiviral activity of AZT?
A: Yes ($p < 0.01$).

Q: Does DPM antagonize the cytotoxicity of AZT?
A: Yes ($p < 0.01$).

Q: Does DPM increase the therapeutic index?
A: Yes ($p < 0.01$) -- a 12.4-fold increase for 1 µM DPM.

where z = num/den = (y-d)/(a-d) is the normalized formazan level. These equations were incorrectly rendered in ref. (3). Here, y is the measured formazan level in natural units; a is the formazan level in the absence of virus and drug; d is the formazan level at indefinitely high drug concentrations; $IC_{50}e$, Be, $PC_{50}e$, and BPe are parameters related to the antiviral efficacy and defined as were their equivalents in the "robust potentiation" model; $IC_{50}t$, Bt, $PC_{50}t$, and BPt are similar parameters related to the cell toxicity; av is the normalized formazan level at zero drug. The above pair of equations may look complex, but they arise naturally from a simple binding model that has quite general application. In this data set, it was important to consider both efficacy and toxicity limbs of the dose-response curve simultaneously since the response variable, an index of cell health, reflects both damage by the virus and damage by the drugs. In other cases, the mixing of viral and toxic effects might be more subtle, for example when cell toxicity diminishes viral production of measured p24 or reverse transcriptase.

This eff-tox analysis indicates a surprising dissociation of DPM's influence on AZT's antiviral and cytotoxic activities. DPM modestly potentiates the antiviral activity of AZT and, at the same time, greatly antagonizes its cytotoxicity. The net effect is to increase the *in vitro* therapeutic index for the CEM-SS cells; These studies suggest that more than one mechanism of action is at work and that the balance of effects may depend on cell type and experimental conditions. Similar complexities are often seen with biological response modifiers. The "eff-tox" profile resembles the biphasic dose-response curves often obtained with those agents, indicating a path for analysis of combinations exhibiting such behavior. Good tools of analysis will clearly be required to put the interactions of biological response modifiers (with themselves and with other therapeutic modalities) into proper perspective. The COMBO algorithms are being used for that purpose.

ACKNOWLEDGEMENTS

We are grateful to L. Muenz for advice on the statistics. We thank O.S. Weislow, J. Szebeni, P. Ashorn, B. Moss, V.K. Chaudhary, D.J. FitzGerald, I. Pastan, and E.A. Berger for permission to use their data to illustrate the analyses here. The work of J.N.W. was supported in part by the National Institutes of Health Intramural Targeted AIDS Antiviral Program.

REFERENCES

1. P. Ashorn B. Moss J. N. Weinstein V. K. Chaudhary D. J. FitzGerald I. Pastan & E. A. Berger (1990). Elimination of infectious human immunodeficiency virus from human T-cell cultures by synergistic action of CD4-Pseudomonas exotoxin and reverse transcriptase inhibitors.*Proc. Natl. Acad. Sci. USA* **87**, 8889-8893.

2. B. Bunow & J. N. Weinstein (1990). COMBO: A new approach to the analysis of drug combinations in vitro.*Annals N.Y. Acad. Sci.* **616**, 490-494.

3. J. N. Weinstein B. Bunow R. F. Schinazi S. M. Wahl L. M. Wahl O. S. Weislow & J. Szebeni (1990). Synergistic drug combinations in AIDS therapy: Dipyridamole-zidovudine in particular and principles of analysis in general.*Annals N.Y. Acad. Sci.* **616**, 367-384.

4. K. L. Hartshorn M. W. Vogt T.-C. Chou R. S. Blumberg R. Byington R. T. Schooley & M. S. Hirsch (1987). Synergistic inhibition of human immunodeficiency virus in vitro by azidothymidine and recombinant alpha A interferon.*Antimicrob. Agents Chemother.* **31**, 168-172.

5. M. C. Berenbaum (1977). Synergy, additivism and antagonism in immunosuppression.*Clin. exp. Immunol.* **28**, 1-18.

6. W. R. Greco H. S. Park & Y. M. Rustum (1990). Application of a new approach for the quantitation of drug synergism to the combination of cis-diamminedichloroplatinum and 1-β-D-arabinofuranosylcytosine.*Cancer Research* **50**, 5318-5327.

7. R. F. Schinazi (1991). Combined chemotherapeutic modalities for viral infections: Rationale and clinical potential. In: T.-C. Chou and D. C. Rideout, Synergism and Antagonism in Chemotherapy, Academic Press, Orlando, FL, 109-181.

8. G. G. Steel & M. J. Peckham (1979). Exploitable mechanisms in combined radiotherapy-chemotherapy: The concept of additivity.*J. Radiation Oncology Biol. Phys.* **5**, 85-91.

9. J. Suhnel (1990). Evaluation of synergism or antagonism for the combined action of antiviral agents.*Antiviral Research* **13**, 23-40.

10. C.-M. Tsai A. F. Gazdar D. J. Venzon S. M. Steinberg R. L. Dedrick J. L. Mulshine & B. S. Kramer (1989). Lack of *in vitro* synergy between etoposide and cis-diamminedichloroplatinum(II).*Cancer Research* **49**, 2390-2397.

11. V. A. Johnson M. A. Barlow T.-C. Chou R. A. Fisher B. D. Walker M. S. Hirsch & R. T. Schooley (1989). Synergistic inhibition of human immunodeficiency virus type 1 (HIV-1) replication in vitro by recombinant soluble CD4 and 3'-azido-3'-deoxythymidine.*J. Infec. Dis.* **159**, 837-844.

12. T.-C. Chou & P. Talalay (1984). Quantitation analysis of dose-effect relationships: the combined effects of multiple drugs or enzyme inhibitors.*Adv. Enz. Regulation* **22**, 27-55.

13. K. C. Syracuse & W. R. Greco (1986). Proceedings of the Biopharmaceutical Section of the American Statistical Association.*Proc. Biopharm. Sec. Amer. Stat. Assoc.* 127-132.

14. M. N. Prichard & C. Shipman Jr. (1991). A three-dimensional model to analyze drug-drug interactions.*Antiviral Research* in press.

15. B. D. Efron (1979). Bootstrap methods: Another look at the jackknife.*Ann. Statistics* **7**, 1-26.

16. B. Efron & G. Gong (1983). A leisurely look at the bootstrap, the jackknife, and cross-validation.*Amer. Statistician* **37**, 36-48.

17. M. C. Berenbaum (1978). A method for testing for synergy with any number of agents.*J. Infect. Dis.* **137**, 122-130.

18. O. S. Weislow R. Kiser D. L. Fine J. Bader R. H. Shoemaker & M. R. Boyd (1989). New soluble formazan assay for HIV-1 cytopathic effects: Application to high-flux screening of synthetic and natural products for AIDS-antiviral activity.*J. Natl. Cancer Inst.* **81**, 577-586.

COMBINATIONS OF LYMPHOCYTE ACTIVATING AGENTS FOR EXPANSION OF TUMOR INFILTRATING LYMPHOCYTES FROM RENAL CELL CARCINOMA

Gilda G. Hillman, Sudha Sud, Eric J. Dybal,
J. Edson Pontes and Gabriel P. Haas

Department of Urology
Wayne State University
Detroit, MI

INTRODUCTION

Metastatic renal cell cancer (RCC) is resistant to most chemotherapeutic agents therefore attempts have been made to activate the patients immune system to induce an anti-tumor response leading to tumor regression. In several clinical trials, patients with metastatic RCC have been treated with immunotherapy consisting of infusions of the lymphokine Interleukin-2 (IL-2) or IL-2 combined with Lymphokine Activated Killer (LAK) cells (1,2). Although some patients responded well to these treatments, the overall rate of anti-tumor responses was relatively low (15-30%) and the therapy was limited by dose-dependent IL-2 toxicity.

Continuing efforts to develop less toxic and more effective therapies focused attention on lymphocytic infiltrates frequently observed within human or murine solid tumors. These Tumor Infiltrating Lymphocytes (TIL) can be isolated from enzymatic digests of tumor specimens and can be selectively expanded in presence of IL-2. TIL infusions have demonstrated dramatic anti-tumor responses in animal tumor models (3,4). In human studies, TIL were isolated and expanded from malignant melanoma (5,6), from renal cell cancer (7) and also from many other histologies (8). Based on these TIL studies, clinical trials with TIL and IL-2 were initiated (9). Dramatic responses were obtained in melanoma patients (9) but initial clinical trials using TIL for the treatment of metastatic RCC showed limited therapeutic efficacy (10). In contrast to TIL expanded from melanoma specimens, TILs expanded from RCC specimens did not demonstrate MHC-restricted specific cytotoxicity against the autologous tumor target. The growth conditions for TIL expansion in culture may select for the generation of killer cells specific for the autologous tumor. RPMI supplemented with human serum has been used in some studies, others have used serum free medium such as AIMV, and it is unclear whether the choice of medium in itself affects the properties of the TIL generated. Therefore, we tested three types of medium and the lymphocyte activating agents IL-2, Interleukin 4 (IL-4), Tumor

Combination Therapies, Edited by A.L. Goldstein and
E. Garaci, Plenum Press, New York, 1992

Necrosis Factor (TNF) and anti-CD3 monoclonal antibody (mAb) for expansion of TIL from RCC specimens. IL-4 has been shown to inhibit the IL-2-induced non MHC-restricted LAK activity (11). IL-4 combined with IL-2 also promoted the growth of melanoma TIL specific for the autologous tumor (12). TNF was found to upregulate expression of MHC antigens and the IL-2 receptor and to synergize with IL-2 in the generation of CD8+ TILs from ovarian cancer (13). Anti-CD3 mAb, a potent T cell mitogen (14), augmented the expansion of TIL with IL-2 (13,15). Here, we report the increased expansion of RCC TIL by addition of IL-4, TNF or anti-CD3 to IL-2. IL-4+IL-2 inhibited the generation of NK/LAK phenotype from these TILs. TNF+IL-2 and anti-CD3+IL-2 showed a tendency to expand CD8+ T cells. The majority of TILs generated under these conditions were T cells capable of mediating high levels of killing of the autologous RCC tumor but also non specific lysis of allogeneic tumors.

MATERIALS AND METHODS

Tumor specimens. Sterile renal tumor specimens, obtained from 7 patients after nephrectomy, were minced with scissors into small pieces and digested with 0.4mg/ml collagenase type IV (Sigma Chemical Co., St Louis, MO) in RPMI 1640 medium supplemented with 2mM glutamine, 10mM hepes buffer, 100 units/ml penicillin/ streptomycin and 0.05mg/ml gentamicin. The mixture was stirred overnight at room temperature and filtered through a wire mesh. The cell suspension was washed twice in Hank's balanced salt solution (HBSS) then separated by Ficoll-Hypaque (Histopaque, Sigma) density gradient centrifugation.

Culture of RCC tumor cells. Cultures of tumor cells isolated from RCC specimens were initiated at $2-4 \times 10^6$ cells/flask in RPMI and 10% Fetal Bovine Serum (FBS). The cultures were incubated at $37^{\circ}C$ in a 5% CO_2 incubator and split when confluent. Cells after 3-4 passages were used as RCC targets for the cytotoxic assays.

Lymphocyte activating agents. Recombinant human IL-2 (specific activity of 3×10^6 units/mg protein) and recombinant TNF (19×10^6 units/mg protein) were kindly supplied by the Cetus Corporation (Emeryville, CA). Recombinant human IL-4 (1.5×10^6 units/100μg/ml) was generously provided by Sterling Drug Inc (Malvern, PA). Anti-CD3 (OKT3) monoclonal antibody (mAb), directed against the CD3 component of the T cell receptor complex was purchased from Ortho Diagnostics, Raritan, NJ.

Culture of tumor-infiltrating lymphocytes. Lymphocytes isolated from RCC tumor specimens were plated at 5×10^5 cells/ml in 6-well culture plates (Costar, Cambridge, MA) in 3 types of culture medium: in RPMI 1640 supplemented with 10% FBS or 10% Human AB Serum (HS) or in serum free medium AIMV (Gibco, Grand Island, NY). TILs were cultured in the presence of 10, 100 or 1000 units/ml IL-2 alone or combined with 1000 units/ml IL-4 or 1000 units/ml TNF. The cultures were incubated at $37^{\circ}C$ in a 5% CO_2 incubator. After 7-10 days, TILs were harvested and resuspended at 2.5×10^5 cells/ml in their respective fresh media supplemented with the same activating agents. Cultures were split once or twice a week according to growth rate and assessed for expansion. TILs stimulated with anti-CD3 mAb were cultured in immobilized anti-CD3 mAb in the presence of 100 units/ml IL-2. Wells were pre-coated with purified anti-CD3 mAb at 10 μg/ml in phosphate buffered saline (PBS) for 1h at 37°C and washed twice with PBS prior to use (14). Three days following initiation of culture, cells were removed from anti-CD3 coated plates, washed and plated at 2.5×10^5 TIL/ml in medium containing 100 units/ml IL-2 alone. The continuous long term expansion of TIL required restimulation with a pulse of anti-CD3 mAb after 2-3 weeks.

Phenotypic analysis. TILs were harvested, washed with PBS and labeled with fluorescent mAbs for 30 min at 4°C (14). Cells were washed twice with PBS and the lymphocyte fraction was analyzed on a FACS 440 flow cytometer (Becton Dickinson, San Jose, CA). The monoclonal antibodies anti-leu4 (CD3) conjugated to fluorescein isothiocyanate (FITC), anti-leu3a (CD4) conjugated to phycoerythrin (PE) and anti-leu2a-FITC (CD8) (which react with the T helper/inducer cells and the T cytotoxic/suppressor cells respectively), anti-leu19-PE (CD56, which reacts with a 220 kD protein expressed on NK cells) were purchased from Becton Dickinson. For two color analysis, cells were double labeled with anti-CD3-FITC and anti-CD56-PE or anti-CD8-FITC and anti-CD4-PE. Gates were set for nonspecific binding using cells labeled with mouse IgG_1-FITC and mouse IgG_1-PE.

Cytotoxicity assay. The RCC tumor lines established from the patients and the NK sensitive K562 target (erythroleukemia line) were used as targets to assess the cytotoxic activity of the TILs. Target cells were labeled with 250 μCi ^{51}Cr for 2 hrs at 37°C in a 5% CO_2 incubator, washed and resuspended in medium. TILs were harvested, plated in triplicate in U-bottomed microtiter plates and serially diluted in 0.1ml medium. Labelled target cells at $5 \times 10^3/0.1ml$ were added to the wells resulting in 4 different effector/target (E/T) ratios. LAK cell control was included in each experiment. Following incubation for 4 hrs at 37°C, the cells were harvested onto a glass fiber filter with a Micromate 196 harvester (Packard Instrument Company, Meriden, CT) and counted in the Packard Matrix 96 to assess the ^{51}Cr retained in the cells. Percent cytotoxicity was calculated using the mean of triplicate wells as follows:

$$\% \text{ cytotoxicity} = \frac{\text{retained total counts} - \text{retained sample counts}}{\text{retained total counts} - \text{non releasable counts}} \times 100$$

Retained total counts were obtained from targets incubated in medium alone while non releasable counts were obtained from targets lysed with 2% cetrimide detergent solution (Sigma). This method gives an assessment of lysis of the target cells by the effector cells that parallels the lysis obtained by the conventional assessment of Cr release (unpublished data). Lytic units (LU) were calculated using 4 E/T ratios as described previously (14). One lytic unit was defined as the number of effector cells causing 20% lysis of 5×10^3 target cells; lytic units are expressed as $LU/10^7$ effector cells.

RESULTS

TIL expansion in RPMI+10%FBS

Expansion of TIL cultures was limited in RPMI+10%FBS as shown in Table 1. Cultures in IL-2 alone at 10, 100 or 1000 units/ml demonstrated poor expansion. The addition of IL-4 to

Table 1. Expansion of TIL on day 32 in RPMI+10%FBS

Conditions	FOLD EXPANSION		
	PATIENT 1	PATIENT 4	PATIENT 5
IL-2: 10	x0.7	x1.3	x0.4
100	x4.6	x0.4	x3.6
1000	x2.4	x4.6	N.T.
1000 IL-4			
+IL-2: 10	x1	x2.6	x1.4
100	x7.2	x0.5	x4.5
1000 TNF			
+IL-2: 10	x12	none	x15
100	x20	x1.4	x23

IL-2 did not improve the proliferation of TIL while addition of
TNF to IL-2 did increase slightly TIL expansion. Most of these
TILs died after 34-40 days.

TIL expansion in RPMI+10%HS and AIMV

    Combination of IL-2 with IL-4. TIL were cultured in 10 or
100 units/ml IL-2 alone or combined with 1000 units/ml IL-4.
Data obtained from a representative patient (#1) are shown in
Figure 1. TIL expanded in RPMI+10%HS showed a poor growth in 10
or 100 units/ml IL-2.   The addition of IL-4 to 10 or 100
units/ml IL-2 augmented TIL expansion.   Although variations
between TIL from different patients were noted, the best growth
was demonstrated by 100 units/ml IL-2 and 1000 units/ml IL-4.
This synergistic effect of IL-4 with IL-2 was less pronounced in
TIL cultured in AIMV medium. TIL growth was greater in AIMV in
100 units/ml IL-2 alone or with IL-4 than in RPMI+10%HS
(Figure 1). Expansion with 10 units/ml IL-2 in AIMV was smaller.

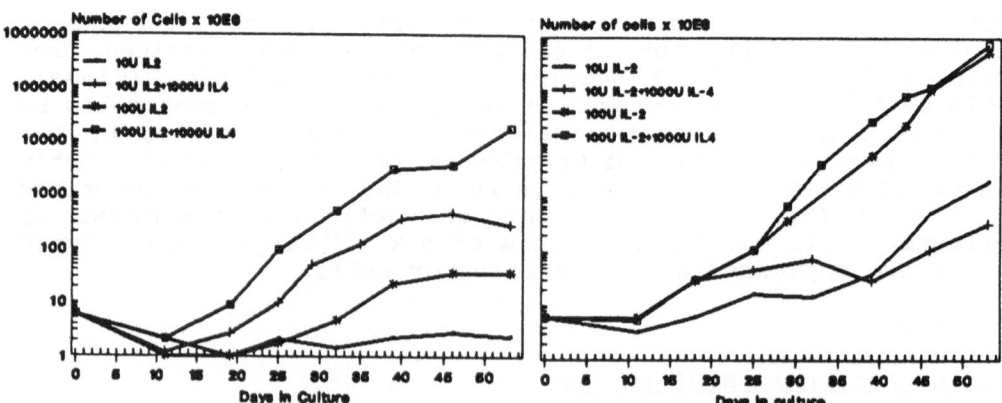

Figure 1. Growth curve of TIL cultured in IL-2+IL-4
in two types of media: RPMI+10%HS and AIMV.

Table 2. Expansion of TIL with IL-2 and TNF in RPMI+10%HS

Patients		TIL FOLD EXPANSION		
TIL	day	1	6	4
10U IL-2	30-32	x0.25	x12	x14
	46-48	x0.4	x339	x38
10U IL-2	30-32	x333	x9.6	x18
1000U TNF	46-48	x834	x44	x425
100U IL-2	30-32	x0.8	x160	x96
	46-48	x6	x4323	x830
100U IL-2	30-32	x820	x61	x128
1000U TNF	46-48	x7804	x1498	x1346
1000U IL-2	30-32	x42	x528	x223
	46-48	x87	x15878	x926

Combination of IL-2 with TNF. The proliferation of TIL stimulated by IL-2 and TNF varied from patient to patient. In cultures established in RPMI+10%HS, addition of TNF to 10 or 100 units/ml IL-2 augmented considerably the expansion of TIL in two patients (# 1,4) to levels greater than 1000 units/ml IL-2 alone (Table 2). The combination of TNF with 100 units/ml IL-2 resulted in greater expansion than with 10 units/ml IL-2. TIL isolated from patient 6 were highly responsive to IL-2 and no additional effect was observed with TNF. This variability of the responsiveness of TIL from different patients to IL-2 and TNF was also seen with TIL cultured in AIMV. Only two patients (# 6,7) from 4 tested showed an additive effect of TNF with 100 units/ml IL-2 (Tables 3,6).

Phenotype

The phenotype of TIL cultured in IL-2 combined with IL-4 or TNF varied from patient to patient both in AIMV and RPMI+10%HS.

Table 3. Phenotype of TIL from patient 7 cultured in AIMV in the presence of IL-2 with IL-4 or TNF

culture conditions	day	expansion (fold)	% cells positive for					
			CD3	CD4	CD8	CD56	CD3/ CD56	CD4/ CD8
10U IL-2	26	x 0.2	96	77	37	2	2	22
1000U IL-4	43	x 0.1	97	31	86	4	4	23
100U IL-2	26	x 4	98	74	31	2	2	15
1000U IL-4	43	x 582	98	64	51	4	4	19
10U IL-2	26	x 2.8	98	48	64	4	3	25
1000U TNF	43	x 2.2	93	18	70	13	13	8
100U IL-2	20	x 18	86	32	65	24	15	18
1000U TNF	26	x 78	95	14	67	27	24	6
	43	x 3129	98	4	94	18	18	2

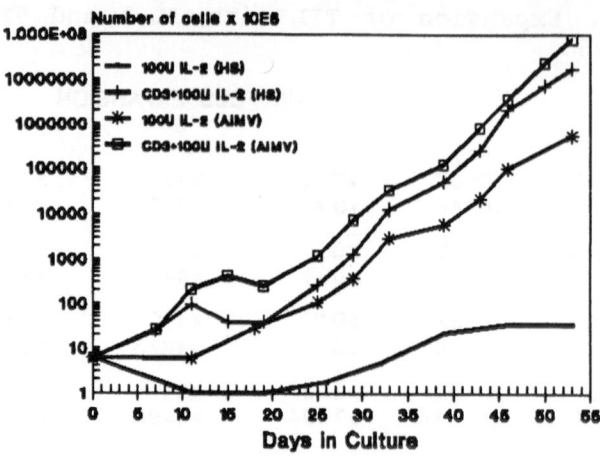

Figure 2. Expansion of TIL from patient 1 cultured
in IL-2 and anti-CD3

In some patients, cells of the NK phenotype (CD56+/CD3-) were
expanded in early cultures of IL-2 or IL-2+TNF but decreased
with time in culture (Table 6).   Other patients showed an
expansion of a CD3+/CD56+ population in IL-2+TNF that was
maintained in longer cultures (Table 3).   In contrast to
cultures containing TNF, CD56+ cells were rare in cultures grown
in IL-4 (Tables 3,6).   All cultures consisted predominantly of
T cells after 3 weeks and maintained this phenotype for the life
span of the culture. A tendency to expand more CD8+ T cells at
the expense of CD4+ T cells was seen with IL-2+TNF combination
in both types of media (Table 3,6).   A more varied T cell
phenotype was observed in TIL stimulated by IL-2+IL-4, some
showing a predominance of CD4+ cells, others of CD8+ cells
(Table 6) and other a mixture of both (Table 3). Moreover IL-
2+IL-4 seem to induce the expansion of a double positive
CD4+/CD8+ T cell population (Table 3,6).

Table 4. Phenotype of TIL from patient 1 stimulated
with anti-CD3 and IL-2.

culture conditions	day	expansion (fold)	CD3	CD4	CD8	CD56	CD3/ CD56	CD4/ CD8
RPMI-10% HS								
100U IL-2	43	x 3.6	94	94	1	7	3	0
anti-CD3	12	x 16	93	63	35	7	N.T.	N.T.
100U IL-2	28	x 215	97	61	50	1	1	14
	43	x 8600	98	27	89	2	2	19
AIMV								
100U IL-2	12	x 1	62	41	21	32	N.T.	N.T.
	28	x 61	97	47	59	7	5	12
	43	x 975	97	17	85	30	30	5
anti-CD3	12	x 34	92	46	46	7	N.T.	N.T.
100U IL-2	28	x 1248	98	75	34	0	0	13
	43	x 20672	99	91	17	0	0	9

44

Expansion of TIL in anti-CD3 combined with IL-2

TIL stimulated by immobilized anti-CD3 mAb and 100 units/ml IL-2 for 3 days then cultured in 100 units/ml IL-2 showed a rapid and extensive proliferation. Data from a representative patient (#1) are shown in figure 2. The difference in TIL growth in 100 units/ml IL-2 and anti-CD3 versus IL-2 alone was considerable in both RPMI+10%HS and AIMV although more pronounced in RPMI+10%HS.

The phenotype of TIL from the same patient (#1) stimulated with anti-CD3 is shown in Table 4 and indicates that anti-CD3 mAb combined with IL-2 induces predominantly CD3+ T cells both in RPMI+10%HS and in AIMV. In RPMI+10%HS, an increase in the CD8+ T cell population was observed with time in culture concomitant with an increase in CD8+/CD4+ population and a decrease in the CD4+ T cells. In AIMV, CD8+ cells seem to decrease with time in culture while CD4+ cells increase.

Lytic activity of TIL

The lytic activity of TIL obtained from patient 6 was tested against its autologous tumor cell line (RCC-6), allogeneic RCC tumor lines (RCC-7 and RCC-8) and K562. TIL cultured in AIMV mediated killing of the autologous RCC-6 tumor already by day 22 of culture. The autologous killing mediated by TIL cultured in 100 units/ml IL-2 and TNF was greater than that mediated by TIL cultured in 100 units IL-2 and IL-4. Both conditions showed a high level of NK activity by day 22 but it was reduced by day 44 of culture while the killing of autologous RCC was maintained. Although killing of allogeneic RCC-7 was lower, killing of RCC-8 was high. Based on LAK control, RCC-8 target seems to be very lysable. Thus, TIL expanded in AIMV in the presence of IL-4 or TNF combined with IL-2 are able to mediate killing of their autologous tumor target but also of allogeneic tumor targets. The phenotype of these TIL showed the presence of CD56+ LAK cells in early cultures in IL-2 or IL-2+TNF that decreased significantly in later cultures (Table 6).

Table 5. Lytic ability of TIL from patient 6 cultured in AIMV

LYTIC UNITS / 10^7 effectors

TIL	day	K562	RCC-6	RCC-7	RCC-8
100u IL-2	44	414	316	N.T.	434
1000u IL-2	22	187	98	30	N.T.
	44	190	193	N.T.	263
10u IL-2	22	261	23	0	N.T.
+1000u IL-4	44	165	213	N.T.	341
100u IL-2	22	1497	164	50	N.T.
+1000u IL-4	44	200	231	N.T.	356
100u IL-2	22	2540	324	177	N.T.
+1000u TNF	44	208	279	N.T.	381

Table 6. Phenotype of TIL from patient 6 cultured in AIMV

TIL	day	expansion (fold)	CD3	CD4	CD8	CD4/ CD8	CD56	CD3/ CD56
			\% Cells Positive for markers					
100u IL-2	14	x4.3	61	53	25	9	41	12
	37	x136	94	30	59	13	4	3
1000u IL-2	14	x7.6	52	43	23	7	46	9
	37	x240	95	68	58	34	4	4
10uIL-2 +1000IL-4	14	x2.5	92	72	45	26	6	1
	37	x563	98	38	93	34	3	3
100u IL-2 +1000u IL-4	14	x3	89	63	42	17	7	2
	37	x529	97	34	90	30	13	13
100u IL-2 +1000u TNF	14	x7	40	37	3	1	48	8
	37	x365	92	33	67	17	7	6

T cells predominated in most cultures with a higher percent of CD8+ cells that may correlate with their lytic ability.

TIL from the same patient (#6) expanded in RPMI+10%HS showed lytic activity against K562 and allogeneic RCC-8 but mediated limited killing of the autologous tumor RCC-6 (0-30 LU) both on day 22 and day 44 of culture (data not shown). This RCC-6 line was lysable by control LAK cells (270 LU) that were generated from normal PBL for 6 days in IL-2 in the same RPMI+10%HS medium and tested together with AIMV or RPMI+10%HS cultured TIL . Thus, the TIL from patient 6 acquired this "lack of recognition" of their autologous tumor during their long term culture in RPMI+10%HS. These TIL presented an unusual high percent of CD4+/CD8+ cells.

DISCUSSION

Tumor Infiltrating Lymphocytes (TIL), isolated from renal cell carcinoma (RCC) specimens and expanded in IL-2, showed limited therapeutic efficacy when reinfused to the patients (10). RCC TIL have demonstrated non MHC-restricted cytotoxicity (7,10) in contrast to TIL expanded from melanoma patients that mediated MHC-restricted specific cytotoxicity against the autologous tumor (5,6). The aim of our study was to test several culture conditions for RCC TIL in an attempt to generate TIL capable to mediate more specific lytic activity against their autologous tumor cells. We found that the medium and the serum used to expand TIL are critical. RPMI medium supplemented with 10%FBS failed to sustain the expansion of RCC TIL. In contrast, RPMI supplemented with 10%HS or AIMV induced a significant expansion of RCC TIL for a long term (up to 3 months). In most of the cultures, AIMV allowed for greater TIL expansion than RPMI+10%HS. The concentration of IL-2 in these cultures was also a limiting factor with 10 units/ml IL-2 being insufficient. The combination of IL-4 or TNF with IL-2 demonstrated a synergistic effect in the expansion of RCC TIL that was greater when 100 units/ml IL-2 was used. The synergy of IL-2 and TNF was generally more pronounced in TIL cultured in RPMI+10%HS than in AIMV. We observed that IL-4 or TNF augmented TIL expansion in AIMV only in cultures which were not responsive to IL-2. This suggests that, for AIMV cultures, the beneficial effect of the addition of IL-4 or TNF to IL-2 depends on the responsiveness of the lymphocytes isolated from different RCC specimens and is not predictable. In contrast, activation of TIL with immobilized anti-CD3 mAb and IL-2 followed by culture in 100 units/ml IL-2 induced a rapid and extensive proliferation of RCC TIL that was consistent both in AIMV and in RPMI+10%HS. TIL generated by anti-CD3+IL-2 were predominantly CD3+/CD56- T cells with a preferential expansion of CD8+ T cells in most cultures. Our findings on the synergy between anti-CD3 mAb and IL-2 confirm previous studies using RPMI and HS medium (13,15) but also document the establishment of long term TIL cultures. The phenotypic analysis of TIL stimulated by IL-2+IL-4 or IL-2+TNF showed variations from patient to patient. However, some findings were consistent in relationship to the combination used. TILs analyzed from early cultures (day 12-15) in IL-2 or IL-2+TNF consisted of a mixture of CD3+ T cells and CD56+ NK cells but became predominantly CD3+ T cells with time in culture. IL-2+TNF showed a tendency to expand more CD8+ T cells in long term cultures. These data contrast with the findings of Yi Li et al (13) who documented an early expansion of CD8+ cells followed later by an increase in CD56+ cells in ovarian tumor TILs cultured also in 100 units/ml IL-2 and 1000 units/ml TNF. NK expansion was minimal in TIL cultured with IL-2+IL-4 while T cells predominated with mixed ratios of CD4+ cells versus CD8+ cells. This indicates that IL-4 inhibits the generation of NK/LAK cells in TIL expanded from RCC similar to previous findings in melanomas (12). Moreover, IL-2+IL-4 induced the expansion of a double positive CD4+/CD8+ T cell population whose functional significance remains to be clarified. The relationship of the phenotype of TILs generated under these conditions and their lytic ability was examined. Preliminary experiments showed that TILs expanded in IL-2 or IL-2 combined with IL-4 or TNF demonstrated a pattern of non MHC-restricted cytotoxicity against RCC tumors and K562. However, only TIL expanded in AIMV serum free medium mediated a high level of killing of their autologous RCC tumor cells while this killing was poor in TILs expanded in RPMI and human serum. LAK cells generated in this human serum were able to kill this particular RCC target indicating that some regulation mediated by factors present in human serum may have occurred at the level of T cell recognition of the autologous tumor.

Cell separation studies are underway to identify specific subpopulations of T cells that could be responsible for the autologous killing mediated by the TIL bulk cultures. These studies indicate that TIL are particularly sensitive to growth conditions and that variations of culture conditions can select for desired expansion, phenotype and lytic activity that may ultimately lead to improved clinical results. The properties of the ideal TIL for adoptive transfer are yet to be defined.

Acknowledgements: We thank M. KuKuruga for flow cytometry analysis at the WSU-Ben Kasle Flow Cytometry Facility. This work was supported by ACS grant # 4-48017.

REFERENCES

1. S.A.Rosenberg, M.T. Lotze, L.M. Muul, A.E. Chang, F.P. Avis, S. Leitman, W.M. Linehan, C.N. Robertson, R.E. Lee, J.T. Rubin, C.A. Seipp, C.G. Simpson and D.E. White. A progress report on the treatment of 157 patients with advanced cancer using

lymphokine-activated killer cells and interleukin-2 or high dose interleukin-2 alone. N Eng J Med. 316:889 (1987).

2. S.A. Rosenberg, M.T. Lotze, J.C. Yang, P.M. Aebersold, W.M. Linehan, C.A. Seipp and D.E. White. Experience with the use of high dose interleukin 2 in the treatment of 652 cancer patients. Ann Surg 210:474 (1989).

3. S.A. Rosenberg, P. Spiess and R. Lafreniere. A new approach to the adoptive immunotherapy of cancer with tumor-infiltrating lymphocytes. Science. 223:1318 (1986).

4. P.J. Spiess, J.C. Yang and S.A. Rosenberg. In vivo antitumor activity of tumor-infiltrating lymphocytes expanded in recombinant interleukin-2. J Natl Cancer Inst. 79:1067 (1987).

5. S.L. Topalian, L.M. Muul and S.A. Rosenberg. Growth and immunologic characteristics of lymphocytes infiltrating human tumor. Surg Forum. 37:390 (1987).

6. K. Itoh, C.D. Platsoucas and C.M. Balch. Autologous tumor-specific cytotoxic T lymphocytes in the infiltrate of human metastatic melanomas: activation by interleukin-2 and autologous tumor cells, and involvement of the t cell receptor. J Exp Med. 168:1419 (1988).

7. A. Belldegrun, L.M. Muul and S.A. Rosenberg. Interleukin 2 expanded tumor-infiltrating lymphocytes in human renal cell cancer: isolation, characterization, and antitumor activity. Cancer Res. 48:206 (1988).

8. G.P. Haas, D.L. Solomon and S.A. Rosenberg. Isolation and characterization of tumor-infiltrating lymphocytes from non-renal urologic malignancies. Cancer Immunol Immunother. 30:342 (1990).

9. S.A. Rosenberg, B.S. Packard, P.M. Aebersold, D. Solomon, S. L. Topalian, S.T. Toy, P. Simon, M.T.Lotze, J.C. Yang, C.A. Seipp, C. Simpson, C. Carter, S. Bock, D. Schwartzentruber, J. Wei and D. White. Use of tumor-infiltrating lymphocytes and interleukin-2 in the immunotherapy of patients with metastatic melanoma: a preliminary report. N Engl J Med. 319:1676 (1988).

10. J. Finke, S. Murthy, J. Alexander, P. Rayman, R. Tubbs, E. Pontes, J. Sergi and R. Bukowski. Tumor infiltrating-lymphocytes in human renal cell carcinoma: Adoptive immunotherapy and characterization of interleukin-2 expanded tumor-infiltrating lymphocytes in: Immunotherapy of renal cell carcinoma, F.M.J. Debruyne, R.M. Bukowski, J.E. Pontes and P.H.M. de Mulder, ed., Springer-Verlag, Berlin, p119 (1991).

11. Y. Kawakami, M.C. Custer, S.A. Rosenberg and M.T. Lotze. IL-4 regulates IL-2 induction of lymphokine-activated killer activity from human lymphocytes. J Immunol. 142:3452 (1989).

12. Y. Kawakami, S.A. Rosenberg and M.T. Lotze. Interleukin 4 promotes the growth of tumor-infiltrating lymphocytes cytotoxic for human autologous melanoma. J Exp Med. 168: 2183 (1988).

13. W. Yi Li, S. Lusheng, A. Kanbour, R.B. Herberman and T.L. Whiteside. Lymphocytes infiltrating human ovarian tumors: Synergy between tumor necrosis factor alpha and interleukin 2 in the generation of CD8+ effectors from tumor-infiltrating lymphocytes. Cancer Res. 49:5979 (1989).

14. G. Weil-Hillman, K. Schell, D.M. Segal, J.A. Hank, J.' Sosman and P. M. Sondel. Activation of human T cells obtained pre and post IL-2 therapy by anti-CD3 monoclonal antibody plus IL-2: implications for combined in vivo treatment. J Immunother. In press, (1991).

15. D.D. Schoof, C.M. Selleck, A.F. Massaro, S.E. Jung and T.J. Eberlein. Activation of human tumor-infiltrating lymphocytes by monoclonal antibodies directed to the CD3 complex. Cancer Res. 50:1138 (1990).

IL-2 BASED COMBINATION THERAPY OF MALIGNANT DISEASE:

SUMMARY OF THE PHASE I EXPERIENCE AT THE CLEVELAND CLINIC

G.T. Budd, S.V. Murthy, J. Finke, R.R. Tubbs,
J. Alexander, S. Gautam, J. Sergi, and R. Bukowski

Cleveland Clinic Foundation
Cleveland, OH 44195

We have performed Phase I trials of rIL-2 in combination with IFNα or doxorubicin (DOX), based upon the independent activity of these agents and preclinical evidence of therapeutic synergy. In a Phase I trial of the combination of doxorubicin (DOX) and rIL-2, myelosuppression prevented dose escalation beyond the MTD of DOX 40 mg/m^2 IV bolus day 1 and rIL-2 3.0 MU/m^2/24 hr IV on days 2-5, 9-12, and 16-19. Significant increases in peripheral blood NK and LAK precursor activities were observed, but no clinical responses were produced in this patient population with largely gastrointestinal malignancies. In other Phase I studies, four week cycles of rIL-2 given by intravenous (IV) bolus injection three times weekly (TIW) have been administered in combination with rHuIFNα2a given intramuscularly (IM) TIW. With aggressive supportive care, the Maximum Tolerated Dose (MTD) of rIL-2 that could be given with rHuIFNα2a 10 MU/m^2 IM TIW was 22.0 x 10^6 BRMP Units (MU)/m^2 IV TIW. Dose limiting toxicities were CNS, pulmonary and cardiovascular. When given with rHuIFNα2a 10.0 MU/m^2 TIW, the MTD of infusion rIL-2 was 3.0 MU/m^2/24 hr x 5 days, weekly x 4. We have also treated pts with RCC and MM in Phase II trials of rIL-2 3.0 MU/m^2/24 hrs D1-4 and rHuIFNα2a 5.0 MU/m^2 SQ D1-4. Overall, 3/7 pts with RCC treated with infusion schedule rIL-2 and rHuIFNα2a have responded in our Phase I study, as opposed to 3/33 pts with RCC treated with bolus schedule rIL-2 and rHuIFNα2a. Of pts with MM, 6/23 pts have responded to bolus schedule rIL-2 and rHuIFNα2a while 0/3 have responded to infusion schedule rIL-2 with rHuIFNα2a in our Phase I studies. We have also entered patients on multi-center Phase II studies utilizing a somewhat less dose-intense schedule of infusion schedule rIL-2 and rHuIFNα2a. Among patients entered on these trials from the Cleveland Clinic, 3/11 pts with RCC have responded, while 2/10 pts with MM have responded. Further studies of the mechanisms by which responses are mediated are needed if IL-2 based therapies are to be improved.

Introduction

Interleukin-2 (IL-2) is an immunoregulatory cytokine which exerts effects on several effector cell populations. IL-2 supports the growth and proliferation of T-cells and other lymphocytes and augments certain effector functions, including antigen-specific and non-specific cytolytic activities [1-5]. IL-2 exerts these effects in a complex milieu comprised of other cytokines and immune regulatory and effector cells. It is not unreasonable to expect that the specific effects of an administered dose of an agent such as IL-2 will depend greatly on the influences of these other immunologic factors. Pre-clinical models have suggested that IL-2 in combination with other agents may have greater anti-tumor effects than single agent treatment. Based upon these observations, we have performed a series of Phase I trials employing IL-2 in combination with other agents.

Phase I Experience with IL-2 and Doxorubicin

The rationale underlying the combination of IL-2 with cytotoxic chemotherapy has been reviewed [6]. The combination of doxorubicin and IL-2 with LAK cells was found to be superior to treatment with either modality alone in the Renca murine renal cell carcinoma model [7]. Gautam has demonstrated similar results in the Renca system in studies combining doxorubicin and IL-2 without LAK cells [8], and doxorubicin was found to augment the antitumor effects of IL-2 in a murine lymphoma system [9]. Based upon these studies, we have performed a Phase I trial of doxorubicin and IL-2 in patients with refractory malignancies [10]. Doxorubicin was administered as an intravenous bolus injection on day one, with rIL-2 (Hoffmann-LaRoche) being administered by continuous intravenous infusion on days 2-5, 9-12, and 16-19 of each 3-4 week treatment cycle. Cycles were repeated as tolerated unless disease progression was noted. The doses studied were doxorubicin 40 mg/m^2 + rIL-2 1.0 x 10^6 U (MU)/m^2/24 hours, doxorubicin 40 mg/m^2 + rIL-2 3.0 MU/m^2/24 hours, and doxorubicin 60 mg/m^2/24 hours + rIL-2 1.0 MU/m^2/24 hours. At this last dose level, 4/5 patients developed NCI Grade 3 neutropenia, 3/5 developed Grade 3 granulocytopenia, and 1 developed Grade 3 thrombocytopenia. The next lower dose level was, therefore, identified as the Maximum Tolerated Dose (MTD): that is, doxorubicin 40 mg/m^2 + rIL-2 3.0 MU/m^2/24 hours. At the MTD, 2/6 patients developed Grade 3 leukopenia, 2/6 patients developed Grade 3-4 neutropenia, and 1/6 patients developed Grade 3 thrombopenia.

Immunologic effects were observed, suggesting that doxorubicin does not abrogate the effects of Il-2 on peripheral blood lytic activity. With doxorubicin 40 mg/m^2, rIL-2 1.0 MU/m^2 produced rises in peripheral blood NK activity to >200 lytic units/10^7 cells (LU) in 4/5 patients, while rIL-2 3.0 MU/m^2 produced rises in this activity to >200 LU in 4/4 patients. Peripheral blood LAK activity was observed during treatment in 2/9 patients; both of these patients were treated with doxorubicin 40 mg/m^2 + rIL-2 1.0 MU/m^2/24 hours. LAK precursor activity in the peripheral blood (assayed by determining the lytic activity of peripheral blood lymphocytes cultured for 3 days with 1000 U/ml of rIL-2) was found to be increased on day 16 of treatment, compared to pretreatment values, in 1/4 patients studied serially after treatment with doxorubicin 40 mg/m^2 + rIL-2 1.0 MU/m^2/24 hours and in 3/4 patients studied after treatment with doxorubicin 40 mg/m^2/24 hours + rIL-2 3.0 MU/m^2/24 hours. Whether these changes are quantitatively different than those that would be produced by treatment with rIL-2 alone cannot be determined in this Phase I study; a controlled trial would be required to address this issue.

No clinical responses were observed among the 17 patients entered in this trial, but it should be noted that 14 of these 17 patients suffered gastrointestinal malignancies, while no patients with renal cell carcinoma or malignant melanoma were entered. Further studies in these "immunoresponsive" tumors or in tumors responsive to doxorubicin might be considered, using the dose identified as the MTD.

Phase I Experience With IL-2 and IFNα

The combination of IL-2 and IFNα has been found to produce greater antitumor effects than either cytokine alone in several preclinical model tumor systems [11-14]. We have performed a series of clinical investigations of this combination, based upon these preclinical studies.

Toxicity of IL-2/IFNα

In our initial trial, rIL-2 (Hoffmann-LaRoche) was administered as an intravenous bolus injection three times weekly and rHuIFNα2a was given intramuscularly on the same days; treatment was continued for four consecutive weeks, followed by a rest period as needed [15]. All possible combinations of doses of rIL-2 0.1, 0.5, or 2.0 MU/m^2 and rHuIFNα2a 0, 0.1, 1.0, or 10.0 MU/m^2 were given to successive cohorts of patients in a traditional Phase I trial design. At the highest doses of the agents (rIL-2 2.0 MU/m^2 with rHuIFNα2a 10.0 MU/m^2), Grade 3 neutropenia was produced in 3/6 patients, determining the MTD as defined in the experimental design of the study.

Because 1) hematologic toxicity was rapidly reversible and asymptomatic, 2) non-hematologic toxicity was mild, and 3) considerable clinical experience had indicated that aggressive supportive measures would allow higher doses of rIL-2 to be given, we performed a second Phase I trial of high dose bolus rIL-2 with IFNα [16]. In this trial, the dose of rIL-2 was escalated in successive cohorts of patients while the dose of rHuIFNα2a was fixed at 10.0 MU/m^2 (with the exception of patients treated with rIL-2 10 MU/m^2, at which dose level doses of rHuIFNα2a of 0.1, 1.0, and 10.0 MU/m^2 were studied). The doses of rIL-2 administered with rHuIFNα2a were 4, 6, 8, 10, 12, 14, 18, 22, and 26 MU/m^2. As in our low dose bolus administration trial, rIL-2 was administered as a rapid intravenous injection three times weekly and rHuIFNα2a was administered intramuscularly three times weekly. Both agents were given for four consecutive weeks, followed by a rest period of at least two weeks. Stable and responding patients were retreated, provided that they had recovered from the toxicity of the previous course and that toxicity had been acceptable. The experimental design called for stopping the trial once 3 or more of 6 patients at a dose level experienced unacceptable toxicity; this would define the next lower dose as the Maximum Tolerated Dose (MTD). In the event of unacceptable toxicity in an individual patient, treatment was held until toxicity had recovered to grade 0-1; treatment was then reinstituted at the next lower dose level. In order to allow dose escalation beyond those used in the low-dose bolus administration trial, modified definitions of unacceptable toxicity were used. Unacceptable toxicity was defined as: serum creatinine >5 mg/dl, serum bilirubin >5 mg/dl, dyspnea at rest, hypotension refractory to pressors, altered mental status or coma, and other toxicities of Grade 3-4 as defined by the NCI Common Toxicity Criteria.

At a dose of rIL-2 of 26 MU/m^2 in combination with rHuIFNα2a 10 MU/m^2 three times weekly, 3 of 3 patients developed unacceptable toxicity, consisting of dyspnea at rest in one patient, central nervous system depression in one patient, and hypotension poorly controlled with phenylephrine in two patients. The next lower dose level, rIL-2 22 MU/m^2 with rHuIFNα2a 10 MU/m^2, then, was identified as the MTD. Hypotension was observed at all dose levels including rIL-2 at doses greater than 8 MU/m^2, but this hypotension was responsive to support with phenylephrine, so that therapy could be continued. Other toxicities included fluid retention, mild dyspnea, fatigue, exfoliative skin rash, diarrhea, oliguria, abnormal renal and hepatic function tests, hypocalcemia, neutropenia, and thrombopenia. Despite these toxicities, therapy was administered on a regular nursing floor.

Because others had reported relatively greater degrees of immunomodulation with infusion as opposed to bolus schedules of IL-2 administration [17,18], and because continuous intravenous infusion was felt to better simulate the pharmacokinetics of the intraperitoneal administration of IL-2 used in some pre-clinical models, we have also studied the administration of rIL-2 by continuous infusion with intramuscular IFNα in a Phase I trial [19]. In this trial, successive cohorts of 4-6 patients were treated with escalating doses of the two agents; rIL-2 was administered as a continuous 120 hour infusion on days 1-5 of four consecutive weeks and rHuIFNα2a was administered intramuscularly three times weekly for four consecutive weeks. The dose levels studied were: 1a) rIL-2 3.0 MU/m^2/24 hours + rHuIFNα2a 5.0 MU/m^2, 1b) rIL-2 3.0 MU/m^2/24 hours + rHuIFNα2a 10.0 MU/m^2, and 2a) rIL-2 4.5 MU/m^2/24 hours + rHuIFNα2a 5.0 MU/m^2. Using the modified toxicity criteria described above, unacceptable toxicity was produced at dose level 2a (rIL-2 4.5 MU/m^2/24 hours + rHuIFNα2a 5.0 MU/m^2). Unacceptable toxicity at that dose level included CNS depression (3/6 patients, including one instance attributed to sepsis) and dyspnea at rest (4/6 patients, including 2 requiring mechanical ventilation). These and other toxicities proved reversible with the discontinuation of therapy. Other side effects included nausea and vomiting, stomatitis, anorexia, fatigue, myalgias, arthralgias, insomnia, diarrhea, neutropenia, thrombopenia, and abnormal liver and renal function. Again, with the exception of those patients requiring temporary intubation, therapy was managed on a regular nursing floor.

Anti-tumor Effects of IL-2/IFNα

In our low dose bolus trial, 3 partial responses of relatively short duration (4-12 weeks) were observed among the 55 patients treated. These responses were observed in malignant melanoma (1/6 patients), renal cell carcinoma (1/12 patients), and breast cancer (1/1 patient) [15]. In the high dose bolus trial, 8 of the 57 treated patients responded [16]. Two partial responses were observed among 21 patients with metastatic renal cell carcinoma, while one of three patients with metastatic breast cancer responded partially. Among 17 patients with metastatic malignant melanoma were observed 2 complete and 3 partial responses; the two complete responses have proven durable, with both patients remaining in unmaintained complete remission for periods exceeding 2 years.

Among the 23 patients treated with infusion rIL-2 in combination with rHuIFNα2a in our Phase I trial, four partial responses were produced [19]. One occurred in the single patient with endometrial cancer who was treated, while the remaining 3 were produced in the 7 patients with metastatic renal cell carcinoma who were entered on this trial. One patient with renal cell carcinoma was rendered disease free by nephrectomy after extensive pulmonary metastases had resolved completely. Although this patient suffered an isolated CNS recurrence over one year post-therapy, this lesion was resected and the patient remains alive in excess of two years after entry on study.

In addition to the Phase I experience discussed above, we have participated in multi-center Phase II trials of rIL-2 3.0 $MU/m^2/24$ hrs given in combination with rHuIFNα2a 5.0 MU/m^2 IM; in these trials, both agents were given for four consecutive days of four consecutive weeks. Thus, this infusion schedule was somewhat less dose intense than the dose-schedule identified by us as the MTD. Among 11 patients with renal cell carcinoma entered on these trials, we have produced responses in 3 patients, while 2/10 patients with melanoma have responded in the Phase II trials [20].

These results suggest that the combination of rIL-2 and rHuIFNα2a can produce objective complete and partial remissions in patients with metastatic malignancy. The data suggest that the infusion schedule may be worthy of investigation in the treatment of renal cell carcinoma. Further studies of the bolus schedule should be performed in patients with malignant melanoma.

Immunologic Effects of IL-2/IFNα Therapy

The combination of rIL-2 and rHuIFNα2a has been found to produce increased NK and LAK activities in the peripheral blood of treated patients in our studies [16,19]. Increases in peripheral blood lymphocytes (PBL's) bearing the NK-cell marker CD56 have also been observed. Although the total number of CD3+ T-cells in the peripheral blood did not change greatly in treated patients, at least at the time points sampled, increases in the number of circulating activated T-cells (CD3+CD25-HLADr+, CD3+CD25+HLADr+) were seen [19]. Also of interest was the lack of infiltration of lymphocytes bearing NK-markers into tumors, despite the observation of changes in NK activity and numbers in the peripheral blood [21]. Both prior to and during IL-2/IFNα therapy, the majority of lymphocytes infiltrating tumors bear the T-cell marker CD3. Although we have been unable to demonstrate reproducible changes in the intensity or phenotypic distribution of this lymphocytic infiltration as a consequence of therapy, the intensity of the CD3+ infiltrate positively correlates with HLA-Dr expression by tumor cells [21].

Conclusion

IL-2 is a powerful immunoregulatory cytokine whose in-vivo effects may be affected by other immunomodulatory influences. In order to advance the state of immunotherapy, it is important that the immunologic events relevant to antitumor response be clarified and that the effects of immunotherapeutic maneuvers on these immunologic parameters be studied. The dichotomy of effects of IL-2 based therapy on peripheral blood and tumor infiltrating lymphocytes suggests that immunologic studies that focus on events occurring at the site of the tumor may be needed in order to adequately understand the mechanisms by which tumor regressions are mediated.

References

1. Stotter H, Rude E, Wagner H. T-cell factor (interleukin-2) allows in vivo induction of T-helper cells against heterologous erythrocytes in athymic (nu/nu) mice. European Journal of Immunology. 10:719-722, 1980.

2. Erard F, Corthesy P, Nabholz M, Lowenthal JW, Zaech P, Plaetinck G, MacDonald HR. Interleukin-2 is both necessary and sufficient for the growth and differentiation of lectin-stimulated cytolytic T lymphocyte precursors. Journal of Immunology. 134:1644-1651, 1985.

3. Henney CS, Kuribayashi K, Kern DF, Gillis S. Interleukin-2 augments natural killer cell activity. Nature. 291:335-338, 1981.

4. Itoh K, Tilden AB, Balch CM. Lysis of human solid tumor cells by lymphokine-activated natural killer cells. Journal of Immunology. 136:3910-3915, 1986.

5. Phillips JH, Lanier LL. Dissection of the lymphokine activated killer phenomenon. Relative contribution of peripheral blood natural killer cells and T-lymphocytes to cytolysis. Journal of Experimental Medicine. 164:814-825, 1986.

6. Mitchell MS. Combining chemotherapy with biological response modifiers in treatment of cancer. Journal of the National Cancer Institute. 80:1445-1450, 1988.

7. Wiltrout RH, Salup RR. Adoptive immunotherapy in combination with chemotherapy for cancer treatment. Prog. Exp. Tumor Res. 32:128-153, 1988.

8. Gautam SC, Chikkala NF, Ganapathi R. Chemoimmunotherapy of established murine renal cell carcinoma with Adriamycin and IL-2. Proc. Amer. Assoc. Cancer Res. 30:361, 1989.

9. Yu PP, Paciucci PA, Jolland JF. Activity of recombinant human interleukin-2 (rIL-2) and doxorubicin in tumor bearing BL/6 mice. Proc. Am. Assoc. Cancer Res. 27:317, 1986.

10. Bukowski RM, Sergi J, Budd GT, Murthy S, Tubbs R, Gibson V, Herzog P, Stanley J, Finke J. Phase I trial of continuous infusion Interleukin-2 and Adriamycin in patients with refractory malignancy. Proc. Amer. Assoc. Cancer Res. 31:204, 1990.

11. Finke J, Lewis I, Yen-Lieberman B, Proffitt M. Anti-tumor activity of IL-2 in combination with FINαA/D in a murine tumor model. Proceedings of the FASEB, 1986.

12. Finke J, Lewis I, Tubbs R, Ganapathi R. Combination of IL-2 and IFNαA/D: antitumor and immunomodulatory activity. Lymphokine Research. 6:1511, 1987.

13. Cameron RB, McIntosh JK, Rosenberg SA. Synergistic antitumor effects of combination immunotherapy with recombinant interleukin-2 and a recombinant hybrid α-interferon in the treatment of established murine hepatic metastases. Cancer Research. 48:5810-5817, 1988.

14. Rosenberg SA, Schwartz SL, Spiess PJ. Combination immunotherapy for cancer: synergistic antitumor interactions of interleukin-2, alfa interferon, and tumor-infiltrating lymphocytes. Journal of the National Cancer Institute. 80:1393-1397, 1988.

15. Budd GT, Osgood B, Barna B, Boyett JM, Finke J, Medendorp SV, Murthy S, Novak C, Sergi J, Tubbs R, Bukowski RM. Phase I Clinical Trial of Interleukin-2 and Interferon-alpha: Toxicity and Immunologic Effects. Cancer Research 49:6432-6436, 1989.

16. Budd GT, Sergi J, Barna B, Finke J, Medendorp S, Murthy S, Tubbs R, Novak C, Bukowski R. Phase I Trial of Interleukin-2 (rIL-2) and IFN-α (rHuIFN-α2a) in Human Malignancy. Proceedings of the American Association for Cancer Research. 30:362, 1989.

17. West WH, Tauer KW, Yannelli JR, et. al. Constant-infusion recombinant interleukin-2 in adoptive immunotherapy of advanced cancer. New England Journal of Medicine. 316:899-905, 1987.

18. Sosman JA, Kohler PC, Hank JA, et. al. Repetitive weekly cycles of interleukin-2. II. Clinical and immunologic effects of dose, schedule, and addition of indomethacin. J Natl Cancer Inst. 80:1451-61, 1988.

19. Bukowski RM, Murthy SR, Sergi JS, **Budd GT,** McKeever S, Medendorp SV, Tubbs R, Gibson V, Fishleder A, Finke J: Phase I trial of continuous infusion recombinant Interleukin-2 and intermittent recombinant Interferon-alpha-2a: Clinical Effects. Journal of Biologic Response Modifiers. 9:538-545, 1990.

20. Budd GT, Sergi J, Finke J, Tubbs R, Murthy S, Gibson V, Medendorp S, Bauer L, Barna B, Boyett J, Bukowski RM. Combination Interleukin-2 and alpha-interferon therapy of metastatic renal cell carcinoma and malignant melanoma. Proceedings of the American Association for Cancer Research. 31:271, 1990.

21. Tubbs R, Budd GT, Finke J, Sergi J, Murthy S, Bukowski RM. Cellular infiltrates in tumor specimens from patients treated with cytokines and adoptive cellular therapy. Proceedings of the American Association for Cancer Research. 31:175, 1990.

THE ROLE OF COMBINATION BIOLOGIC THERAPY IN THE IMMUNOTHERAPEUTIC APPROACH TO THE TREATMENT OF RENAL CELL CARCINOMA

Robert A. Figlin*, Antoine S. Abi-Aad, Arie Belldegrun,
Jean B. deKernion

(*)Department of Medicine, Division of Hematology-Oncology;
Department of Surgery, Division of Urology, UCLA School of
Medicine

INTRODUCTION

Renal cell carcinoma (RCC) is the most common malignancy of the kidney accounting for approximately 3% of all adult cancers. The tumor is more common among urban dwellers and males, and occurs primarily in the fifth to seventh decades of life. Overt symptoms accompanying RCC are often associated with advanced local or distant disease. Approximately two-thirds of the all locally confined renal tumors are found incidentally (1). Surgical extirpation is the cornerstone of therapy of localized RCC. In spite of years of research and many clinical trials, the management of metastatic disease remains undefined.

NATURAL HISTORY

The etiology of RCC is unclear and little evidence is available to incriminate any specific etiologic agent. It has been proposed that loss of a gene or genes with tumor suppressor function might be associated with the development of RCC (2). Recent evidence indicates that deletions and translocations involving the short arm of chromosome 3 are important for the oncogenesis and tumor progression of RCC (3). Transforming growth factor (TGF)-alpha and beta are two tumor-produced regulatory growth factors that may be related to the development of RCC (4). These studies could lead to further understanding of the pathogenesis of RCC and highlight the genetic propensity to either enhanced metastatic spread or spontaneous degeneration.

The natural history of RCC is not always predictable. Some of the tumors remain silent and are only discovered postmortem. Careful postmortem studies in a series of 16,294 autopsies performed in Malmo, Sweden, revealed 350 cases of RCC, 235 of which had been unrecognized during life(5). These otherwise clinically occult tumors are now being detected with increasing frequency, due to the increased use of ultrasound, computed tomography and magnetic resonance imaging. Because RCC outcome may be capricious, the impact on the ultimate survival in this group of patients is yet to be determined.

Haematogenous spread of RCC is the most important and most frequent route to metastatic disease. Tumor extension through Gerota's fascia, lymph node involvement, extension to contiguous organs, multiple distant metastases, and certain histological features (ie. high grade, aneuploidy, cell type), have all been associated with poor prognosis (6). Ritchie et al. has reported that the incidence of metastases at the time of presentation in 3159 patients with RCC was 23% (7). The reported survival in the presence of metastatic disease is 73% at 6 months, 48% at 1 year and 9% at 5 years (8).

MANAGEMENT OF METASTATIC RENAL CELL CARCINOMA

The urologist and medical oncologist are often faced with the perplexing problem of the patient with advanced renal cell carcinoma, including those who present with metastases at the time of diagnosis and those in whom the metastases develop after radical surgery. In our practice at UCLA those 2 groups combined account for approximately half of the patients with the diagnosis of renal cell carcinoma. Surgery, chemotherapy, hormonal therapy, and immunotherapy with or without surgery can be proposed as options for management in such patients.

Nephrectomy

Nephrectomy in the presence of unresectable local or distant metastases has not been of proven benefit. Golimbu et al. (9) reported 92 patients with disseminated disease who underwent nephrectomy. The 5-year survival rate of 2.2 % was no better when compared to the survival of untreated stage IV patients. After adjunctive nephrectomy regression can be expected to occur in less than 1 % of patients (10), with most regressions short-lived and the mortality rate from the surgery ranging from 2 to 15 percent, depending largely upon patient selection. It therefore, seems impossible to support the routine practice of adjunctive nephrectomy in patients with metastatic disease. Adjunctive nephrectomy, in order to reduce tumor load or to initiate experimental therapy represent in our opinion the only indication for surgery in asymptomatic patients with unresectable metastases. To this end, the Southwest Oncology Group has initiated a randomized trial addressing the role of nephrectomy in patients presenting with metastatic disease.

Hormone Therapy

As currently used, endocrine therapy is of only marginal benefit in metastatic RCC. In vitro, progesterone is the only agent that has shown antitumor effect. Hrushesky and Murphy (11) noted that the early enthusiasm for androgenic and progestational therapies was generated by the lack of strict response criteria. In a review of 110 patients at our institution, no patient had an objective response to progestational agents (12).

Chemotherapy

Cytotoxic drugs remain the cornerstone of treatment of advanced solid tumors, either alone or in combination. However, despite the remarkable advances made in the treatment of some tumors, RCC remains one of the tumors most refractory to standard chemotherapy. In a recent review by Yagoda (13), the results of 39 agents evaluated in 2,120 patients were disappointing. Only 8.7 percent of the patients achieved complete or partial response, mostly of short duration, 5 months. At UCLA, vinblastine was the most potent cytotoxic agent though no patient achieved a complete response (14). The basis for this multidrug resistance (MDR) appears related to a transmembrane glycoprotein (P-glycoprotein, P170) encoded by the MDR1 gene that functions as an energy dependent drug efflux pump (15).

IMMUNOTHERAPY

Metastatic RCC has been a target for a variety of treatment protocols involving experimental agents or procedures, more commonly referred to as biological response modifiers (BRMs). The broad spectrum of biologic activities displayed by these agents has stimulated considerable interest in the oncologic community because of their potential application in the treatment of malignant disease. This enthusiasm is mainly due to the recent advances achieved in immunology and molecular biology. Most of the clinical studies for RCC have a common rationale for BRM application, including the peculiar behavior of metastatic RCC where instances of spontaneous regression of established lesions have been well documented. Biological response modifiers represent a broad class of agents that may affect tumor cells or host cells in a variety of ways other than non-specific cytotoxicity. This may include, but is not limited to, the regulation of the immune system and tumor cell differentiation.

This approach to treatment can be classified into active and passive categories. Passive or adoptive immunotherapy involves the transfer to the tumor-bearing host of active immunologic reagents, such as cells with anti-tumor reactivity, that can mediate either directly or indirectly, anti-tumor effects. Active immunotherapy refers to the immunization of the tumor-bearing host with agents that attempt to induce in the host a state of immune responsiveness to the tumor. Non-specific immune stimulators include Bacillus Calmette (BCG) vaccine, monoclonal antibodies, autologous tumor cells or antigens, autologous tumor-specific vaccines, activated lymphocytes and a variety of cytokines. The cytokines, referred to as lymphokines when produced by lymphocytes, are proteins which among other activities, regulate various aspects of lymphocyte and macrophage proliferation and differentiation. The first of these lymphokines to receive clinical use were the interferons, which were discovered more than 30 years ago.

Interferons

The interferons constitute a complex family of inducible cellular glycoproteins. The major species of interferon are designated alpha, beta, and gamma according to antigenic type. The development of recombinant DNA techniques has enabled the production of large quantities of purified lymphokines. Interferons initiate biological activity by binding to specific membrane receptor sites on the cell surface. The mechanism of in vivo anti-cancer proliferation is not well understood, but it could stem from a number of cellular events, including direct cytotoxic or cytostatic effects, and modulations of host-tumor immune interactions mainly conveyed by natural killer (NK) cells and other cytotoxic subpopulations of effector cells. In addition, malignant proliferation may be slowed by the inhibition of oncogene expression (16).

In 1983, the UCLA (17) and M.D. Anderson group (18) in independent studies reported on the regression of metastatic renal cell carcinoma with partially purified human leukocyte interferon. Objective responses (complete and partial response) occurred in 16.5% and 26% of patients, respectively. Following this initial report numerous phase II trials with interferon-alpha have confirmed a reproducible objective response rate of 15-20 percent (19,20). Responses appear independent of the interferon-alpha preparation utilized and correlate with prior nephrectomy, good performance status, a long disease free interval and lung predominant disease. Patients with these favorable prognostic variables have a higher overall response rate (21). In the majority of patients a 3-month course of rIFNa treatment is sufficient to judge whether or not a patient is going to respond.

Combination of interferon with vinblastine resulted in an overall efficacy similar to that achieved by interferon alone, and demonstrated added toxicity, without improving the overall response rate (22). The Recombinant Human Interferon Gamma Research Group reported a trial of patients with metastatic RCC in which a 9.4 % objective response rate was seen in patients treated by continuous rIFNg infusion and a 20 % response rate in patients administered rIFNg intermittently over 8 weeks (23).

Interleukins

The discovery of the T-cell growth factor, Interleukin-2 (IL-2) has revolutionized the field of cancer immunotherapy and opened new prospects for the treatment of RCC. Natural interleukin-2 is a lymphokine which is produced and secreted by T lymphocytes. This glycoprotein molecule is intimately involved in the induction of virtually all immune responses in which T cells play a role (24). The antitumor effect of IL-2 has been documented in tumor-bearing animal models (25). Interleukin-2 was reported to produce objective response in some patients. Of the 54 evaluable patients treated at the NCI with RCC, 4 CR and 8 PR were achieved, for a total (CR+PR) of 22 percent (26). The regimen used included high doses of IL-2 which resulted in frequent and severe toxicity. However, in contrast, some studies (27) using high-dose bolus of rIL-2, demonstrated no objective responses. The authors suggest that this disparity compared to other results (26,28,29) was due to the small number of patients treated and not ideal patient characteristics. It has been shown that IL-2 can be administered at lower doses as a continuous intravenous infusion, in an attempt to decrease the incidence and severity of toxicities (30).

Recombinant IL-2 has moderate-to-severe toxic effects, but can be administered over a prolonged period of time with appropriate dose reductions (29). The possibility that a decrease in the dose intensity of rIL-2 may decrease its efficacy is, however, only theoretical in renal cell carcinoma. The duration of response, beyond 20 months in some series (29,31), is significant and noteworthy when compared to other treatment modalities used for metastatic RCC.

COMBINATION BIOLOGIC THERAPY

The ability of the immune system to mediate antitumor effects may depend on a series of immunoregulatory signals. If this hypothesis is true, then therapy with a combination of BRMs administered in combination may prove to be beneficial for cancer patients and RCC patients in particular. Combinations of cytokines have shown direct antitumor effect in vitro that are both additive and synergistic (32).

Interferon Combination

The use of the combination of rIFNa and recombinant interferon gamma (rIFNg)in the treatment of patients with metastatic RCC was based on the following observations: rIFNa has a distinct and separate receptor from that of rIFNg (33,34); rIFNg can modulate the rIFNa receptor; IFNa enhances the expression of major histocompatibility complex (MHC) class I antigens, while IFNg primarily enhances MHC class II(35); and IFNa with IFNg have synergistic antiproliferative effects in vitro (32). Although these observations provide a rationale for the combined administration of these agents, the schedule, dose and sequence have not been optimized. In preliminary trials (36) the combination of rIFNa and rIFNg administered concomitantly did not prove to be superior to rIFNa alone, and toxicity was increased. However in a recent report (37) rIFNa and rIFNg administered sequentially induced clinical response in eight (2 CR and 6 PR) of 30 assessable patients. The results of this study suggest that the efficacy and toxicity profile associated with combination IFN therapy can be reduced by administering these agents sequentially as opposed to simultaneously.

Interleukin-2 and Interferon

In an attempt to achieve an improved therapeutic index there has been interest in combining interferon with IL-2. In experimental murine models the combination of IL-2 and interferon-alpha resulted in better antitumor effects than the administration of either agent alone (38,39). There are many reports in the literature (40-42) utilizing rIL-2 and rINFa. These were phase I trials which utilized different administration schedules of rIL-2 (continuous infusion or bolus) and different doses of either cytokine. In an effort to exploit the in vitro synergy of the IL-2/INF combinations and the potentially lower toxicity profile of continuous infusion of IL-2 (28,30), we have performed a phase II trial in metastatic renal cell carcinoma. To date, 30 patients with measurable disease RCC have been treated at UCLA with rIL-2 (2MU/M2) by continuous intravenous infusion on days 1 through 4 and Roferon-A (6MU/M2) IM or SC on days 1 and 4 of each treatment week. Each 4 week treatment period (1 course) was followed by a two week rest. A 4 week course was repeated until disease progression, unacceptable toxicity, or a maximum of 6 courses. One complete response (3.3%) and eight (27%) partial responses were observed for a total response rate of 30 percent. Two patients had a surgical complete response following a salvage nephrectomy. Three patients had pathologically confirmed complete remissions following clinical partial remissions in peripheral and mediastinal lymph nodes and a recurrent renal fossa mass respectively. Patients responses were noted in lung, mediastinum, lymph nodes, kidney and renal fossa. All pathologic complete remissions are on going. Grade IV toxicity occurred in only 3 patients (10%). A grade IV cardiac toxicity occurred in one patient, whose death was considered possibly treatment related. Grade III toxicity was observed in 14 patients (46%). Ten patients (33%) required dose attenuation (43,44). In a phase I trial of a very similar regimen Hirsh et al. (45) reported objective responses in six of 12 assessable (3 CR and 3 PR) patients with metastatic RCC who as in the UCLA study received the majority of their treatment on an outpatient basis. Atzpodien et al. (46) has observed similar activity in patients receiving long term administration of subcutaneous IL-2 and interferon-alpha.

At this relatively early stage of clinical investigation, little objective information can be extracted from the literature with regard to the role of prior nephrectomy in IL-2 based therapy. In our institution, two patients who were treated with IL-2 and IFNa became free of distant metastatic lesions while the primary tumor was in situ. Nephrectomy resulted in a surgical complete response of these two patients. In addition, responses to combination biologic therapy are not predominantly limited to lung lesions as was commonly the case with prior IFNa alone trials.

Interleukin-2 and LAK

The incubation of resting lymphocytes in IL-2 for 3-4 days results in the generation of cells capable of lysing a variety of fresh, NK-resistant tumor cells, but not normal cells. This phenomenon was termed lymphokine activated killing or LAK (47). Renal cell cancer patients, like normal donors, generated good LAK effector cells with broad antitumor specificity against autologous tumors and a variety of allogenic tumors. The treatment regimens, results, and toxicities of the combination therapy with IL-2 and LAK have been reported (26,48-50). Of seventy-two patients with RCC receiving LAK and high-dose IL-2 immunotherapy at the NCI eight patients experienced CR and 17 patients had PR, for a total response (CR+PR) of 35 percent (26). However in some reports, the addition of LAK cell infusions to IL-2 regimens did not cause a noticeable change in antitumor response rate, when compared to IL-2 alone, but did cause more severe toxicity (48). Thus, the contribution of LAK to the clinical responses associated with high dose IL-2 remains undefined.

FUTURE PROSPECTIVE

A new promising application of IL-2 is in combination with tumor infiltrating lymphocytes (TIL). TIL are grown selectively from single-cell tumor suspensions cultured in IL-2 (51). Whereas LAK cells are mainly activated NK cells, TIL are activated cytotoxic T cells and show greater specificity in their targets. In experimental systems TIL are 50-100 times as powerful as LAK (52). Many trials including our own at UCLA are ongoing with encouraging preliminary results. Current efforts are in progress to enhance the therapeutic efficacy of TIL such as with in-vivo priming with interferon-alpha, and by selecting subpopulation of TIL as potentially more potent effector cells (53). Innovative approaches with the insertion of specific genes coding for specific biological response modifiers are the focus of present studies with the hope of improving the therapeutic potency of activated immune cells. Adoptive immunotherapy is an approach that can ideally be combined with chemotherapy, radiation therapy, or many of the new biologic response modifiers.

CONCLUSION

Although the treatment of metastatic renal cell carcinoma remains a difficult and frustrating problem for the surgical and medical oncologist, there is a window of hope through the use of combination biologic therapy. Although combination immunotherapy remains experimental, it seems promising in selected groups of patients. Adoptive immunotherapy and combined cytokine administration appears to be the most promising. However, their current use must be restricted to clinical trials until their efficacy and toxicity are well established.

Major problems remain that must be overcome if therapy with BRMs is to be widely used. Clinical studies designed to increase the therapeutic effect and decrease the toxicity profile are needed, including further investigation of dose modification and treatment schedules, the use of repetitive treatments in responding patients, and the extension of those treatments to the adjuvant patient.

Patient selection is yet another important issue. In addition to identifying important clinical predictors of survival in patients with recurrent or metastatic RCC (54), molecular biology studies are underway in an attempt to better recognize suitable candidates for more aggressive forms of therapy.

REFERENCES

1. I. M. Thompson and M. Peek, Improvement in survival of patients with renal cell carcinoma, The role of serendipitously detected tumor, J Urol, 140:487 (1988).
2. B. Ponder, Gene losses in human tumors, Nature 335:400 (1988).
3. G. Kovacs and S. Frisch, Clonal chromosome abnormalities in tumor cells from patients with sporadic renal cell carcinoma, Cancer Res 49:651 (1989).
4. L. G. Gomella, E. R. Sargent, T. P. Wade, P. Anglard, W. M. Linehan, and A. Kasid, Expression of transforming growth factor a in a normal

adult kidney and enhanced expression of transforming growth factors a and Bi in renal cell carcinoma, Cancer Res 49:6972 (1989).

5. S. Hellsten, T. Berge, and L. Wehlin, Unrecognized renal cell carcinoma: Clinical and diagnostic aspects, Scand J Urol Nephrol 8:269 (1981).

6. J. B. deKernion, Management of renal adenocarcinoma, in: "Genitourinary Cancer Management", J. B. deKernion and D. B. Paulson ed., Lea and Febiger , Philadelphia (1987).

7. A. W. S. Ritchie and J. B. deKernion, The natural history and clinical features of renal carcinoma, Sem Neph 7:131 (1987).

8. J. D. Maldazys and J. B. deKernion, Prognostic factors in metastatic renal carcinoma, J Urol 136:376 (1986).

9. M. Golimbu, P. Joshi, A. Sperber, A. Tessler, S. Al-Askari and P. Morales Renal cell carcinoma: Survival and prognostic factors, Urology 27:291 (1986).

10. J. B. deKernion and D. Berry, The diagnosis and treatment of renal cell carcinoma, Cancer 45:1947 (1980).

11. W. J. Hrushesky and G. P. Murphy, Current status of the therapy of advanced renal carcinoma, J Surg Oncol 9:277 (1977).

12. J. B. deKernion, K. D. Ramming, and R. B. Smith, The natural history of metastatic renal cell carcinoma: A computer analysis, J Urol 120:148 (1978).

13. A. Yagoda, Chemotherapy of renal cell carcinoma: 1983-1989, Sem Urol 7:199 (1989).

14. J. B. deKernion, Treatment of advanced renal cell carcinoma. Traditional and innovative approaches, J Urol 130:2 (1983).

15. Y. Kakehi, H. Kanamaru, O. Yoshida, H. Ohkubo, S. Nakanishi, M. M. Gottesman, and I. Pastan, Measurement of multidrug resistance messenger RNA in urogenital cancers; Elevated expression in renal cell carcinoma is associated with intrinsic drug resistance, J Urol 139:862 (1988).

16. J. M. Kirkwood and M.S. Ernstoff, Interferons in the treatment of human cancer, J Clin Oncol 2:336 (1984).

17. J. B. deKernion, G. Sarna, R. A. Figlin, A. Lindner, and R. B. Smith, The treatment of renal cell carcinoma with human leukocyte alpha interferon, J Urol 130:1063 (1983).

18. J. R. Quesada, D. A. Swanson, A. Trindade, and J. U. Gutterman, Renal cell carcinoma: Antitumor effects of leukocyte interferon, Cancer Res 43:940 (1983).

19. T. Umeda and T. Nijiima, Phase II study of alpha interferon on renal cell carcinoma, Cancer 58:1231 (1986)

20. R. A. Figlin, J. B. deKernion, E. Mukamel, A. V. Palleroni, L. M. Itri, and G. Sarna, Recombinant interferon alpha-2a in metastatic renal cell carcinoma: Assessment of antitumor activity and anti-interferon antibody formation. J Clin Oncol 6:1604 (1988).

21. G. Sarna, R. A. Figlin, and J. B. deKernion, Interferon in renal cell carcinoma: The UCLA experience, Cancer 59:610 (1987).

22. R. A. Figlin, J. B. deKernion, J. Maldazys, and G. Sarna, Treatment of renal cell carcinoma with alpha (human leukocyte) interferon and vinblastine in combination: a phase I-II trial, Cancer Treat Rep 69:263 (1985).

23. Recombinant Human interferon gamma (S-6810) research group on renal cell carcinoma. Phase II study of recombinant human interferon gamma (S-6810) on renal cell carcinoma. Summary of two collaborative studies. Cancer 60:929 (1987).

24. J. J. Farrar, W. R. Benjamin, M. L. Hilfiker, M. Howard, W. L. Farra, and J. Fuller-Farrar, the Biochemistry, biology, and role of interleukin-2 in the induction of cytotoxic T-cell and antibody-forming B cell responses, Immunological Rev 63:129 (1982).

25. S. A. Rosenberg, J. J. Mule, P. J. Spiess, C. M. Reichart, and S. L. Schwarz, Regression of established pulmonary metastasis and

subcutaneous tumor mediated by the systemic administration of high-dose recombinant interleukin-2, J Exp Med 161:1169 (1985).

26. S. A. Rosenberg, M. T. Lotze, J. C. Yang, P. M. Aebersold, W. M. Linehan, C. A. Seipp, and D. E. White, Experience with the use of high-dose Interleukin-2 in the treatment of 652 cancer patients, Ann Surg 210:474 (1989).

27. J. S. Abrams, A. A. Rayner, P. H. Wiernik, D. R. Parkinson, M. Eisenberger, F. R. Aronson, R. Gucalp, M. B. Atkins, and M. J.Hawkins, High-dose recombinant interleukin-2 alone: A regimen with limited activity in the treatment of advanced renal cell carcinoma, J Natl Cancer Inst 82:1202 (1990).

28. J. A. Sosman, P. C. Kohler, J. Hank, K. H. Moore, R. Bechhofer, B. Storer and P. M. Sondel, Repetitive weekly cycles of recombinant human interleukin-2: responses of renal carcinoma with acceptable toxicity, J Natl Cancer Inst 80:60 (1988).

29. R. M. Bukowski, P. Goodman, E. D. Crawford, J. S. Sergi, B. G. Redman, and R. P. Whitehead, Phase-II trial of high-dose intermittent inter-leukin-2 in metastatic renal cell carcinoma: A Southwest Oncology Group Study, J Natl Cancer Inst 82:143 (1990).

30. W. N. West, K. W. Tauer, J. R. Yannelli, G. D. Marshall, D. W. Orr, G. B. Thurman, and R. K. Oldham, Constant infusion recombinant interleu-kin-2 in adoptive immunotherapy of advanced cancer. N Engl J Med 316:898 (1987).

31. S. R. Rosenberg, M. T. Lotze, L. M. Muul, A. E. Chang, F. P. Avis, S. Leitman, W. M. Linehan, C. N. Robertson, R. E. Lee, J. T. Rubin, C. A. Seipp, C. G. Simpson, and D. E. White, A progress report on the treatment of 157 patients with advanced cancer using lymphokine-acti-vated killer cells and interleukin-2 or high-dose interleukin alone, N Engl J Med 316:889 (1987).

32. A. J. Beniers, W. P. Peelen, and B. T. Hendricks, Effect of alpha- and gamma-interferon and tumor necrosis factor on colony formation of two human renal tumor xenografts in vitro. Sem Surg Oncol 4:195 (1988).

33. J. A. Langer, J. R. Ortaldo, and S. Pestka, Binding of human alpha-interferon to natural killer cell, J Interferon Res 6:97 (1986).

34. S. J. Littman, C. R. Faltynek, and C. Baglioni, Binding of human recom-binant I E125-interferon gamma receptors on human cells, J Biol Chem 260:1191 (1985).

35. T. Stewart ed., "The Interferon System", San Diego, Academic (1979).

36. J. Reinhart, L. Malspeis, D. Young, and J. Neidhart, Phase I-II of human recombinant beta-interferon serine in patients with renal cell carci-noma, Cancer Res 46:5364 (1986).

37. M. S. Ernstoff, S. Nair, R. R. Bahnson, L. M. Miketic, B. Banner, W. Gooding, R. Day, T. Whiteside, T. Hakala, and J. M. Kirkwood, A phase 1A trial of sequential administration recombinant DNA-produced inter-ferons: Combination recombinant interferon gamma and recombinant interferon alfa in patients with metastatic renal carcinoma, J Clin Oncol 8:1637 (1990).

38. M. J. Brunda, D. Bellantoni, and V. Sulich, In vivo antitumor activity of combinations of interferon-a and interleukin-2 in a murine model. Correlation of efficacy with the induction of cytotoxic cells resem-bling natural killer cells, Int J Cancer 40:365 (1987).

39. R. B. Cameron, J. K. McIntosh, and S. A. Rosenberg, Synergistic anti-tumor effects of combination immunotherapy with recombinant interleu-kin-2 and recombinant hybrid alpha-interferon in the treatment of established murine hepatic metastases, Cancer Res 48:5810 (1988).

40. R. M. Bukowski, S. Murthy, J. Sergi, T. Budd, S. McKeever, S. V. Medendorp, R. Tubbs, V. Gibson, and J. Finke, Phase I trial of contin-uous infusion recombinant interleukin-2 and intermittent recombinant interleukin-alph2a: Clinical effects, J Biol Response Mod 9:538 (1990).

41. K. H. Lee, M. Taplaz, J. M. Rothberg, J. L. Murray, N. Papadopoulos, C. Plager, R. Benjamin, D. Levitt, and J. Gutterman, Concomitant adminis- tration of recombinant human interleukin-2 and recombinant inter- feron-alpha2a in cancer patients: a phase I study, <u>J Clin Oncol</u> 7:1726 (1989).

42. S. A. Rosenberg, M. T. Lotze, J. C. Yang, M. Linehan, C. Seipp, S. Calabro, S. E. Karp, R. M. Sherry, S. Steinberg, and D. E. White, Combination therapy with interleukin-2 and alpha interferon for the treatment of patients with advanced cancer, <u>J Clin Oncol</u> 7:1863 (1989).

43. R. A. Figlin, M. Citron, R. Whitehead, J. deKernion, M. Desner, A. Smith, G. Jones, and D. Levitt, Low dose continuous infusion recombi- nant human interleukin-2 and Roferon-A; An active outpatient regimen for metastatic renal cell carcinoma, <u>Proceedings of ASCO</u> 9:142 (1990).

44. A. Belldegrun, A. S. Abi-Aad, J. B. deKernion, and R. A. Figlin, Con- comitant administration of recombinant human interleukin-2 in metasta- tic renal cell carcinoma: A UCLA Phase II pilot study, <u>Proceedings of the AUA</u>, in press, (1991).

45. M. Hirsh, A. Lipton, H. Harvey, E. Givant, K. Hopper, G. Jones, J. Zeffren, and D. Levitt, Phase I study of interleukin-2 and interferon alfa-2a as outpatient therapy for patients with advanced malignancy, <u>J Clin Oncol</u> 8:1657 (1990).

46. J. Atzpodien, A. Korfer, C. R. Franks, H. Poliwoda, and H. Kirchner, Home therapy with recombinant interleukin-2 and interferon-alpha2b in advanced human malignancies, <u>Lancet</u> 335:1509 (1990).

47. S. A. Rosenberg, Lymphokine-activated killer cells: A new approach to the immunotherapy of human cancer, <u>Cancer</u> 55:1327 (1985).

48. M. R. Albertini, J. A. Sosman, J. A. Hank, K. H. Moore, A. Borchert, K. Schell, P. C. Kohler, R. Bechhofer, B. Storer, and P. M. Sondel, The influence of autologous lymphokine-activated killer cell infusion on the toxicity and antitumor effect of repetitive cycles of interleu- kin-2, <u>Cancer</u> 66:2457 (1990).

49. J. W. Clark, J. W. Smith II, R. G. Steis, W .J. Urba, E. Crum, R. Mill er, J. McKnight, H. C. Stevenson, S. Creekmore, M. Stewart, K. Con- lon, M. Sznol, P. Kremers, P. Cohen, and D. L. Longo, Interleukin 2 and lymphokine-activated killer cell therapy: Analysis of a bolus interleukin 2 and a continuous infusion interleukin 2 regimen, <u>Can- cer Res</u> 50:7343 (1990).

50. E. R. Gaynor, G. R. Weiss, K. A. Margolin, F. R. Aronson, M. Sznol, P. Demchak, K. M. Grima, R. I. Fisher, D. H. Boldt, J. H. Doroshow, M. H. Bar, M. J. Hawkins, J. W. Mier, and G. Caliendo, Phase I study of high-dose continuous-infusion interleukin-2 and autologous lympho- kine-activated killer cells in patients with metastatic or unresec- table malignant melanoma and renal cell carcinoma, <u>J Natl Cancer Inst</u> 82:1397 (1990).

51. A. Belldegrun and S. A. Rosenberg, Adoptive immunotherapy of urologic tumors, <u>in</u>: "Urologic Oncology", H. Leporand T. L. Ratliff eds., Kluwer Academic Publishers, Boston (1989).

52. P. J. Spiess, J. C. Yang, S. A. Rosenberg, In vivo activity of tumor- infiltrating lymphocytes expanded in recombinant interleukin-2, <u>J Natl Cancer Inst</u> 79:1067 (1987).

53. A. S. Belldegrun, R. A. Figlin, A. S. Abi-Aad, and J. B. deKernion, Adoptive immunotherapy of renal carcinoma using tumor infiltrating lymphocytes: From basic science to clinical practice, <u>Proceeding of AUA Western Section</u>, in press, (1991).

54. P. J. Elson, R. S. Witte, and D. L. Trump, Prognostic factors for sur- vival in patients with recurrent or metastatic renal cell carcinoma, <u>Cancer Res</u> 48:7310 (1988).

MAINTENANCE TREATMENT WITH RECOMBINANT INTERFERON ALFA-2b PROLONGS REMISSION AND SURVIVAL IN PATIENTS WITH MULTIPLE MYELOMA RESPONDING TO INDUCTION CHEMOTHERAPY

Franco Dammacco, Giuseppe Avvisati*, Mario Boccadoro§,
Vito Michele Lauta, Rita Di Stefano, Alessandro Pileri§,
Franco Mandelli*

Department of Biomedical Sciences and Human Oncology,
Section of Internal Medicine,
University of Bari Medical School;
* Department of Human Biopathology, Section of Hematology,
University "La Sapienza", Rome;
§ Department of Experimental Hematology and Oncology,
Section of Hematology,
University of Turin

Experimental studies of myeloma cells have shown that interferon can decrease both the labeling index of such cells and the capacity for self-renewal in myeloma-forming cells[1]. However, when IFN was used as a single induction agent in previously treated or untreated patients with MM, an overall response rate of approximately 20% has been found[2-5].

We decided to evaluate whether recombinant interferon (rIFN)-α2b is effective as maintenance therapy for prolonging response and survival in patients with multiple myeloma (MM) responding to induction chemotherapy.

PATIENTS AND METHODS

105 patients with MM, diagnosed at three participating institutions (Bari, Rome and Turin), were enrolled in the study. They had responded to induction chemotherapy consisting of 12 monthly courses of orally administered melphalan plus prednisone (MP) for 7 days or a combination regimen of vincristine, melphalan, cyclophosphamide, and prednisone (VMCP) alternating with a regimen of vincristine, BCNU, doxorubicin, and prednisone (VBAP). Criteria to define "objective response" or "disease stabilization" were described elsewhere[6].

Of the 105 patients admitted, 80 achieved an objective response and 25 disease stabilization. 4 patients dropped out so that a total number of 101 patients entered the study. After stratification based on their

Combination Therapies, Edited by A.L. Goldstein and
E. Garaci, Plenum Press, New York, 1992

first-line induction therapy, patients were randomized to receive IFN as maintenance treatment (50 patients) or no therapy (51 patients). rIFN-α2b (Essex Italia-Schering Corp.) was given s.c. three times a week in a dose of 3 MU/m^2/body surface area until relapse. Although patients were not allowed to take corticosteroids throughout the study, they were free to use acetaminophen to reduce side-effects. Clinical and laboratory features were assessed in all patients at monthly intervals. On these same occasions serum samples were collected and deep-frozen until they were thawed and assayed for the occurrence of antibodies to IFN.

Patients were defined as having relapse in the presence of one or more of the following parameters: a) an increase of 25% or more in the serum level of the M-component above the nadir; b) an increase in the urinary output of the M-protein to 2g/day; c) the reappearance of the M-component in serum and/or urine; d) an increase in the size or number of osteolytic lesions.

The durations of response and survival for both the IFN group and control group were plotted as Kaplan-Meier curves, and differences between the curves were analyzed using the log-rank test.

RESULTS

No significant differences were detected in the two study groups as regards their clinical and laboratory features, including isotypes of the M-component, disease stage, serum β2-microglobulin level, and labeling

Table 1. Follow-up of patients

	IFN GROUP (N. 50)	CONTROL GROUP (N. 51)
Patients died	14 (28%)	23 (45%)
Patients relapsed	25 (50%)	41 (80%)
Patients still alive and responding to first treatment	21 (42%)	8 (16%)
Median duration of response	26 months	14 months *
Median duration of survival (from randomization)	52 months	39 months **
Median duration of survival (from relapse)	35 months	16 months

* p = 0.0002
** p = 0.0526

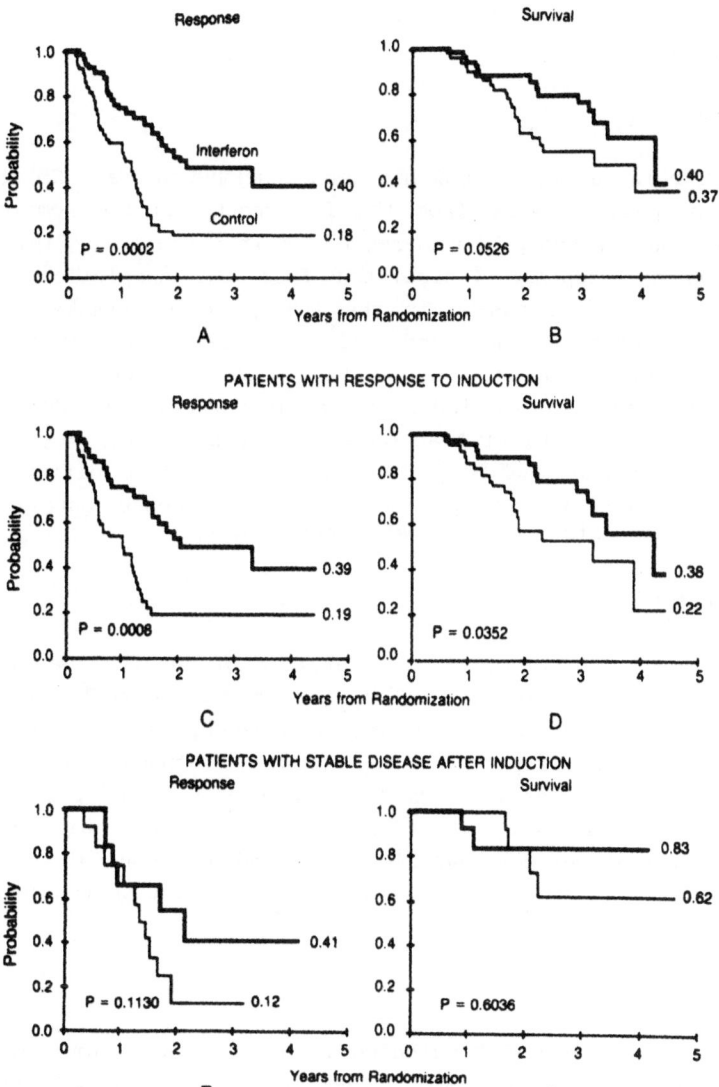

Fig. 1. Response and survival of patients belonging to the interferon group or control group, evaluated by Kaplan-Meier curves (reproduced from New Engl. J. Med. 322: 1430, 1990, with permission).

index. In addition, the type of response to induction treatment, namely objective response or disease stabilization, was also similar in the two groups.

Because of poor compliance, only 2 patients were drop-outs and discontinued IFN therapy. During follow-up death was recorded in 37 patients (36.6%) : 14 of them (28%) belonged to the IFN group and 23 (45%) to the control group (Table 1). As expected, disease progression was the most frequent cause of death in both groups (10 patients and 21 patients, respectively).

Assessment of Relapse

An overall relapse rate of 65% has been observed so far. 25 (50%) of the 66 relapsing patients were from the IFN group and the remaining 41 (80%) from the control group. Furthermore, as it appears in Fig. 1, the median duration of response (calculated from the completion time of induction therapy) was 26 months in the IFN group as compared with 14 months in the control group, and this difference is statistically significant (p=0.0002). However, when patients were grouped on the basis of the type of response to induction chemotherapy, the duration of response among patients achieving an objective response was significantly better in the IFN group (p=0.0008). On the contrary, no difference was observed between the two groups in terms of response duration when patients with disease stabilization were compared.

Analysis of Survival

When lastly evaluated, the median duration of survival was found to be 52 months in the IFN group and 39 months in the control group. This difference was not significant (p=0.0526). However, it was found again that patients who had achieved an objective response to induction chemotherapy and had been assigned to the IFN group showed a significantly longer duration of survival (p=0.0352). Conversely, no difference in survival was observed between the IFN group and the control group when patients with disease stabilization at the end of induction treatment were considered.

Toxicity

Antibodies to IFN were not detected in any of the serum samples. At the dose of 3 MU/m^2 s.c. three times a week toxic reactions were mild and usually limited to an influenza-like syndrome which gradually faded after 3 to 4 weeks of treatment.

DISCUSSION

The present study clearly indicates that maintenance therapy with IFN is effective in controlling the reappearance of the plasma cell tumor and that among patients who had achieved an objective response to first-line induction chemotherapy, those receiving rIFN-α2b showed a significantly longer overall response and a longer survival as compared to the group of untreated control patients[6].

It seems likely that IFN is capable of decreasing the cell-growth rate, thus explaining the effectiveness of the drug in controlling the plateau phase in chemotherapy-responsive patients, in whom the tumor mass is obviously reduced. On the contrary, and as it would be expected on the basis of this hypothesis, the durations of response and survival were not significantly different among patients achieving disease stabilization, irrespective of whether they received maintenance IFN treatment or not.

Although additional explanations are obviously conceivable, the observation made by Bergsagel et al[7]. (1986) seems worth mentioning: these Authors have indeed found that IFNs can inhibit the capacity of myeloma cells for self-renewal, thus resulting in a prolongation of the plateau phase. It seems, therefore, reasonable to suggest that, under the condition of this study, rIFN-α2b can exert both immunomodulating properties and inhibitory effects on the proliferation of myeloma plasma cells.

It has been established that the bone marrow plasma cell labeling index (LI %) and the serum level of β2-microglobulin (β2m) have undisputable prognostic significance[8], in that a LI $\geqslant$2% and/or a β2m level $\geqslant$509 nmol/l imply a poor prognosis and a very short survival. Although patients were not prospectively stratified according to these prognostic criteria, patients with a LI $\geqslant$2% and/or with β2m levels $\geqslant$509 nmol/l were equally distributed between the two study groups.

With a standardized dose of 3 MU/m^2 of IFN s.c. three times a week, the level of toxicity was acceptable, the most common side-effect being an influenza-like syndrome of mild to intermediate severity which faded gradually after 3 to 4 weeks of treatment. Hematologic toxicity was also absent or moderate and in none of the patients receiving this dose was it necessary to discontinue IFN administration.

On the basis of our experience, it can be concluded that maintenance treatment with rIFN-α2b is capable of significantly prolongig the durations of response and survival in patients with MM responding to induction chemotherapy.

REFERENCES

1. G. Brenning, The in vitro effect of leucocyte alpha-interferon on human myeloma cells in a semisolid agar culture system, Scand. J. Haematol. 35: 178 (1985)
2. H. Mellstedt, A. Ahre, M. Björkholm, G. Holm, B. Johansson, H. Strander, Interferon therapy in myelomatosis, Lancet 1: 245 (1979)
3. R. Alexanian, J. Gutterman, H. Levy, Interferon treatment for multiple myeloma, Clin. Haematol. 1: 211 (1982)
4. J.J. Costanzi, M.R. Cooper, J.H. Scarffe, et al., Phase II study of recombinant alpha-2 interferon in resistant multiple myeloma, J. Clin. Oncol. 3: 654 (1985)
5. J.R. Quesada, R. Alexanian, M. Hawkins, et al., Treatment of multiple myeloma with recombinant alpha-interferon, Blood 67: 275 (1986)
6. F. Mandelli, G. Avvisati, S. Amadori, M. Boccadoro, A. Gernone, V.M.

Lauta, F. Marmont, M.T. Petrucci, M. Tribalto, M.L. Vegna, F. Dammacco, A. Pileri, Maintenance treatment with recombinant interferon alfa-2b in patients with multiple myeloma responding to conventional induction chemotherapy, New Engl. J. Med. 322: 1430 (1990)

7. D.E. Bergsagel, R.H. Haas, H.A. Messner, Interferon alfa-2b in the treatment of chronic granulocytic leukemia, Semin. Oncol. 13: Suppl. 2: 29 (1986)

8. B.G. Durie, S.E. Salmon, T.E. Moon, Pretreatment tumor mass, cell kinetics, and prognosis in multiple myeloma, Blood 55: 364 (1980)

COMBINATION OF FLUOROURACIL AND INTERFERON: MECHANISMS OF INTERACTION

AND CLINICAL STUDIES

Richard Pazdur

Division of Medicine, The University of Texas M. D.
Anderson Cancer Center, Houston, Texas

INTRODUCTION

Recombinant DNA technology has provided the clinician with a variety of biological response modifiers (BRMs) to combine with conventional cytotoxic agents. Preclinical models have suggested interactions between particular BRMs and cytotoxic agents ranging from antagonistic to synergistic. These conflicting preclinical results reflect variations in cell lines, assays, concentrations, duration of the regimen, and sequence of exposure.[1] The bases for developing combination chemotherapy regimens, such as increasing dose intensity and combining drugs that have independent antitumor activity, may not apply to those for combining BRMs and cytotoxic drugs. Thus, the rationale for adding BRMs to chemotherapy may be more complex than for combining chemotherapy drugs.

The following discussion addresses possible mechanisms of interaction between BRMs and chemotherapeutic agents and presents a clinical example in which recombinant interferon alfa-2a (rIFN-2a) was used with 5-fluorouracil (5-FU) in the treatment of advanced colorectal carcinoma.

MECHANISMS OF INTERACTION

Most clinical studies of BRMs combined with chemotherapeutic agents have been designed empirically, frequently without a clear understanding of the interaction between these agents. Little is known, for example, about the dosages of BRMs required to achieve the desired biological effects or about the proper sequencing of the biological and cytotoxic agents. Possible mechanisms of interaction include the following:

1. A BRM and a chemotherapeutic agent used together may lead to greater tumor reduction because of the direct, independent, antitumor activity of each agent.

Combination Therapies, Edited by A.L. Goldstein and
E. Garaci, Plenum Press, New York, 1992

2. Biological agents may provide protection against the toxicities of chemotherapy. One example of this interaction is the use of granulocyte-macrophage colony-stimulating factors to reduce the duration of chemotherapy-induced neutropenia. In addition, interferon decreased 5-FU toxicity in a murine model.[3]

3. A BRM may alter the pharmacokinetics of the chemotherapeutic agent. In a recent study, for example, 5-FU plasma clearance decreased in the presence of rIFN-2a.[3]

4. BRMs may modulate the action of chemotherapeutic agents on key enzymes. In the adenocarcinoma 38 and HL-60 cell lines, enhanced accumulation of 5-fluoro-2-deoxyuridine 5-monophosphate (FdUMP) was observed in interferon-treated cells after exposed to 5-FU.[4] FdUMP inhibits thymidylate synthase (TS); as a result, DNA synthesis is inhibited.

5. BRMs may alter the drug resistance mechanisms of chemotherapeutic agents. For instance, 5-FU may acutely induce TS, thereby decreasing 5-FU sensitivity. Gamma interferon can reverse the development of resistance to 5-FU in the H630 cell line by inhibiting the overexpression of TS resulting from previous 5-FU therapy.[5]

6. The increased immunomodulating actions of both the cytotoxic agent and the BRM on natural killer cells may enhance their antitumor activity.[6]

7. The BRM activates host defense mechanisms that, when combined with the cytotoxic action of the chemotherapeutic agent, may lead to enhanced antitumor activity.

8. BRMs may alter cell-cycle kinetics, which may lead to increased cytotoxicity of the chemotherapeutic drug.

In addition to these possible mechanisms, chemotherapeutic agents may function independently as immunomodulators. For example, at doses of 300-500 mg/m^2, cyclophosphamide selectively depletes suppressor T-cell populations.[7]

The mechanisms by which BRMs and chemotherapeutic agents work together to enhance antitumor activity are thought to be one or several of the above; the actual mechanisms, however, remain to be identified. The following clinical example of rIFN-2a and 5-FU used together to treat advanced colorectal carcinoma may provide insight into the problems of combining these agents.

CLINICAL TRIALS

Introduced into clinical practice over 30 years ago, 5-FU has remained the major chemotherapeutic agent in the treatment of metastatic colorectal carcinoma. Yet although a variety of doses and schedules have been used, 5-FU has not altered the survival rate of patients with metastatic disease.[8] Recent attempts to modulate 5-FU biochemically by adding folinic acid (calcium leucovorin) have been successful, allowing improved response rates in comparison with single-agent 5-FU. Several trials have indicated a small yet statistically significant survival advantage.[9,10]

Recombinant interferon alfa 2-a is an active neoplastic agent against a variety of neoplasms, including renal cell carcinoma, chronic myelogenous leukemia, and hairy cell leukemia. However, clinical trials examining the use of rIFN-2a alone in metastatic colorectal carcinoma have failed to demonstrate antitumor activity.[11]

Investigators from the Albert Einstein Cancer Center initiated clinical studies based on preclinical data that suggested a synergistic relationship between rIFN-2a and 5-FU. Their first trial demonstrated a response rate of 76%, with 13 of 17 previously untreated patients responding.[12] Since clinical trials using 5-FU with folinic acid have generally provided response rates of only 30-35%, investigators from other institutions also became interested in this combination.

Presented below are the results of four clinical trials examining the use of 5-FU with rIFN-2a. These clinical trials all employed the following treatment regimen: 9×10^6 U of rIFN-2a was administered subcutaneously three times weekly throughout the treatment; 750 mg/m^2 of 5-FU was administered daily for 5 consecutive days as a continuous intravenous infusion, followed by a weekly bolus administration of 750 mg/m^2 of 5-FU. None of the patients in these trials had been previously treated with chemotherapy, and all had measurable disease. The differences in the response rates and frequencies and severity of the toxicities observed in these studies may reflect different patient characteristics, such as performance status and degree of metastatic hepatic involvement, as well as the different dose modifications for toxicity that were used.

Response Rates[13-16]

Investigators at the Albert Einstein Cancer Center extended their study with the above combination to treat 32 patients with advanced colorectal carcinoma who were previously untreated with chemotherapy. In all patients, the cancer had metastasized to either the visceral organs, the abdominal wall, or the pelvis. A response rate of 63% (95% confidence interval: 46,79%) was observed. Twenty patients experienced a partial response. At a median follow-up of 8 months, 23 of the 32 patients were still alive.

Fifty-two patients were enrolled in a clinical trial of this regimen at The University of Texas M. D. Anderson Cancer Center. Fifty-one patients were evaluable for toxicity, and 45 were evaluable for response. Fifteen patients experienced partial responses, and one achieved a complete clinical response, for an overall response rate of 35% (95% confidence interval: 22, 50%). The median response duration was 7 months. The median survival was 16 months. At a median follow-up of 18 months (with a range of 16-24 months), 60% of the patients had died.

In a study of 34 evaluable patients treated at Memorial Sloan-Kettering Cancer Center, 9 patients (26%) (95% confidence interval: 11,41%) had partial responses, and 7 had minor responses; 9 had stable disease. A median response duration of 7.5 months was reported.

In a multi-institutional Eastern Cooperative Oncology Group (ECOG) trial of 38 patients with advanced colorectal carcinoma, an objective response rate of 42% (95% confidence interval: 27,58%) was observed. Of 36 evaluable patients entered in this trial, 14 experienced partial responses, and one had a complete clinical response.

Toxicity (13-16)

In these four trials, similar types of toxicities were reported; the frequency and severity of the toxicities, however, appeared to differ. Serious toxicities included leukopenia, diarrhea, oral mucositis, infection, rash, and neurological toxicity. A syndrome of profuse, watery diarrhea with subsequent neutropenia was observed in three patients, whose subsequent deaths were treatment related. A fourth treatment-related death was attributed to bilateral interstitial pneumonitis. Fevers and myalgias ascribed to rIFN-2a were observed in all patients.

Mucositis, generally occurring after the continuous infusion of 5-FU, was the most prominent toxicity observed in the M. D. Anderson Cancer Center trial. Grade 3 mucositis--confluent oral ulcerations with severe symptoms--was observed in 37% of the patients. It was observed in 40% of the patients in the Albert Einstein trial, but only 9% developed grade 3 mucositis. In the ECOG trial, 31% of the patients developed mucositis, and in the Memorial Sloan-Kettering trial, it was reported in 10%.

In the Memorial Sloan-Kettering trial, neurological toxicity was the most common serious toxicity leading to major dose modifications. Twelve patients (34%) developed neurological toxicities, including gait disturbances, dizziness, dementia, confusion, and memory loss. Investigators from M. D. Anderson observed drug-related seizures in two patients. In the Albert Einstein trial, one person with a previous seizure disorder experienced a complex partial seizure, and another was hospitalized for stupor, which resolved upon discontinuation of rIFN-2a. Two patients in the ECOG trial developed slurred speech and gait disturbances.

The degree of myelosuppression differed among the trials. Grade 3-4 leukopenia was noted in 16% of the patients treated in the Albert Einstein Cancer Center. At Memorial Sloan-Kettering, grade 3 leukopenia occurred in 6% of the patients treated. In the M. D. Anderson study, 18% of the patients developed grade 4 granulocytopenia (<500/mL), and 25% developed grade 3 granulocytopenia (500-900/mL); six of these patients required hospitalization for granulocytopenic fevers. In the ECOG trial, 16% of the patients developed grade 4 granulocytopenia.

These clinical experiences suggest greater toxicity of 5-FU when combined with rIFN-2a; thus, the observations conflict with the preclinical observation that interferon protects against 5-FU toxicity. This relationship was observed when the interferon inducer polyinosinic-polycytidylic acid and 5-FU were coadministered to mice bearing colon tumor 26, allowing the dose of 5-FU to be increased significantly, thus increasing tumor reduction.[2]

In contrast to the results of cytotoxic combination chemotherapy, higher doses of rIFN-2a may not lead to greater antitumor activity. In a phase I clinical study of 5-FU and rIFN-2a conducted at the Albert Einstein Cancer Center, the maximum tolerated dose of rIFN-2a when combined with 5-FU was $15-18 \times 10^6$ U three times weekly. The dose-limiting toxicity of the regimen was fatigue. The maximum antitumor responses, however, were observed in patients treated with $6-9 \times 10^6$ U of rIFN-2a three times weekly.[17]

CONCLUSION

Because the mechanisms of interaction between biological agents and chemotherapeutic agents are poorly understood, the schedules and doses of these agents have been empirically derived. A clear relationship may not exist between maximum tolerated dose and optimal therapeutic dose for biological agents. Preclinical animal tumor systems may not accurately predict a clinical situation.

Whether the addition of rIFN-2a to 5-FU in this schedule represents an advance in the treatment of metastatic colorectal carcinoma remains to be seen. Similar response rates and survival data have been observed with intensive single-agent 5-FU and with regimens of 5-FU plus folinic acid. Current randomized trials comparing this regimen with 5-FU and with 5-FU in combination with folinic acid may clarify the effectiveness of 5-FU with rIFN-2a.

REFERENCES

1. Wadler S, Schwartz EL. Antineoplastic activity of the combination of interferon and cytotoxic agents against experimental and human malignancies. Cancer Res 1990;50:3473-3486.

2. Stolfi RL, Martin DS, Sawyer RC, Spiegelman S. Modulation of 5-fluorouracil-induced toxicity in mice with interferon or with the interferon inducer, polyinosinic-polycytidylic acid. Cancer Res 1983;43:561-566.

3. Grem JL, Allegra CJ, McAtee N, Balis FM, Sartor O, Goldstein LJ, Murphy RF, Sorensen JM, Hamilton JM. Phase I study of interferon alfa-2a, 5-fluorouracil and high-dose leucovorin in metastatic gastrointestinal carcinoma (abstr). Proceedings of the American Society of Clinical Oncology 1990;9:70.

4. Elias L, Crissman HA. Interferon effects upon the adenocarcinoma 38 and HL-60 cell lines: anti-proliferative responses and synergistic interactions with halogenated pyrimidine antimetabolites. Biochem Biophys Res Comm 1989;163: 867-874.

5. Mitchell MS, Kempf RA, Harel W, Shau H, Boswell WD, Lind S, Bradley EC. Effectiveness and tolerability of low-dose intravenous interleukin-2 in disseminated melanoma. J Clin Oncol 1988;6:409-424.

6. Chu E, Zinn S, Boarman D, Allegra CJ. Interaction of gamma interferon and fluorouracil in the H630 human colon carcinoma cell line. Cancer Res 1990;50:5834-5840.

7. Matheson DS, Green BJ, Friedman SJ, Hoar DI. Studies on the mechanism of activation of human natural killer function by interferon and inhibitors of thymidylate synthesis. Cell Immunol 1988;111:118-125.

8. Einhorn LH. Improvements in fluorouracil chemotherapy? J Clin Oncol 1989;7:1377-1379.

9. Poon MA, O'Connell MJ, Moertel CG, Wieand HS, Cullinan SA, Everson LK, Krook JE, Mailliard JA, Laurie JA, Tschetter LK, Wiesenfeld M. Biochemical modulation of fluorouracil: evidence of significant improvements of survival and quality of life in patients with advanced colorectal carcinoma. J Clin Oncol 1989;7:1407-1418.

10. Erlichman C, Fine S, Wong A, Elhakim T. A randomized trial of

fluorouracil and folinic acid in patients with metastatic colorectal carcinoma. J Clin Oncol 1988;6:469-475.

11. Gutterman JU, Fein S, Quesada J, Horning SJ, Levine JF, Alexanian R, Bernhardt L, Kramer M, Spiegel H, Colburn W, Trown P, Merigan T, Dziewanowski Z. Recombinant leukocyte A interferon: pharmacokinetics, single-dose tolerance, and biologic effects in cancer patients. Ann Intern Med 1982;96:549-556.

12. Wadler S, Schwartz EL, Goldman M, Lyver A, Rader M, Zimmerman M, Itri L, Weinberg V, Wiernik PH. Fluorouracil and recombinant alfa-2a-interferon: an active regimen against advanced colorectal carcinoma. J Clin Oncol 1989;7:1769-1775.

13. Wadler S, Wiernik PH. Clinical update on the role of fluorouracil and recombinant interferon alfa-2a in the treatment of colorectal carcinoma. Semin Oncol 1990;17:16-21.

14. Pazdur R, Ajani JA, Patt YZ, Winn R, Jackson D, Shepard B, DuBrow R, Campos L, Quaraishi M, Faintuch J, Abbruzzese J, Gutterman J, Levin B. Phase II study of fluorouracil and recombinant interferon alfa-2a in previously untreated advanced colorectal carcinoma. J Clin Oncol 1990;8:2027-2031.

15. Kemeny N, Younes A, Seiter K, Kelsen D, Sammarco P, Adams L, Derby S, Murray P, Houston C. Interferon alpha-2a and 5-fluorouracil for advanced colorectal carcinoma: assessment of activity and toxicity. Cancer 1990;66:2470-2475.

16. Wadler S, Lembersky B, Kirkwood J, Atkins M, Petrelli N. Phase II trial of fluorouracil and recombinant alfa-2a interferon in patients with advanced colorectal cancer: an Easternn Cooperative Oncology Group (ECOG) Study (abstr). Proceedings of the American Society of Clinical Oncology 1991;10:136.

17. Wadler S, Goldman M, Lyver A, Wiernick PH. Phase I trial of 5-fluorouracil and recombinant alfa-2a interferon in patients with advanced colorectal carcinoma. Cancer Res 1990;50:2056-2059.

COMBINATION CHEMOTHERAPY AND CYTOKINES IN THE TREATMENT OF

ADVANCED PRIMARY LUNG CANCER: CONTROLLED CLINICAL TRIAL

THREE YEAR RESULTS

G.S. Del Giacco, G. Mantovani, V. Arangino. F.
Locci, A.C. Scanu and G. Pusceddu

Department of Clinical Medicine and Department
of Medical Oncology, University of Cagliari and
"R. Binaghi" Hospital, Cagliari, Italy

INTRODUCTION

Nowadays primary lung cancer is the most frequent
malignant tumor in males and one of the most frequent in
females: It is probably one of the most serious malignancies around.

Until now post-surgical adjuvant polychemotherapy or
combination chemotherapy in advanced cancers have failed to
amegliorate the prognosis and, moreover, their undesired side
effects represent one of the main obstacles to further
improvement of these treatments. The same can be said of
radiotherapy as treatment in itself or combined with surgery
and/or chemotherapy.

These facts have suggested the use of immunological
procedures (immunotherapy) in the treatment of primary lung
cancer: BCG, Levamisole, Corynebacterium parvum and other
substances have been used alone or as aids to other therapies (surgery, chemo-radiotherapies). However, to date
results are inconclusive. A number of studies have failed to
shown that the efficacy of chemoimmunotherapy is superior to
chemotherapy alone (1,2,3). However, some comparative clinical trials with chemoimmunotherapy in lung cancer have
produced favourable results (4,5).

Among immunomodulators, Thymic factors or hormones have
been widely used in primary and secondary immunodeficien-
cies, because of their ability and activation of T-cells. In
advanced tumors a secondary immunodeficiency is quite inva-
riably present and this can induce an increased frequency of
infections, an impairment of bone marrow cells to undergo
complete maturation and perhaps an enhancement of ability to
give metastases of primitive malignant cells, as demonstrated
in experimental animals. This justifies the use of biological immunomodifiers like Thymic hormones. These have been
isolated, prepared and synthesized (6,7) and many of them
are well characterized (alpha and beta-thymosins, thymopoietin and its 32-36 synthetic derivative pentapeptide, thymic
serum factor, thymic humoral factor) while others (like
thymostimulin from bovine thymus) have been widely employed

in various clinical trials. As far as lung cancer is concerned, few trials have so far been undertaken using thymic hormones, whereas no clinial trials have been as yet reported using Interferons (IFN_s) in lung cancer.

MATERIAL AND METHODS

Our group began, four years ago, a randomized clinical 0trial to evaluate the effects of the addition of thymostimulin (TS) to surgery and/or chemotherapy of patients with primary lung cancer. Preliminary results and in progress reports have been already presented elsewhere (8,9).
The present study was undertaken in April 1988 to evaluate the effects of the addition of the beta IFN, the activity of which is well known in other, mainly haematological, malignancies, as well as also a powerful immunomodulating agent, to our previous chemoimmunotherapy regimen, including chemotherapy plus TS. In the present study, the patients were randomly assigned to one of three different arms (treatments), as follows:
In the first arm (A Regimen): chemotherapy (CH) + TS were given.
In the second arm (B Regimen): the same as A regimen plus intermittent beta IFN were given.
In the third arm (C Regimen): the same as A regimen plus continuous beta IFN were given.

Patients. Twenty patients (16 men and 4 women; mean age 56.1 years; range 41-68) were enrolled in the study: 18 had non small cell lung cancer (NSCLC) (Stage I: 1, Stage II: 1, Stage III A: 11, Stage III B: 2, Stage IV: 3), which in 13 patients was squamous cell carcinoma (ca.), in 2 patients an adenoca., in 1 patient large cell ca. and in 2 patients was not histologically defined and 2 had small cell lung cancer (SCLC) (Limited disease: 1, Extended disease: 1).

Combination chemotherapy. (the same in all 3 Regimens):
Cisplatin 70 mg/sqm/i.v. day 1,VP 16 (Etoposide) 120 mg/sqm/days 1,3,5 every 4 weeks for 3 subsequent cycles (induction therapy). If an objective clinical response was obtained, then 2 more cycles were administered. In the event of disease progression, the following alternative non cross-resistant regimen was administered: Epirubicin 55 mg/sqm/i.v., Vindesine 3 mg/sqm/i.v., Cytoxan 500 mg/sqm/i.v. and CCNU 30 mg/sqm/p.o., all the first day every 24 days until progression and in any case for at least 5 cycles.
The patients surviving beyond one year, to whom the total doses foreseen of drugs had been overcome, were given an alternative regimen containing Mytomicin C and Lonidamine.

Immunotherapy. TS (TP 1, Serono). A calf thymus extract (10), was administered at a dosage of 1 mg/Kg/i.m. every day starting eight days before chemotherapy and for 8 subsequent days, then stopped during chemotherapy administration and restarted at the end of chemotherapy thrice weekly until the day preceding the next chemotherapy cycle.
Intermittent Beta IFN (Frone,Serono). The beta IFN, Frone,

an human IFN obtained by cultured fibroblasts, was administered at a dosage of $1x10^6$ I.U./sqm/i.m. days 7,15,23 for the first month of treatment, $2x10^6$ I.U./sqm/i.m. the same days for the second month, $3x10^6$ I.U./sqm/i.m. the same days for the third month and then at the same dosage of the third month for the subsequent months.

Continuous Beta IFN. Frone was administered at a dosage of $1x10^6$ I.U./sqm/i.m. every day from fifth to twentieth sixth day for the first month of treatment, $2x10^6$/U/sqm/i.m. in the same days for the second and the third month, $3x10^6$ I.U./sqm/i.m. days 7,15,23 for the fourth and the subsequent months.

After the diagnosis an immunological evaluation has been performed, consisting of in vitro response of peripheral blood mononuclear cells (PBMC) to polyclonal mitogens, to Interleukin 2 (IL 2) and to PHA + IL 2 and in vivo response (skin tests response to recall antigens). These tests have been controlled every six months. Routine tests for haemoglobin, leucocyte and platelet counts, serum albumin and protein electrophoresis have been also made. All the patients gave their informed consent to enter the trial.

All the twenty patients enrolled were evaluable for the study: six patients were assigned to A Regimen (Group A),eight patients to B Regimen (Group B) and six patients to C Regimen (Group C).

RESULTS

The clinical characteristics of patients are shown in Tables 1-3.

TABLE 1. CLINICAL CHARACTERISTICS OF PATIENTS OF GROUP A (CHEMOTHERAPY + TP1)

PATIENTS SEX	AGE	HISTOLOGIC TYPE	TNM	STAGE	DEAD/ ALIVE	SURVIVAL (MONTHS)	CHEMOTH. (No. OF CYCLES)	IMMUNOTH. (No. OF CYCLES)	BEST OBJECTIVE RESPONSE	TIME TO PROGRESSION (MONTHS)	CLINICAL STATUS (MARCH,1991)
C.M.A.♀	63	EC G1	$T_3N_1M_o$	IIIA	D	8	8	8	NC	4	-
S.S. ♂	64	N T	$T_2N_1M_o$	II	D	13	8	7	PR	4	-
M.S.A.♂	41	EC G1	$T_3N_2M_o$	IIIA	D	4	5	5	P	-	-
V.G. ♂	68	EC G3	$T_3N_1M_o$	IIIA	D	8	10	10	PR	7	-
P.P. ♂	59	EC	$T_3N_2M_1B$	IV	A	24(+)	17	26	PR	14	P
B.G. ♂	67	N T	$T_4N_1M_o$	IIIB	D	6	6	6	P	-	-

MEAN:10.5

TABLE 2. CLINICAL CHARACTERISTICS OF PATIENTS OF GROUP B (CHEMOTHERAPY + TP1 + INTERMITTENT β INTERFERON)

PATIENTS SEX	AGE	HISTOLOGIC TYPE	TNM	STAGE	DEAD/ ALIVE	SURVIVAL (MONTHS)	CHEMOTH. (No. OF CYCLES)	IMMUNOTH. (No. OF CYCLES)	BEST OBJECTIVE RESPONSE	TIME TO PROGRESSION (MONTHS)	CLINICAL STATUS (MARCH,1991)
S.S. ♂	53	SC	$T_2N_2M_o$	L.D.	D	8	8	6	NC	3	-
V.G. ♂	61	EC G1	$T_3N_oM_o$	IIIA	D	20	21	21	PR	8	-
C.A. ♂	64	EC G1	$T_3N_1M_o$	IIIA	D	6	5	5	NC	4	-
C.A. ♂	55	EC G2	$T_3N_2M_o$	IIIA	D	19	8	8	-	-	-
F.G. ♂	62	EC G2	$T_3N_1M_o$	IIIA	A	32(+)	26	32	PR	20	P
U.F. ♂	62	EC	$T_3N_2M_o$	IIIA	A	36(+)	18	27	PR	32	P
P.A. ♀	44	SC	$T_3N_2M_o$	E.D.	D	7	5	4	P	-	-
C.S. ♀	46	LC	$T_4N_2M_1$	IV	D	1.5	1	1	P	-	-

MEAN: 16

81

PATIENTS	AGE	HISTOLOGIC TYPE	TNM	STAGE	DEAD/ ALIVE	SURVIVAL (MONTHS)	CHEMOTH. (N. OF CYCLES)	IMMUNOTH. (N. OF CYCLES)	BEST OBJECTIVE RESPONSE	TIME TO PROGRESSION (MONTHS)	CLINICAL STATUS (MARCH, 1991)
C.L. ♂	63	EC G3	$T_3N_1M_0$	IIIA	D	12	12	12	PR	10	-
M.E. ♂	63	EC G2	$T_3N_1M_0$	IIIA	D	10	8	8	NC	6	-
M.F. ♂	45	AC	$T_3N_2M_0$	IV	D	9	3	1	P	-	-
O.F. ♀	50	AC	$T_3N_2M_0$	IIIA	D	10	8	8	NC	6	-
S.M. ♂	44	EC G1	$T_4N_2M_0$	IIIB	D	4	2	2	P	-	-
M.E. ♂	48	EC G3	$T_3N_2M_0$	IIIA	D	21	15	20	NC	4	-

MEAN: 11

EC: EPIDERMOID CARCINOMA   B : BONE
AC: ADENOCARCINOMA   NC: NO CHANGE
LC: LARGE CELL CARCINOMA   P : PROGRESSION
SC: SMALL CEL LUNG CANCER   PR: PARTIAL RESPONSE
NT: NOT TYPED

Survival. The evaluation was made in March, 1991 at 3 years from start of the study. The clinical outcome was: 3 patients (15%) are still alive (1 of Group A, 2 of Group B).

The best objective response has been achieved in the group B (2 alive, at 32 and 36 months, 3 PR) as compared to group A (1 alive at 24 months, 3 PR) and to group C (no alive, 1PR). The disease was in progression in all patients. The comprehensive mean survival was of 12.5 months (+): the mean survival in Group A was of 10.5 months (+), in Group B of 16 months (+) and in Group C of 11 months.

Treatment's toxicity. The haematological toxicity was very mild: there were 2 cases of anemia and 1 case of severe (Grade 3 WHO) toxicity, with fast recovery. The performance status remained good (> 70 according to Karnofsky and Burchenal score) for the most part of the disease, except obviously for the terminal phase, so that all patients could undergo all the chemotherapy cycles, except the first, as outpatients.

Immunological findings. As far as the PBMC response to polyclonal mitogens, IL 2 and PHA + IL 2 is concerned, the best response was obtained in Group A, while in the other two Groups the responses did not change substantially after therapy as compared to the pre-therapy values (Figure 1). As far as it concerns the in vivo immune response, i.e. skin tests to recall antigens, 5/20 (25%) patients showed a shift of the response from the negative to positive, 5 showed no change (3 remained +, 2 remained -), 7/20 (39%) from positive became negative and 3 were not evaluable (Table 4).

Infections. The infectious episodes were very rare in all groups, with the peak incidence (5 cases) in the Group B: with reference to this, the results of our previous study are to be stressed (11), showing a striking difference in incidence of infections, mainly pulmonary, between the group of patients treated with chemoimmunotherapy and that of patients treated with chemotherapy only.

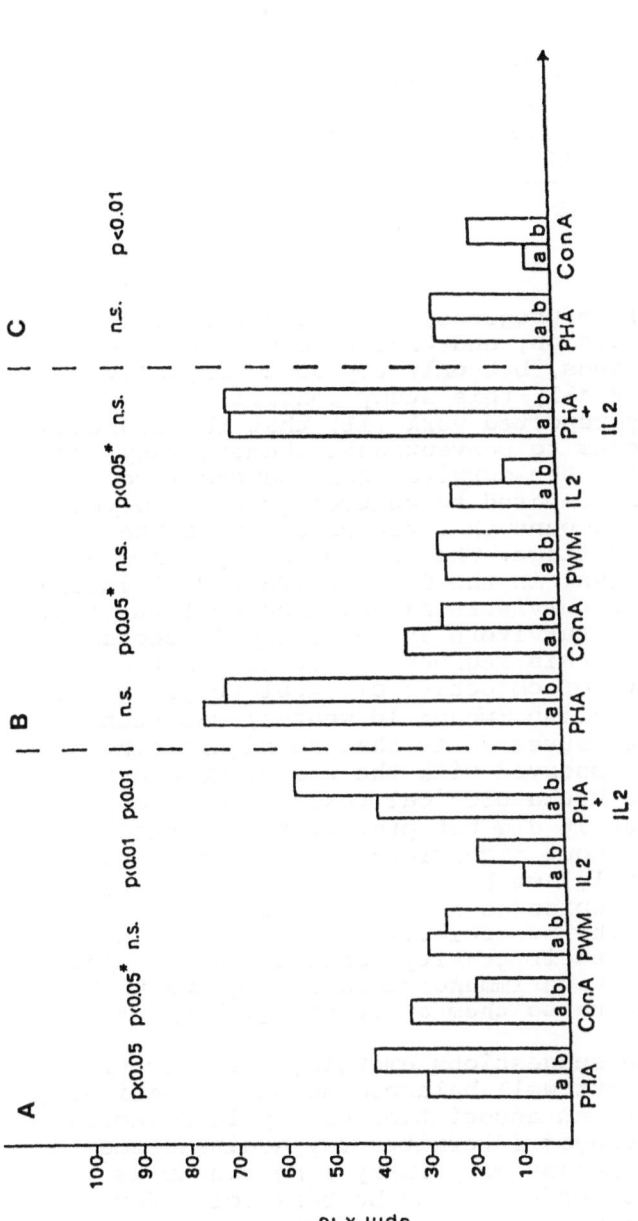

A:Chemotherapy+TP1 B:Chemotherapy+TP1+intermittent β-IFN C:Chemotherapy+TP1+continuous β-IFN

a: before treatment
b: during or after treatment

FIGURE 1. Responsiveness to mitogens PHA, Con A, PWM, to IL 2 and to PHA + IL 2 of PBMC from 20 patients with primary lung cancer.

TABLE 4. In vivo immunological evaluation:
skin tests (comprehensive results).

No. OF PATIENTS		RESPONSE before after treatment		
3	FROM	−	TO	+
2	FROM	±	TO	+
3	FROM	+	TO	+
2	FROM	+	TO	±
2	FROM	+	TO	−
3	FROM	±	TO	−
2	FROM	−	TO	−
3	ND			

ND: NOT DONE

DISCUSSION

The trial is still in progress, because the follow-up
of the alive patients goes on, and therefore we cannot draw
here definitive conclusions, but only try some temptative
considerations. First of all, this study confirms the results of our previously reported work (11) that the addition
of immunomodulating agents to conventional chemotherapy does
not improve significantly the survival nor induces more
prolonged remissions as compared to control group. However,
it is to be taken into account that the majority of the
patients was in advanced stage. The present study, showing a
trend for a better survival in the Group B (CH + TS + intermittent beta IFN) with 2 survivors as compared to 1 survivor
in the Group A and to no survivors in the Group C, seems to
suggest a superiority of this regimen. Moreover, in the
Group B the highest rate of objective clinical responses (3
PR) with the longest duration (mean: 16 months) was found.
An important point to be stressed is that no significant
side effects have been observed with the use of TS and of
beta IFN. Moreover, the haematological toxicity of chemotherapy was reduced so that it did not prevent the planned
schedule of therapy, without significant difference between
the three groups. Finally, we have to consider the very low
incidence of infectious episodes in all groups, with a mild
prevalence in Group B. The possibility of preventing infections and of decreasing their gravity seems to be an important goal to reach in giving immunomodulating agents to this
kind of patients, allowing to them a better "quality of
life".

In conclusion, the suggestions emerging from our trial,
carried out on a small but well balanced number of patients,
are that the addition of an association of thymic hormones
plus beta IFN at low dosages intermittently administered to
the conventional chemotherapy of primary lung cancer is
lacking of untoward side effects, can be beneficial for
controlling a further immune depression induced by treatments and for protecting the patients from severe opportunistic pulmonary infections.

ACKNOWLEDGEMENTS

Work supported by CNR,P.F. Oncologia,Grant N. 88. 00624.44.

REFERENCES

1. Amery, W., and Gough, D.A., 1981, Levamisole and immunotherapy: some theoretic and practical considerations and their relevance to human disease, Oncology, 38: 168.

2. Ludwig Cancer Study Group., 1978, Search for the possible role of "immunotherapy" in operable bronchial non-small cell carcinoma (stage I and II): A phase I study with Corynebacterium parvum intrapleurally, Cancer Immunol. Immunother., 4: 69.

3. Rosso, R., Nobile, M.T., Brema, F., Porcile, G., Cinquegrana, A., De Palma, M., and Rubagotti, A., 1982, Randomized trial of chemoimmunotherapy in advanced non-oat-cell lung cancer, Tumori, 68: 527.

4. Gutterman, J.U., Mavligit, G.M., and Hersh E.M., 1976, Chemoimmunotherapy of human solid tumors, Med. Clin. North Amer., 60: 441.

5. Dimitrov, N.V., Conray, J., Suhrland, L.G., Singh, T., and Teitlebaum, H., 1978, Combination therapy with Corynebacterium parvum and doxorubicin hydrochloride in patients with lung cancer, in: "Immunotherapy of Cancer: Present Status of Trial in Man", W.D. Terry, and D. Windhorst, eds., Raven Press, New York, 181.

6. Goldstein, A.L., Low, T.L.K., McAdoo, M., McClure, J., Thurman, G.B., Rossio, J., Lai, C.Y., Chang, D., Wang, S.S., Harvey, C., Ramel A.H., and Meienhofer J., 1977, Thymosin alpha I: isolation and sequence analysis of an immunologically active thymic polypeptide, Proc. Nat. Acad. Sci., USA, 74: 725.

7. Goldstein, G., 1976, Radioimmunoassay for thymopoietin, J. Immunol. 117: 690.

8. Del Giacco. G.S., Cengiarotti, L., Mantovani, G., Pusceddu, G., Di Tucci, A., Pischedda, A., and Vespa, F., 1984, Advanced lung cancer treated with combination chemotherapy with or without thymostimulin, in, "Thymic factor therapy", N.A. Byrom and J.R. Hobbs, eds., Serono Symposia Publ., Raven Press, New York, 321.

9. Del Giacco, G.S., Mantovani, G., Cengiarotti, L., Pusceddu, G., Pischedda, A., Di Tucci, A., and Vespa, F., 1984, Secondary immunodeficiency in advanced lung cancer: effect of chemotherapy plus thymostimulin in immunodepressed patients, Int. J. Tiss. Reac. 6: 499.

10. Falchetti, R., Bergesi, G., Eshkol, A., Cafiero, C., Adorini, L., and Caprino L., 1977, Pharmacological and biological properties of a Calf Thymus extract (TP-1), Drugs Exp. Clin. Res., 3: 39.

11. Del Giacco, G.S., Mantovani, G., Piludu, G., Locci, F., Loy, M., Piras, M.C., Cengiarotti, L., Lo Presti, M., Meloni, G., Montaldo, E, and Pusceddu G., 1988, Thymic factors in lung cancer, in: "Thymus Hormones in Oncology", G. Nagel, G. Schioppacassi, and P. Schuff-Werner, eds., Serono Symposia Review No. 19, Rome, 149.

TUMOR IMMUNOTHERAPY WITH COMBINED INTERLEUKINS INJECTED

PERILYMPHATICALLY: EXPERIMENTAL AND CLINICAL FINDINGS

Cristina Jemma*, Stefania Vai*, Tiziana Musso*,
Massimo Geuna#, Guido Valente# and Guido Forni@

*Institute of Microbiology,
#Department of Biomedical Sciences and Human Oncology,
University of Turin, and
@Immunogenetics and Histocompatibility Center,
CNR, Turin, Italy

Tumor growth is often perceived by the immune system. Weak cellular reactivity can be shown in the early stages, both in man and in experimental models. In preimmunisation experiments in mice, the immune system has proved capable of inhibiting syngeneic tumor growth[1], while lymphocytes from cancer patients have been shown to react with autologous tumor cells in vitro in proliferation and cytotoxicity assays[2,3]. Nevertheless, most spontaneous or transplanted tumors grow and kill their host. Tumor cells can directly suppress host reactivity by secreting soluble mediators, and actively trigger specific or non- specific suppressor mechanisms that block both natural and adaptive host resistance[4].

One of the greatest clinical problems is the difficulty of starting therapy as soon as a tumor begins to develop. By contrast with animal models, immunotherapy in man is initiated much later, after a tumor has become implanted, and its eradication is less likely. For this reason, the prime goal of optimal cancer immunotherapy is to potentiate the patient's immune system, eliminate the minimal residual disease, and prevent metastasis and recurrences, rather than primary tumor eradication or prevention.

Preclinical studies demonstrate that tumor immunogenicity and activation of a specific host T-cell response against an autologous tumor are crucial for successful cancer therapy. The non-immunogenicity of most human tumors, and the difficulty of identifying tumor-specific or tumor- associated antigens on the membrane of spontaneous tumors, so as to be able to generate a sufficient number of tumor-specific effector cells, have strongly limited the development of this approach.

The "discovery" in 1982[5] of lymphokine activated killer (LAK) activity, distinct from NK and T-mediated lytic functions, opened fresh approaches to cancer immunotherapy. New protocols were developed, based on the encouraging results obtained in mice[6]. Patients with advanced cancer, were injected intravenously with autologous LAK cells, generated and expanded in vitro from PBL, in combination with high doses of recombinant IL-2 (rIL-2). With this treatment, it was demonstrated, for the first time, that an exclusive immunologic therapy can induce the complete regression of large tumors in some patients, after the failure of standard therapy[7]. The use of IL-2 and LAK cells is a good example of how a therapy developed in animal models can be transferred to man with some success. It also illustrates some of the pitfalls. IL-2, in fact, has a much greater toxicity than experiments in the mouse suggested[7].

Cellular adoptive immunotherapy has shown many disadvantages. It is laborious, time-consuming, and expensive. Significant clinical responses have only been obtained in a few types of malignancy and a small proportion of patients, while the great majority of those with frequently occurring tumors (i.e. colon, lung, breast, and prostatic carcinoma) rarely benefit from any of the current immunotherapeutic manipulations[7]. Yet the positive results obtained by the LAK approach and the systemic administration of high doses of IL-2 alone show that even the immune system of a neoplastic patient can be effectively activated to mount such an efficent immune response that large tumor burdens are rapidly destroyed[8]. In this case, IL-2 behaves as a new kind of in vivo immunomodulator. Its pleiotropic activity, as detected in vitro, becomes even more evident in vivo because of the highly interactive nature of the immune system, where a signal delivered by an activated cell affects many others. The efficacy of IL-2 in vivo may in fact rest on induction of this cascade of interconnected effector functions, each affecting neoplastic growth with different mechanisms. In this context, special emphasis is placed on the role of the host's specific T-cell immunity as a key mechanism in cancer rejection, and its possible amplification by cytokines and other biological response modifiers.

THE "HELPER" APPROACH IN CANCER IMMUNOTHERAPY

We believe that the immune system of a neoplastic host can be "helped" to recognize and actively react against poorly immunogenic or non-immunogenic tumors, as most human tumors are. In contrast to the activation of a single effector mechanism, as in the LAK approach, the IL-2 based "helper" strategy utilises IL-2 to interfere with the control mechanisms of the immune system. Its efficacy rests on the repertoire of effector mechanisms activated. It allows the induction of a cascade of interconnected functions leading to tumor growth inhibition through many different cellular and humoral reaction mechanisms[9,10].

Lymphocytes from mice bearing poorly immunogenic tumors do not display any in vitro antitumor reactivity, in terms of release of IFNγ, proliferative or cytotoxic activity against tumor cells; moreover, they are not able to inhibit specific tumor growth in vivo in a Winn type neutralization assay[11]. We therefore studied the possibility of activating an effective T reactivity through the addition of exogenous lymphokines. Several transplantable murine tumors with poor or no immunogenicity were injected sc. A small, but consistent tumor inhibition was obtained following ten daily injections of only 10-20 U of IL-2 around the tumor growing area. By contrast, almost complete inhibition was obtained when IL-2 was injected in mice challenged with tumor cells admixed with spleen cells from tumor bearing mice[12]. Some features of this effective association of a low IL-2 dose with non-reactive lymphocytes were then studied in detail. First, criss-cross type experiments showed that it is not a tumor-specific phenomenon. Depletion studies demonstrated that the lymphokine-induced reactivity rests on two cell populations: T-helper lymphocytes and NK cells. Irradiated lymphocytes can still mediate the phenomenon, whereas it does not take place in irradiated normal or nude mice, showing that the host immune system plays a crucial role, while proliferation and persistent survival of lymphocytes locally admixed with the tumor is not required. Mice in which tumor inhibition mediated by local lymphokine injections took place 30 days earlier display a tumor-specific delayed type hypersensitivity, and a significant number of animals acquire a tumor-specific immune memory[13]. The stream of events leading to tumor inhibition starts when the low doses of IL-2 activate the lymphocytes artificially admixed wih tumor cells. Rather than becoming LAK cells and killing the tumor directly, experimental data show that their major role is to secrete and efficently deliver various lymphokines. In this way, they recruit several host lymphocyte populations, mainly T-helper and NK cells, that can directly destroy the tumor or, in their turn, further amplify the anti-tumor reaction by releasing other lymphokines and chemotactic factors by which they boost endogenous NK activity, activate T-killer cells, and macrophages, attract and activate granulocytes, and finally induce a specific T cell reactivity. The cascade reaction triggered by these non-reactive lymphocytes can be induced by local injection of different lymphokines. It is thus possible to build up a helper system which is fully defined at the molecular level. For this purpose, we first considered the use of IL-1, and in parallel we tested the activity of a highly hydrophilic nonapeptide fragment (163-171 peptide) synthesized by Centro Ricerche Sclavo, Siena, Italy, which retains most of the immunomodulatory activities of the entire IL-1β molecule without its inflammatory activity[14]. Ten daily peritumoral injections of picograms of IL-1β produced a marked inhibition of tumor takes, whereas a small, but statistically significant reduction was obtained in mice injected with micrograms of the 163-171 peptide. The effect of combination with other lymphokines was tested by injecting the 163-171 peptide first, then IL-2 or IFNγ 4 hours later. Efficient tumor inhibition was obtained with the peptide + IL-2 association, whereas both molecules are rather ineffective when injected alone. By contrast, IFNγ is a peptide antagonist[15].

More recently, lymphokines have been injected around the tumor-draining lymph nodes (TD-LN), rather than intralesionally. With this new approach, IL-4 proved more effective than IL-2, IL-1β and IFNγ, and its activity was clearly evident without the addition of lymphocytes. Even low doses triggered an efficient immune recognition of poorly immunogenic tumors. Combined injection of IL-4 with IL-2, IL-1β or IFNγ had no synergistic effect on tumor inhibition, while the establishment of a tumor-specific memory was enhanced by the IL-4 and IL-1β combination[16]. Following the local injection of lymphocytes + lymphokines, or lymphokines alone, the tumor growth area is heavily infiltrated by mononuclear cells and granulocytes. Eosinophils are frequent and mostly in close contact with both lymphocytes and tumor cells, suggesting that their cytotoxic activity is induced by factors secreted by activated lymphocytes. TD-LN show progressive enlargment with expansion of cortical and paracortical zones. Intensive traffic of lymphocytes to and from the lymph nodes (LN) takes place through the wall of epithelioid venules. The non-specific immunity dominating the initial reaction phase creates a favorable environment for local activation of a few tumor-specific T-lymphocytes.

The passage from early, non-specific to late tumor-specific immunity is of clinical significance in overcoming the suppressive activity impairing immunotherapy "a priori". Lymphokine induced tumor inhibition is a new way of looking at immune antitumor therapy, whereby direct reaction to the tumor is elicited by piloting a self-enhancing lymphokine cascade.

PERILYMPHATIC INJECTION OF IL-2 IN HEAD AND NECK TUMORS

The experimental results in mice have promoted the development of clinical trials in patients with local tumors easily accessible to lymphokine injections.

A set of pilot trials was initiated with patients with advanced primary or recurrent head and neck squamous cell carcinomas (HNSCC). These tumors are a rational choice for evaluation of the effectiveness of a local lymphokine treatment for several reasons:
1. Patients with HNSCC, particularly those of the oral cavity and oropharynx display a higher incidence of immunosuppression than patients with other tumors[17,18]. This is mostly due to the emergence of suppressor cells, and made worse by surgery, radiotherapy and chemotherapy. Most have a poor prognosis, due, inter alia, to residual and micrometastatic disease, often related to the degree of immune depression.
2. HNSCC are usually well open to manipulation from the outside through surgical infiltration, are surrounded by the body's thickest lymph node network, and have a typical locoregional progression.
Treatment based on local stimulation of the immune reactivity of TD-LN cells thus appears to be a simple and rational immunotherapeutic approach by which the inability of conventional therapies to control tumor growth and prevent local recurrences can be overcame.

Two categories of HNSCC were selected: a) recurrences no longer open to effective treatment with conventional methods. Here perilymphatic injections of IL-2 are a single, isolated treatment; b) primary tumors of the oral cavity and oropharynx, with IL-2 both before and after surgery to enhance its effect.

In the first trial, 20 patients with recurrent inoperable HNSCC were treated with natural IL-2 (nIL-2) produced by the Jurkat T cell line, and purified by reverse-phase HPLC. Ten daily injections of 200 U of nIL-2 in 0.5 ml of saline plus 10% human serum albumin were given 1.5 cm from the insertion of the sternocleidomastoid muscle on the mastoid at a depth of 1.5 cm. Lymphographic studies had shown that injection of radioopaque substances at this point ensures excellent visualization of the neck lymphatic network[19]. The tumor side was chosen in patients with functional lymph nodes still draining the tumor area, and on the opposite side in those with only residual contralateral functioning lymph nodes, and those who had undergone bilateral TD-LN dissection. When possible, the course was repeated at 45-day intervals. The clinical parameters considered were: reduction or disappearance of the tumor mass; disease-free interval; sensitivity of tumor relapse to further courses of IL-2; effect of the treatment on progression. A response was considered to be complete (CR) if no tumor was evident on direct or optical fiber inspection, partial (PR) if the sum of the products of the longest perpendicular diameters of all lesions decreased by >50%, and minor (MR) if this decrease was <50%.

Several progress reports have been published[20,21,22]. None of the side-effects commonly described after systemic administration of massive doses of IL-2 were observed. Only slight lymph node swelling on the injection side, and slight pain in the tumor mass or in metastatic LN were occasionally reported. In the 20 patients treated, 3 CR (15%), 3 PR(15%), and 8 MR (40%) were found. These subjects presented lymph node enlargement, necrotic sputum and a decrease of the tumor mass. No appreciable clinical effects were detected in patients with a rather poor performance status or LN metastases attached to the deep planes, nor in those who had undergone bilateral LN dissection. By contrast, clinical responses were observed after a single IL-2 course in patients with still functional TD-LN. An interesting observation is that even the presence of contralateral neckn LN only was sufficient to induce tumor shrinkage. A direct toxic effect of IL-2 on tumor cells can be ruled out, since no clinical effects were obtained in patients without functional TD-LN, and the IL-2 injections were not intratumoral. Immunologic studies performed on PBL from 9 patients before and after IL-2 did not reveal any dramatic effect on peripheral immune reactivity. After the first course, an increase of CD 25[+] and of HLA class II[+] cells was found in 4 and 3 patients respectively; in 6 cases, slight variations of other membrane antigens were found. The high individual variability of NK activity in these patients made it difficult to determine any modulation by IL-2. A decrease was none the less observed in 75% of patients after the first course. LAK activity was generally absent or very low in all patients, and slightly increased in 45%.

This study provides one of the first demostrations[20,23], that massive tumor necrosis and disappearance can be achieved by perilymphatic injections of low doses of IL-2 in patients with recurrent HNSCC not subjected to preventive bilateral neck dissection. These biological findings, however, require a few important clinical qualifications. Both CR and PR were temporary. Subsequent recurrences are less sensitive to IL-2. Regression does not prolong survival and is in any case obtained with small recurrent tumors only[24]. When the same IL-2 protocol was applied to 15 far-advanced, non-pretreated HNSCC patients, no tumor shrinkage was observed[25].

In another group of trials, patients with advanced primary HNSCC still open to surgical management were treated. Here IL-2 injected perilymphatically is a therapeutic maneuver added to the best conventional protocol, i.e. surgery and radiotherapy. The aim of this study was to evaluate to what extent local treatment with low doses of IL-2, injected before and after surgery, affects the surgical procedure and scar healing, and influences the disease-free interval. Moreover, histochemical and immunologic studies were performed on surgical LN and tumor specimens to evaluate local immunoreactivity. In a initial study, performed in Rome, 200 U n IL2 were injected both around the mastoid and peritumorally in 4 patients. Histologic and ultrastructural examination of the surgical specimens showed a markedly uniform reaction pattern. In many instances neoplastic cells were intermingled with numerous lymphocytes and eosinophils. This massive infiltration was often associated with degenerated tumor cells or even necrosis. LN displayed hyperplasia of both cortical and paracortical areas, and epithelioid venules with a thick endothelium infiltrated by lymphocytes and granulocytes. In a few cases, a decrease or disappearance of neoplastic lesions was also documented both clinically and histologically[26]. Electron microscopy showed a similar pattern. Immune reactivity, in terms of proliferative response to IL-2 or mitogens, NK and LAK cytotoxic activity, was tested in LN lymphocytes obtained at surgery and in PBL, before and after IL-2. Despite the strong cell reaction detected histologically, the in vitro reactivity of LN lymphocytes and PBL was only slightly or not influenced by IL-2 local injection. LAK activity was not elicited, most probably because the IL-2 doses were too low.

A recent multicentric randomized trial with rIL-2, (Glaxo), coordinated by the Otorhinolaryngology Clinic of the University of Turin, has made a comparative study of tumors and local LN from treated and untreated patients with primary HNSCC. Eighteen patients underwent surgery only, while 15 patients received ten daily injections of 5000 U rIL-2 prior to surgery, and at 45-day intervals starting 45 days after surgery. IL-2 was injected at two points: half the dose was injected near the mastoid, as in recurrent patients, and the other half submentally, 1.5 cm under the mylohyoid muscle. Surgical specimens were investigated immunohistochemically, immunologically and by molecular biology. Variable amounts of eosinophils or neutrophils were seen in both the tumor and the peritumoral stroma after IL-2 treatment. Slight (no more than 10%) necrosis, was found in 50% of cases. Untreated tumors generally displayed less marked infiltration by eosinophils and lymphocytes and less extensive edema[27]. Immunophenotypic examination of TIL showed that CD3+ and CD2+ lymphocytes largely predominated, but no significant differences were found in the amount and distribution of CD4+ and CD8+ cells in treated and untreated patients. By contrast, a consistent significant increase of CD25+ lymphocytes, particularly close to the neoplastic sheets was found in treated tumors (fig.1). A similar histologic pattern was found by other authors in bioptic specimens after IL-2 injections[28].

A thorough histologic, phenotypic and functional analysis was made on TD-LN. No substantial histologic differences were noted between treated and untreated cases, suggesting that the reactivity of the lymphoreticular tissue was not appreciably modified by IL-2, at least from a morphologic point of view. Flow cytometry was performed with a wide panel of monoclonal antibodies on single cell suspensions obtained from the same TD-LN. The only consistent and significant difference observed was an increase of CD3+DR+ lymphocytes in IL-2 treated patients. TD-LN from 4 treated and 3 untreated patients were evaluated for the presence of m-RNA for the IL-2 receptor p55 chain. A marked amount of IL-2R m-RNA of 3.5 and 1.5 kb was only detected in the treated group, despite the weak CD25 positivity revealed by immunofluorescence. Some functional parameters of lymphocytes from ipsilateral and contralateral TD-LN were tested in 9 treated and 5 untreated patients. Spontaneous proliferative and cytotoxic activities were generally lower in TD-LN closer to the neoplasia or tumor-invaded. Basal NK activity was always higher in treated TD-LN. Moreover, LAK

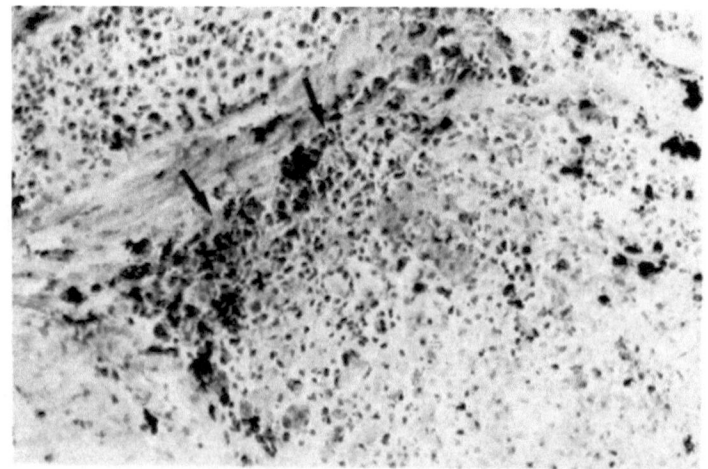

Fig.1 IL-2-treated HNSCC of the oropharynx: the stroma close to the neoplastic sheets is infiltrated by numerous CD25+ lymphocytes (arrows). ABC immunoperoxidase. 230x.

activity (absent in untreated TD-LN), was detected in the ipsilateral TD-LN of 3 treated patients.

In vitro culture of TD-LN lymphocytes with 500 U/ml rIL-2 elicited a marked proliferative response, NK and LAK activity in both treated and untreated cases, while other lymphokines (IL-1 and IL-4) alone or in combination with IL-2 did not produce any distinct effect[29]. No significant release of IL-1, IL-2 and IL-4 was detected in fresh TD-LN cells from either group.

In addition to the absence of any side-effects, no surgical complications have arisen following IL-2 injections. One of the main targets of this trial, besides the study of local immune reactivity, is to evaluate if the pre- and post- surgery IL-2 treatment can extend the disease-free interval. Forty patients have so far been enrolled, but it is still too early to evaluate this aspect.

Several conclusions can be drawn from these studies on HNSCC patients. The histologic findings show that IL-2 induces an active leukocyte traffic in TD-LN, and modifies the cell reaction to the tumor by triggering an inflammatory response, documented by massive infiltration of the tumor area by eosinophils and activated T lymphocytes, with a variable degree of necrosis. The efficacy of this reaction pattern may well be high, as shown by the several instances of regression[20]. Yet, the in vitro reactivity of TD-LN lymphocytes is very poor, and only slightly influenced by in vivo IL-2 injections. The reason for this discrepancy between the histologic and functional in vitro data is not clear.

Infiltration of eosinophils associated with the involution of human tumors has long been described, and is a sign of a favourable prognosis[30]. However, apart from the immediate CR and PR in recurrent HNSCC, an efficient antitumor reactivity is apparently not achieved, since patients relapse after a short time. This feature is different to the outcome in murine models, where persistent reactivity takes place after IL-2 activated tumor inhibition. The discrepancy may depend on differences in the immunogenicity of murine and human tumors. Moreover, In effect, induction of a marked immunosuppression is a major issue in HNSCC patients. Low doses of IL-2 may not be effective in fully overcoming this negative control exerted either by the tumor itself or by suppressor T cells[31]. It should also be remembered that these HNSCC were established, advanced tumors. The efficacy of immune reactivity becomes marginal under these conditions, one reason being the marked immunosuppression induced by HNSCC.

A new protocol based on combined local treatment with IL-2 and αIFN in HNSCC is being elaborated and will soon be introduced. The murine models show in fact, that cytokines can interact in an additive or synergistic manner[15,16,32]. The most impressive clinical results offered by combined cytokines treatment have recently been described by Rosenberg's group in patients with advanced cancer, treated with IL-2 and αIFN[33].

For tumors confined to a certain organ or body compartment, a loco regional administration of cytokines may prove effective, with fewer side effects, as reported by clinical studies with a variety of tumors following IL-2 +/- LAK cell administration intraperitoneal[34], intrapleurally[35], intravescically[36], and intracerebrally[37]. Administration of cytokines peritumorally, intratumorally or perilymphatically, in addition to reducing systemic toxicity, requires much lower doses. Local treatments are not adequate, however, against disseminated forms.

Quite apart from the comparative effectiveness of killer and helper strategies, we believe that in most cases helper manoeuvres alone constitute the most rational approach, and perhaps the only way to achieve significant in vivo manipulation of the immune reactivity to neoplasia; moreover, unlike killer therapy, it can lead to a tumor-specific immune memory, as shown in murine models.

ACKNOWLEDGMENTS

This work was supported by grants from the Associazione italiana per la Ricerca sul cancro (AIRC), MPI 40%-60%, and the ISS Italy-Usa special project in tumor immunotherapy. We thank Dr. J. Iliffe for careful review of the manuscript.

REFERENCES

1. F.J. Foley, Antigenic properties of methylcholantrene- induced tumors in mice of the strain of origin, Cancer Res. 13:835 (1953).
2. G. Parmiani, A. Anichini, and G. Fossati, Cellular immune response against autologous human malignant melanoma: are in vitro studies providing a framework for a more effective immunotherapy?, J. Natl. Cancer Inst. 82:361 (1990).
3. A. Uchida, M. Moore, and E. Klein, Autologous mixed lymphocyte-tumor reaction and autologous mixed lymphocyte reaction.I.Proliferation of two distinct T-cell subsets, Int. J. Cancer 40:165 (1987).
4. G. Forni, L. Varesio, M. Giovarelli, and G. Cavallo, Dynamic state of spontaneous immune reactivity towards a mammary adenocarcinoma, in: "Tumor Associated Antigens and their Specific Immune Response," F. Spreafico, and R. Arnon, eds., Academic Press, London (1980).
5. E.A. Grimm, and S. Rosenberg, The human lymphokine-activated killer cell phenomenon, Lymphokines 9:279 (1983).
6. J.J. Mule', S. Shu, S.L. Schwarz, and S.A. Rosenberg, Adoptive immunotherapy of established pulmonary metastases with LAK cells and reconbinant interleukin-2, Science 225:1487 (1984).
7. S.A. Rosenberg, Immunotherapy of cancer using interleukin-2: Current status and future prospects, Immunol. Today 9:58 (1988).
8. W.H. West, K.W. Tauer, J.R. Jannelli, G.D. Marshall, D.W. Orr, G.B. Thurman, and R.K. Oldham, Costant infusion recombinant interleukin-2 in adoptive immunotherapy of advanced cancer, N. Engl. J. Med. 316:898 (1987).
9. G. Forni, G.P. Cavallo, M. Giovarelli, G. Benetton, C. Jemma, M.G. Barioglio, A. De Stefani, M. Forni, A. Santoni, A. Modesti, G. Cavallo, P. Menzio, and G. Cortesina, Tumor immunotherapy by local injection of interleukin 2 and non-reactive lymphocytes, Prog. exp. Tumor Res. 32:187 (1988).
10. G. Forni, H. Fujiwara, F. Martino, T. Hamaoka, C. Jemma, P. Caretto, and M. Giovarelli, Helper strategy in tumor immunology: expansion of helper lymphocytes and utilization of helper lymphokines for experimental and clinical immunotherapy, Cancer Metastasis Rev. 7:289 (1988).
11. G. Forni, and M. Giovarelli, In vitro re-educated T helper cells from sarcoma bearing mice inhibit sarcoma growth in vivo, J. Immunol. 132:527 (1984).
12. G. Forni, M. Giovarelli, M. Forni, A. Modesti, A. Santoni, Lymphokine- activated tumor inhibition (LATI) in vivo, Lymphokines 14:335 (1987).
13. G. Forni, M. Giovarelli, A. Santoni, A. Modesti, and M. Forni, Interleukin-2 activated tumor inhibition in vivo depends on the systemic involvement of host immunoreactivity, J. Immunol. 138:4033 (1987).

14. D. Boraschi, L. Nencioni, L. Villa, S. Censini, P. Bossu', P. Ghiara, R. Presentini, F. Perin, D. Frasca, G. Doria, G. Forni, T. Musso, M. Giovarelli, P. Ghezzi, R. Bertini, H.O. Besedovsky, A. del Rey, J.D. Stipe, G. Antoni, S. Silvestri, A. Tagliabue, In vivo stimulation and restoration of the immune response by the noninflammatory fragment 163-171 of the human IL-1 beta, J. Exp. Med. 168:675 (1988).

15. G. Forni, T. Musso, C. Jemma, D. Boraschi, A. Tagliabue, and M. Giovarelli, Lymphokine activated tumor inhibition (LATI) in mice: ability of a nonapeptide of the human Interleukin-1 to recruit antitumor reactivity in recipient mice, J. Immunol. 142:712 (1989).

16. M.C. Bosco, M. Giovarelli, M. Forni, A. Modesti, S. Scarpa, L. Masuelli, and G. Forni, Low doses of IL-4 injected perilymphatically in tumor-bearing mice inhibit the growth of poorly and apparently nonimmunogenic tumors and induce a tumor-specific immune memory, J. Immunol. 145:3136 (1990).

17. J. Lundy, H. Wanebo, C. Pinsky, E. Strong, and H. Oetthen, Delayed hypersensitivity reaction in patients with squamous cell cancer of the head and neck, Am. J. Surgery 128:530 (1974).

18. G. Cortesina, B. Morra, F. Beatrice, G.P. Cavallo, M. Bussi, V. Di Fortunato, E. Poggio, M. Vercellino, and A. Sartoris, Evaluation of blocking mechanisms against immunological response in patients with laryngeal carcinoma, The Laryngoscope 94:6 (1984).

19. L. Traissac, Cervical Lymphography:Difficultes and advantages, Rev. Laryng. 898:81 (1968).

20. G. Cortesina, A. De Stefani, M. Giovarelli, M.G. Barioglio, G.P. Cavallo, C. Jemma, C. and G. Forni, Treatment of recurrent squamous cell carcinoma of head and neck with low doses of interleukin-2 (IL-2) injected perilymphatically, Cancer 62:2482 (1988).

21. G. Forni, G.P. Cavallo, M. Giovarelli, G. Benetton, C. Jemma, M.G. Barioglio, A. De Stefani, M. Forni, A. Modesti, G. Cavallo, P. Menzio, and G. Cortesina, Tumor immunotherapy by local injection of interleukin-2 and non-reactive lymphocytes, Prog. Exp. Tumor Res. 32:187 (1986).

22. G. Forni, M. Giovarelli, C. Jemma, M.C. Bosco, P. Caretto, A. Modesti, A. Santoni, M. Forni, G. Cortesina, A. De Stefani, G.P. Cavallo, E. Galeazzi, P. Musiani, E. De Campora, S. Valitutti, F. Castellino, C.V. Calearo, G. Fontana, and G. Sesia, Perilymphatic injection of cytokines: a new tool in active cancer immunotherapy. Experimental rationale and clinical findings, Ann. Ist. Super. Sanita' 26:397 (1990).

23. T. Saito, H. Kakiuti, K. Kuki, M. Yokota, T. Jinnin, T. Kimura, K. Fujiwara, J. Yoda, M. Kunimoto, and H. Arai, Clinical evaluation of local administration of RIL-2 in head and neck cancer, Nippon Jibiinkoka Gakkai Kaiho, 92:1265 (1989).

24. C. Cortesina, A. De Stefani, E. Galeazzi, G.P. Cavallo, C. Jemma, M. Giovarelli, S. Vai, and G. Forni, Interleukin-2 injected around tumor-draining lymph nodes in head and neck cancer, Head and Neck 769 (1991), in press.

25. V. Mattijssen, P.H. De Mulder, J.H. Schornagel, J. Verweij, P. Van den Broek, A. Galazka, S. Roy, and D.J. Ruiter, Clinical and immunopathological results of perilymphatically injected recombinant interleukin-2 in locally far advanced,nonpretreated head and neck squamous cell carcinoma, J. Immununotherapy 10:63 (1991).

26. P. Musiani, E. De Campora, S. Valitutti, F. Castellino, C. Calearo, G. Cortesina, M. Giovarelli, C. Jemma, A. De Stefani, and G. Forni, Effect of low doses of interleukin-2 injected perilymphatically and peritumorally in patients with advanced primary head and neck squamous cell carcinoma, J. Biol. Resp. Mod. 8:571 (1989).

27. G. Valente, A. De Stefani, C. Jemma, M. Giovarelli, M. Geuna, G. Cortesina, G. Forni, and G. Palestro, Infiltrating leucocyte populations and T-lymphocyte subsets in head and neck squamous cell carcinoma from patients receiving perilymphatic injections of recombinant interleukin-2. A pathologic and immunophenotypic study, Modern Pathology 3:702 (1990).

28. T. Saito, T. Kawaguti, J. Yoda; T. Kimura, and T. Tabata, Immunohistology of tumor tissue in local administration of recombinant interleukin-2 in head and neck cancer, Nippon Jibiinkoka Gakkai Kaiho 92:1271 (1989).

29. G. Cortesina, A. De Stefani, E. Galeazzi, M. Bussi, C. Giordano, G.P. Cavallo, C. Jemma, S. Vai, G. Forni, and G. Valente, The effect of preoperative local interleukin-2 (IL-2) injections in patients with head and neck squamous cell carcinoma, Acta Otolaryngol (Stockh), 111:428 (1991).

30. T.P. Pretlow, E.F. Keith, A. Cryar Keith, A.A. Bertolucci, A.M. Pitts, T.G. Pretlow II, P.M. Kimball, and E.A. Boohaker, Eosinophil infiltration of human colonic carcinoma as a prognosis indicator, Cancer Res. 43:2997 (1983).

31. F. Cozzolino, M. Torcia, A.M. Carossino, R. Giordani, C. Selli, G. Talini, E. Reali, A. Novelli, V. Pistoia, and M. Ferrarini, Characterization of cells from invaded lymph nodes in patients with solid tumors. Lymphokine requirement for tumor-specific lymphoid proliferative response, J. Exp. Med. 166:303 (1987).

32. F. Belardelli, V. Ciolli, U. Testa, E. Montesoro, D. Bulgarini, E. Proietti, P. Borghi, P. Sestili, C. Locardi, C. Peschle, and I. Gresser, Antitumor effects of interleukin-2 and interleukin-1 in mice transplanted with different syngeneic tumors, Int. J. Cancer 44:1108 (1989).

33. S.A. Rosemberg, M.T. Lotze, J.C. Yang, W. Marston Linhean, C. Seipp, S. Calabro, S.E. Karp, R.M. Sherry, S. Steimberg, and D.E. White, Combination therapy with interleukin-2 and α-interferon for the treatment of patients with advanced cancer, J. Clin. Oncol. 7:1863 (1989).

34. W.J. Urba, J.W. Clark, R.G. Steis, M.A. Bookman, J.W. Smith II, S. Beckner, A.E. Maluish, J.L. Rossio, H. Rager, J.R. Ortaldo, and D.L. Longo, Intraperitoneal lymphokine-activated killer cell/interleukin-2 therapy in patients with intra-abdominal cancer: immunologic considerations, J. Natl. Cancer Inst. 81:602 (1989).

35. K. Yasumoto, K. Miyazaki, A. Nagashima, T. Ishida, T. Kuda, T. Yano, K. Sugimachi, and K. Nomoto, Induction of lymphokine-activated killer cells by intrapleural instillation of recombinant interleukin-2 in patients with malignant pleurisy due to lung cancer, Cancer Res. 47:2184 (1987).

36. G. Pizza, G. Severini, D. Menniti, C. De Vinci, and F. Corrado, Tumour regression after intralesional injection of interleukin-2 in bladder cancer. Preliminary report, Int. J. Cancer 34:359 (1984).

37. S. Yoshida, R. Tanaka, N. Takai, and K. Ono, Local administration of autologous lymphokine-activated killer cells and recombinant interleukin-2 to patients with malignant brain tumor, Cancer Res. 48:5011 (1988).

COMBINATION THERAPIES WITH CYTOKINES AND ANTI-CYTOKINES IN MURINE OPPORTUNISTIC INFECTIONS

Luigina Romani, Simonetta Mocci, Franca Campanile, Paolo Puccetti, and Francesco Bistoni

Department of Experimental Medicine and Biochemical Sciences, University of Perugia, Via del Giochetto, 06100 Perugia, Italy

INTRODUCTION

Systemic administration of purified recombinant cytokines has been performed in various animal models and clinical trials for the treatment of neoplasia, infectious disease, hemapoietic failure and immunosuppression. In particular, in infectious disease, cytokines have radically changed our understanding of the mechanisms of resistance, and have also provided new clues to the elucidation of the mechanisms of both resistance and pathology, such that the use of cytokines or anti-cytokines appears to be extremely promising for treatment of conditions associated with microbial infection.

Two major characteristics of cytokines are pleiotropy, (i.e., each cytokine mediates more than one function) and redundancy (i.e., more than one cytokine mediates the same or similar function). The reasons for pleiotropy and redundancy of the cytokines are unclear but there are several levels of control to consider (1). Firstly, not all cytokines are produced in response to a given antigen. Secondly, not all target cells are available at a given immune site. Thirdly, the effect of a cytokine depends not only on the phenotype of the target cell but also on the presence of other stimuli. Finally, most cytokines are interactive in either synergism or antagonism. Due to the peculiar immunobiology of the cytokines, the challenge remains to provide a rational basis for the clinical enhancement or suppression of immune responsiveness by manipulation of endogenous cytokine synthesis or by cytokine administration (2).

We will summarize recent data from our laboratory on the possible role of cytokines in two different infection models, one fungal and the other bacterial. In a murine <u>Candida albicans</u> infection model, evidence will be provided that protective immunity relies on the production of a particular panel of cytokines, the Th1 cytokines. In addition, it will be shown that host susceptibility to infection can be modulated by treatment with anti-cytokine antibody. In a bacterial <u>Pseudomonas</u> infection model, treatment with cytokines will be shown to reduce the need for antibacterial chemotherapy in neutropenic mice.

Combination Therapies, Edited by A.L. Goldstein and
E. Garaci, Plenum Press, New York, 1992

1. Role of Cytokines and Cytokine Producing Cells in Acquired Immunity

Specific anti-Candida immunity can be induced in mice by vaccination with a low-virulence Candida variant strain. This procedure results in chronic infection of mice, associated with the persistent colonization of different organs (3), and results in enhanced antimicrobial resistance at about two weeks post-infection, possibly mediated by activated macrophages (4-9). In this model, the in vivo administration of antibodies directed to either the L3T4 or Lyt2 surface antigens greatly affects the outcome of subsequent challenge with virulent Candida cells (10,11). In one experiment, anti-Lyt2 mAb, alone or in combination with anti-L3T4 antibodies were injected for five consecutive days into Candida-immune mice starting 24 hours before systemic challenge with virulent Candida cells. In alternative, a group of mice received antibodies to murine IFN-γ. At 4, 10 and 20 days after challenge viable yeast cells were titrated in the kidneys. Table 1 shows that anti-Lyt2 mAb treatment, alone or in combination with anti-L3T4 mAb, greatly enhanced the animals' susceptibility to challenge in that significantly more yeast cells were recovered from the organs of treated mice. Neutralization of endogenous IFN-γ by specific mAb led to decreased anticandidal resistance, with a yeast titer in the kidneys much higher than in control mice on day 10 after infection.

Table 1. Effect of anti-Lyt2 treatment on mouse reactivity to C. albicans challenge in immunized mice.

Treatment [a]	Log_{10} yeast units in kidneys on day:		
	4	10	20
None	4.2	3.8	2.9
Anti-Lyt2	5.1*	4.8*	3.3*
Anti-Lyt2 + anti-L3T4	5.7*	5.3*	3.4*
Anti-IFN-γ	4.8*	4.6*	2.9

a) Fourteen day immune mice were challenged i.v. on day 0 with virulent Candida. On days 4, 10 and 20, the yeast titer in the kidneys was measured (6).
* P< 0.01 to 0.05 (antibody treated versus control mice).

This experiment provides evidence for the involvement of the two major T cell populations in acquired immunity to Candida. In addition, IFN-γ seems to have a definite and important role in the control of reinfection with virulent Candida cells in mice, once immunity has developed. This contention is also supported by in vitro studies showing that purified lymphocytes of both T-cell populations could produce IFN-γ in response to Candida antigens presented by appropriate antigen presenting cells (APC) (11).

2. Cytokine Production by Candida-Immune T Cells

It is known that IFN-γ is a product of a particular subset of L3T4+ cells, the Th1 subset. Several in vitro studies have shown that two distinct functional types of L3T4+ cells can be defined, the Th1 and

Th2 subsets (12). Th1 lymphocytes seem to be primarily involved in determining protective immunity in most infection models with intra-cellular pathogens through their ability to release cytokines that result in macrophage activation and development of delayed type hypersensitivity (DTH) reaction to microbial antigens. Th1 cells are characterized by secretion of a particular pattern of cytokines, of which IFN-ɣ and IL-2 are the prototypes. Therefore, in a series of experiments we addressed the question whether Th1 cells and Th1 cytokines participate in the development and maintenance of protective immunity to Candida albicans. Table 2 shows the profile of cytokine production by L3T4+ cells from vaccinated mice. Unfractionated splenic lymph, ytes or positively selected L3T4+ cells mixed with syngeneic macrophages as APC were cultured for 20 hours with Candida cells before culture supernatants were tested for cytokine activity.

Table 2. Cytokine production by Candida immune lymphocytes.

Source of supernatant[a]	Cytokine activity (U/ml)[b]			
	IFN-ɣ	LT	IL-2	GM-CSF
Nonimmune spleen cells	< 2	5	0	20
Immune, unfractionated	35	250	909	350
L3T4+ cells	160	604	4,810	1,560

a) Heat inactivated yeast cells were cocultured with unfractionated spleen cells or a mixture of L3T4+ cells and APC for 20 hours prior to collection of supernatants.
b) Supernatants were tested for cytokine activity in functional assays as described (10).

It is apparent that L3T4+ cells produced Th1-specific cytokines, namely IL-2, IFN-ɣ, lymphotoxin (LT) and also the Th1-preferential cytokine, granulocyte/macrophage colony stimulating factor (GM-CSF). In experiments not reported here (10,11), we also found that both DTH and resistance to C. albicans infection were depressed in immunized mice treated for five consecutive days with anti-L3T4 mAb. These results indicate that all functions predicted to be mediated by Th1-like cells are present in protective immunity to C. albicans.

3. Immune Regulation in Candida Infection

Most immune responses are the result of a fine balance between activation of Th1 and Th2 cell subsets. It is also true that in different experimental conditions and disease states selective activation of either one of the L3T4+ cell subsets may occur. The Th2 functional set is the major source of help in antibody responses and is believed to be primarily involved in immunosurveillance against extracellular pathogens. These cells make a distinct panel of cytokines; IL-4 is a characteristic member. To evaluate the contribution of Th2 cell function in Candida infection, we infected mice with two low-virulence variant strains of C. albicans obtained by mutagenesis of the virulent strain. The ability of the two mutagenized variants to confer protection against subsequent challenge with virulent Candida cells was then evaluated. Our results showed that the two mutagenized variants differed in their ability to confer protection against challenge with virulent Candida cells. In particular, vaccination with the variant Vir- 3 resulted in the induction of protective immunity to challenge with virulent <u>Candida</u>. Protection correlated with the appearance of strong candidacidal activity in the spleens and development of strong DTH reaction to <u>Candida</u> cells. On the contrary, mice vaccinated with the variant Vir- 13 were unable to survive challenge with virulent <u>Candida</u> cells, and did not develop candidacidal activity in the spleens although exhibited a moderate DTH reaction to intra-footpad challenge. To verify whether the protective and non-protective immune states correlated with a different pattern of cytokine production, L3T4+ splenocytes from vaccinated mice were tested in vitro for cytokine production in response to mitogens or inactivated <u>Candida</u> cells. The results in Table 3 show that the protective immunity elicited by vaccination with Vir- 3 variant cells was associated with an increasing production of Th1 cytokines, IL-2 and IFN-γ. The non-protective state associated with Vir- 13 infection resulted in the production of high amounts of Th2 cytokines, IL-4 and IL-6.

Table 3. Pattern of cytokine secretion in protective (Vir- 3) and non-protective (Vir- 13) immunity induced in mice by vaccination with two different mutagenized <u>C. albicans</u> variants.

Cytokines from L3T4+ cells	Days post-infection					
	+3		+7		+14	
	Vir- 3	Vir- 13	Vir- 3	Vir- 13	Vir- 3	Vir- 13
IL-2	+	+	++	+	++	±
IFN-γ	+	+	++	+	++	±
IL-4	-	-	-	+	±	++
IL-6	-	-	-	-	±	++

All together these data can be taken to indicate that activation of both Th1 and Th2 T cell subsets may occur in murine <u>C. albicans</u> infection. Therefore, mechanisms seem to exist for the regulation of the functional nature of immune anticandidal responses at the level of selective activation of Th1 and Th2 cell functions. One such mechanism may be represented by the reciprocal regulation of Th1 and Th2 cells. Several features of immune responses suggest that Th1 and Th2 cells are mutually inhibitory and that at least some of these effects are mediated by soluble cytokines (12). This inhibition may operate at the levels of effector function, cytokine synthesis and proliferation.

Figure 1 shows some possible regulatory mechanisms between Th1 and Th2 cells that may occur in murine <u>Candida</u> infection. In particular, it is shown that IFN-γ may inhibit the growth of Th2 cells in response to IL-2 or IL-4, and Th2 cells may inhibit Th1 cytokine production through release of the "cytokine synthesis inhibitory factor" (CSIF) (12).

THE <u>PSEUDOMONAS AERUGINOSA</u> INFECTION MODEL

1. <u>Combination Chemotherapy with Cytokines in Neutropenic Mice</u>

Although most microbial infections are usually treated successfully with chemotherapeutic agents, some infections are still difficult to control by chemotherapy alone, such as in the case of severe opportunistic infections in immunocompromised hosts. It is indeed known that the efficacy of chemotherapy depends not only on the intrinsic properties of an agent, but also on the host immunological status. In this respect, IL-1 (a cytokine produced by a variety of host cells in response to infectious, inflammatory and immunological stimuli (13)) has been shown to augment the resistance of intact or immunodepressed mice to a variety of experimental microbial infections (14). For this reason, we have recently begun to investigate the ability of human recombinant IL-1 beta to synergize with antipseudomonal chemotherapy in mice rendered neutropenic by cyclophosphamide and challenged with live P. aeruginosa cells.

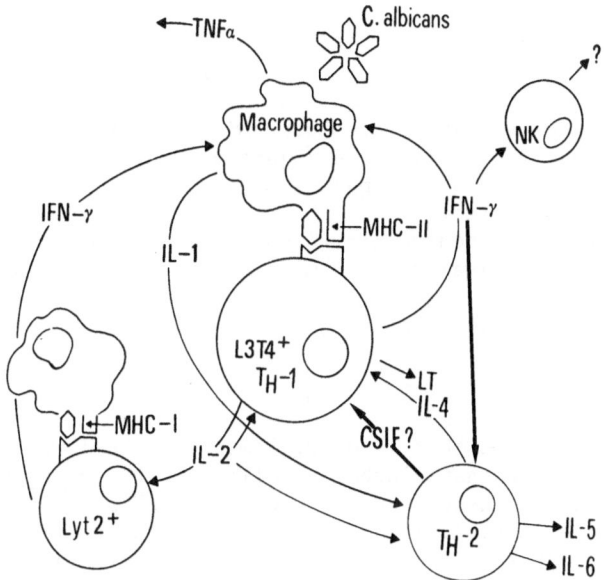

Figure 1. Proposed mechanism of immune regulation in C. albicans infection in mice.
The lines indicate positive effects. Inhibitory effects are indicated by the darker lines.

2. Combined Effects of Gentamicin and IL-1 Treatment

We have tested IL-1 for immunostimulant activity in the Pseudomonas infection model by injecting the cytokine at .7 or .07 micrograms/kg four days after cyclophosphamide treatment, i.e., 24 hours before bacterial challenge. Additional groups of mice received .7 or .07 micrograms/kg of IL-1 in three doses of 5.3 or 0.53 ng each, respectively, administered on days 1, 2, and 4 following myelosuppression. At 1 and 5 hours post-infection, the animals treated with .07 micrograms/kg of IL-1 were also given gentamicin chemotherapy. The results obtained (Table 4) clearly demonstrate that IL-1 increased the survival rate of infected mice in a dose- and schedule-dependent manner.

Table 4. Effect of IL-1 administration on survival of granulocytopenic[a] mice challenged with P. aeruginosa.[b]

IL-1 treatment				
Dose	Day [c]	MST	D/T	%Survivors
-	-	1	0/9	0
0.7	1	1	7/9	22
0.7	4	-	4/8	50
0.7	1,2,4(*)	-	2/8	75
0.07	1	1	0/8	0
0.07	4	1	7/8	12.5
0.07	1,2,4(*)	1.5	5/8	37.5
0.07	1,2,4(*)[d]	-	1/8	87.5

a) Animals were treated with cyclophosphamide on day 0.
b) 10^{10} live pseudomonas cells were injected i.p. on day 5.
c) IL-1 was administered as a single i.p. injection or in 3(*) divided doses on days indicated.
d) The animals received gentamicin (4 mg/kg) 1 and 5 hr after bacterial challenge. The survival rate of mice treated with gentamicin alone was 25%.
MST, median survival time (days). D/T, dead animals over total animals challenged.

This table shows that .7 micrograms/kg of IL-1 was effective in protecting animals against lethal challenge with P. aeruginosa when given one day before inoculation of bacteria (50% survival rate versus 0% of untreated controls). In contrast, the administration of the same dosage of the cytokine one day after myelosuppression gave poorer results. Interestingly, the repeated exposure of mice to an overall IL-1 dosage of .7 micrograms/kg during the four days after myelosuppression was found to optimally restore the animals antibacterial resistance (75% survival rate). A regimen of .07 micrograms/kg of IL-1 administered as a single injection 24 hours before microbial challenge yielded a 12.5% survival rate. However, considerable protection was achieved when the same overall dosage of IL-1 was administered in multiple doses at different times before challenge (37.5% survival rate). This effect was maximized by concurrent administration of gentamicin. In fact, mice treated with both IL-1 and gentamicin had a survival rate of 87.5% in comparison with 25% rate of mice injected with gentamicin alone. Therefore, these results indicate that the restorative effects of IL-1 are largely dependent on treatment schedule and are synergistic with chemotherapeutic agents.

CONCLUSIONS

During the past several years, much progress has been achieved in the characterization of the biological activity and chemical composition of cytokines and their receptors (15). A clear picture of the cytokine network has emerged from the concept that cytokines often have multiple cellular targets and functions. It is also apparent that many of the cytokines are produced by a variety of tissues.

The roles of IFN-ɣ and IL-1 in infectious disease are now beginning to be adequately appreciated. However, it is also known that the interaction between various cytokines and their target cells is considerably complex. Studies reported thus far deal primarily with established infections. To gain further insight regarding the contribution of various cytokines and their regulatory roles in the immune response during the early phases of infection requires detailed analysis of the dynamic state of cells involved in the response to pathogens (15). This approach, as we have attempted to illustrate in the present paper, would benefit from further studies of the interaction between Th1 and Th2 cells. The direct application of results generated in the experimental models to clinical counterparts would be a logical extention in this area of research, such as in the case of the combined effects of anti-bacterial chemotherapy and cytokine administration in immunosuppressed hosts. Undoubtedly, such application should proceed with caution because of the complexity in the outbred populations in humans and the differences that exist between target cells sensitive to murine and human cytokines.

ACKNOWLEDGMENT

Invaluable secretarial help by E. Mahoney is gratefully acknowledged.

REFERENCES

1. F. R. Balkwill and F. Burke, The cytokine network, Immunol. Today 10:229 (1989).
2. N. Kelso, Cytokines: structure, function and synthesis, Curr. Opin. Immunol. 2:215 (1989).
3. A. Vecchiarelli, R. Mazzolla, S. Farinelli, A. Cassone, and F. Bistoni, Immunomodulation by Candida albicans: crucial role of organ colonization and chronic infection with an attenuated agerminative strain of C. albicans for establishment of anti-infectious protection. J. Gen. Microbiol. 134: 2583 (1988).
4. A. Vecchiarelli, G. Verducci, S. Perito, P. Puccetti, P. Marconi, and F. Bistoni, Involvement of host macrophages in the immunoadjuvant activity of amphotericin B in a mouse fungal infection model, J. Antibiotics 39:846 (1986).
5. F. Bistoni, A. Vecchiarelli, E. Cenci, P. Puccetti, P. Marconi, and A. Cassone, Evidence for macrophage-mediated protection against a lethal Candida albicans infection, Infect. Immun. 51:668 (1986).
6. F. Bistoni, G. Verducci, S. Perito, A. Vecchiarelli, P. Puccetti, P. Marconi, and A. Cassone, Immunomodulation by a low virulent agerminative variant of Candida albicans. Further evidence for macrophage activation as one of the effector mechanisms of non-specific anti-infectious protection, J. Med. Veter. Mycol. 26: 285 (1988).
7. E. Blasi, S. Farinelli, L. Varesio, and F. Bistoni, Augmentation of GG2EE macrophage cell line-mediated anti-Candida activity by gamma interferon, tumor necrosis factor, and interleukin-1, Infect. Immun. 58:1073 (1990).

8. E. Cenci, A. Bartocci, P. Puccetti, S. Mocci, E. R. Stanley, and F. Bistoni, Macrophage colony stimulating factor in murine candidiasis: serum and tissue levels during infection and protective effect of exogenous administration, Infect. Immun. 59:868 (1991).

9. A. Vecchiarelli, E. Cenci, M. Puliti, E. Blasi, P. Puccetti, A. Cassone, and F. Bistoni, Protective immunity induced by low-virulence Candida albicans. Cytokine production in the development of the anti-infectious state, Cell. Immunol. 124:334 (1989).

10. E. Cenci, L. Romani, A. Vecchiarelli, P. Puccetti, and F. Bistoni, Role of L3T4+ lymphocytes in protective immunity to systemic Candida albicans infection in mice, Infect. Immun. 57:3581 (1989).

11. E. Cenci, L. Romani, A. Vecchiarelli, P. Puccetti, and F. Bistoni, T cell subsets and IFN-γ production in resistance to systemic candidosis in immunized mice, J. Immunol. 144:4333 (1990).

12. T. R. Mosmann and R. L. Coffman, Heterogeneity of cytokine secretion patterns and functions of helper T cells, Adv. Immunol. 46:111 (1989).

13. C. A. Dinarello, Interleukin-1 and its biologically related cytokines, Adv. Immunol. 44:153 (1989).

14. F. Campanile, L. Binaglia, D. Boraschi, A. Tagliabue, M.C. Fioretti, and P. Puccetti, Antibacterial resistance induced by recombinant interleukin 1 in myelosuppressed mice: effect of treatment schedule and correlation with colony-stimulating activity in the bloodstream, Cell. Immunol. 128:256 (1990).

15. S. M. Fu, The role of cytokines in infection, Curr. Opin. Infect. Dis. 3:361 (1990).

TREATMENT AND PHARMACOKINETICS OF LIPOSOMAL-AMPHOTERICIN B

PATIENTS WITH SYSTEMIC FUNGAL INFECTIONS

Gabriel Lopez-Berestein and Michael G. Rosenblum

Departments of Medical Oncology and Clinical Immunology
The University of Texas M. D. Anderson Cancer Center
Houston, TX

INTRODUCTION

Opportunistic infections occur frequently in immunocompromised patients and in patients with cancer.[1-3] In this latter group, systemic mycoses are one of the most frequent causes of infection-related morbidity and mortality.[4-6] Intensive chemotherapy, the prolonged use of broad spectrum antibiotics, and inherent defects in host immunity related to the underlying disease are among the major predisposing factors for opportunistic infections in general.[7-8] Early histologic diagnosis of systemic mycoses is often difficult in patients with hematologic malignancies due to thrombocytopenia. Delays in histologic and cultural diagnoses lead to delays in initiation of therapy. Antifungal therapy begins when empirically prompted by persistent fever in neutropenic patients in spite of the use of broad spectrum antibiotics.[9-10] The drug of choice for most fungal infections is Amphotericin B (AmpB, Fungizone®) which is particularly effective in non-neutropenic patients and often ineffective in the neutropenic patient.[11,12]

Nephrotoxicity, chills, fever, nausea and vomiting are frequent side effects associated with the administration of AmpB, leading to inadequate dosing or early discontinuation of therapy.[13,14] AmpB, like all polyenes antibiotics, interacts with sterols in membranes which results in the formation of transmembrane pores.[15,16] Although AmpB displays a high degree of selectivity for ergosterol containing membranes, such as fungal membranes, the therapeutic index is not enhanced. AmpB toxicity is related to its membrane permeabilizing effects which allowing the for escape of vital intracellular constituents. However, evidence indicates that membrane permeabilization may not be the only mechanism involved in the lytic effects of AmpB, and that oxidant damage is related to lytic activity and not to permeability changes.

Liposomes are phospholipid-based particles that can be composed of naturally-occurring lipids. Like most particulates, liposomes are taken up preferentially by the Mononuclear Phagocyte System (MPS) which can, in turn, also be the target of fungal infections. Several investigators have used liposomes to serve as synthetic carrier vehicles for a various antimicrobial and anticancer drugs.

Combination Therapies, Edited by A.L. Goldstein and
E. Garaci, Plenum Press, New York, 1992

Table 1. General Patient Characteristics

Number of patients	46
Underlying disease	
Leukemia	31
Lymphoma	2
Other neoplasia	11
No underlying disease	2

Adapted from reference 25

Liposomal-AmpB (L-AmpB) is far less toxic and more active than free AmpB in experimental candidiasis[17-20] and leishmaniasis.[21]

L-AmpB has been used for patients with systemic fungal infections who either failed to respond to AmpB or had adverse side effects (allergy or nephrotoxicity that precluded the use of AmpB.[22-24] We consistently observed L-AmpB to be better tolerated than the conventional form of AmpB. Review of our experience and further follow-up of the treated patients are reported here.

PATIENTS AND METHODS

Forty-six patients with systemic fungal infections were registered in this study and treated with L-AmpB after an informed consent was obtained according to institutional guidelines.[24] All patients were evaluable for response to treatment: 17 patients had hepatosplenic candidiasis, 19 had Aspergillosis, and 3 had agents of mucormycosis (table 1). When L-AmpB therapy began, 4 patients with Aspergillosis also had granulocytopenia. All patients had been treated previously with AmpB and had evidence of disease progression. Six patients did not receive more than the initial dose of AmpB; of these, 4 had rapidly deteriorating renal function and 2 had a history of allergy to AmpB. In all patients, the diagnosis of progressive fungal infection was confirmed by histologic or cultural assay immediately before L-AmpB treatment began, and response to treatment was confirmed by histologic assay. Pharmacokinetics studies were carried out in 3 patients.

Laboratory and Laboratory Analysis. Evaluations of liver function (serum glutamic oxalacetic transaminase, alkaline phosphatase, lactic dehydrogenase, and total bilirubin), kidney function (blood urea nitrogen [BUN], creatinine, creatinine clearance), serum electrolytes, serum lipids (cholesterol, phospholipids, triglycerides), complete blood counts, and radiologic examinations of the sites of infection were performed before treatment and weekly during treatment.

Treatment-Response Criteria

Complete response was defined in two ways: First, a complete resolution of all signs and symptoms of infection was required for a minimum follow-up period of 6 months. A few patients showed persistent abnormalities on radiological examination, but all signs and symptoms had completely resolved. Second category, 5 patients died from causes other than fungal infection before 6 months and showed no evidence of fungal infection at postmortem examination.

Lipids and Drugs. Chromatographically pure dimyristoyl phosphatidyl-choline (DMPC) and dimyristoyl phosphatidylglycerol (DMPG) were purchased from Avanti Polar Lipids (Birmingham, AL) and deoxycholate-free AmpB was obtained from E. R. Squibb & Sons (Princeton, NJ).

Preparation of Liposomes Containing AmpB. AmpB was incorporated into liposomes as previously described.[25] Drug formulation and analysis were conducted out in our laboratory. Deoxycholate-free AmpB was dissolved at a concentration of 40 µg/mL of methanol and added to a phospholipid-chloroform solution in a 1:14 AmpB to lipid ratio. The organic solvents were evaporated in a rotary evaporator, sterile NaCl solution was added to the dried lipid films, and liposomes were formed by mixing the solution vigorously by hand. Phospho-lipid content of the resulting suspension was determined by measuring the organic phosphorus in the preparation and AmpB content was determined by high-performance liquid chromatography.[25] Liposome size distribution was assessed in a Coulter Channelizer (Coulter Electronics, Hialeah, FL). Liposome diameters ranged from 0.5 to 6.0 µm, with 60% measuring between 0.5 and 3.0 µm. Sterility was determined both by radiometry (Bactec; Johnston Laboratories, Cockeysville, MD) and by direct inoculation onto blood and chocolate agar plates. All cultures were incubated at 37°C for 2 weeks before being considered negative for growth and before liposomes were used. Endotoxin, if present, measured lower than 0.25 ng/mL, as assessed by the Limulus amebocyte lysate assay. The liposome preparation used throughout this study was composed of DMPC and DMPG in a 7:3 molar ratio. The PL: AmpB of the total preparation was 14:1. However, the heterogeneity of PL:AmpB ratios was reflected in the structural heterogeneity of the liposomes which varied from multilamellar structures to PL:AmpB complexes not displaying typical lamellar forms. L-AmpB (2 mg AmpB; 28 mg/lipid/mL) was resuspended in pyrogen-free 0.9% NaCl solution and kept at 4°C until used. L-AmpB is stable for more than 12 months at 4°C (PL and AmpB analysis). Each batch contained between 1.5-2.0 G AmpB. All analytical parameters were consistent in all batches.

Treatment Regimen. Treatment was initiated in all patients within 2 weeks after persistence of fungal infection was confirmed. L-AmpB was administered by IV at dosages between 0.4 and 5.0 mg/kg of body weight. The initial treatment schedule was 0.4 mg AmpB/kg of body weight every other day. The protocol provided for dose escalations of 1 mg AmpB/kg every 3 doses based on patient tolerance, judged by the absence of significant clinical toxicity such as fever, chills and changes in K+, Mg++ or serum creatinine.

Table 2. Patient Characteristics

Patient No.	Age/ Gender	Underlying Disease	Fungal Disease	Main Site of Infection	Dose of AmpB (mg/kg)	Creatinine Clearance (cc/min)	Alk. Phosphatase (U/dl)
1	2/F	None	*Aspergillus*	Rhinocerebral	51	106	121
2	34/M	AML	*Candida*	Liver	86	79	>350
3	8/M	ALL	*Candida*	Liver	30	54	>350

Abbreviations: ALL, acute lymphocytic leukemia; AML, acute myelogenous leukemia.

Table 3. Response to Treatment

Fungal Diagnosis Infection Site	Number of Patients	Complete Response	Failures
Candidiasis	21	14	7
Aspergillus	19	8	11
Agents of mucormycosis	3	1	2
Other	3	1	2

After preliminary experience with the phase I trial, the dose schedule was modified. At present, patients are started at 2 mg AmpB/kg body weight. Once the starting dose is tolerated for 3 days, the dose is escalated by 1 mg AmpB/kg every 3 days until 5 mg/kg is reached. The 5 mg AmpB/kg dose will be continued until a cumulative dose of 75 mg AmpB/kg is reached. This dose was based on our experience with complete responders whose mean cumulative dose was 75 mg AmpB/kg. In most patients a biopsy is repeated 4 weeks following the completion of therapy.

Pharmacokinetic and distribution studies. A dose of 2 mg L-AmpB/kg body weight was given to the 3 patients we studied (table 2). Blood samples (5 mL total volume) were obtained prior to administration, immediately after the end of the infusion, and at 1, 3, 5, 10, 15, 20, 30, 40, 60, 90, 120, 180, 240 minutes and at 5, 12, 24, and 48 hours. After each withdrawal, the catheter was flushed with 0.9% NaCl solution containing 0.1% heparin. Pharmacokinetic parameters, volume of distribution and half-lives (β and α) were calculated by nonlinear regression analysis.

RESULTS

Response to Therapy. Of the 46 patients, 24 responded completely and 22 patients did not (table 3).

Complete responders. Thirteen of the 17 patients with hepatic candidiasis and either of the 19 patients with Aspergillosis showed a complete response. Of the 17 patients with hepatic infection, three were also treated with chemotherapy for relapsing leukemia. In spite of prolonged bouts of neutropenia, a complete response of fungal infection was achieved. In the patients with aspergillus sinusitis, objective response was observed within 2 to 3 days after initiation of therapy.

Fever and chills, when they occurred, presented within 1 to 2 hours of administration and were mostly mild to moderate, and responded readily to traditional measures. Potassium supplementation was required but did not complicate administration. L-AmpB was not discontinued in any patient due to toxicity, and no major alterations in the treatment protocol were required. No evidence of chronic renal, central nervous system, or hepatic toxicity was observed. Cumulative doses of up to 2.9 G phospholipid were administered with no evidence of hepatic toxicity.

Table 4. Pharmacokinetic Summary of Liposomal AmpB

Patient No.	t 1/2 (hours)			CXT Vd (1)	Clp (μg/mlxh)	Mean (μg/mlxmin)	Residence Time (hrs)
	α	β	γ				
1	0.047	--	7.1	24.0	9.6	207.9	9.9
2	0.016	--	4.6	45.5	3.3	607.9	6.6
3	0.088	0.121	8.9	14.4	32.8	61.0	11.7
x±S.E.M.	0.05±0.02	---	6.9±1.3	28±9	15.2±9	292±163	9.4±1.5

Pharmacokinetics. The pharmacokinetic results are summarized in Table 4. The V_D in patient number 1 who had no overt liver function abnormality was 13.5 l. His distribution phase was 17 min and his elimination phase was 992 min. In contrast, patients 2 and 3 who presented with disseminated hepatosplenic candidiasis and markedly altered liver functions had a comparatively increased V_D (24 and 30.5 l., respectively). In addition, their t $1/2$ β was shorter than while the elimination phase was similar to all other patients.

The plasma clearance closely fit a two-compartmental model in two patients and a three-compartmental model in one patient. The a phase half-life was 0.05 hours; however, the terminal phase half-life was 6.9 ± 1.3 hours. The volume of distribution was variable (14.4 ± 45.5 l., means 28 ± 9 liter) and appeared similar to the total body water compartment. Patient 1 demonstrated no overt liver function abnormality; however, patients 2 and 3 presented with disseminated hepatosplenic candidiasis and markedly altered liver function tests. The wide disparity between the pharmacokinetics absent in patient 1 and patients 2 and 3 may be due, in part, to the hepatic dysfunction absent; however, wide variabilities in AmpB pharmacokinetics have been observed in previous studies.[26, 27]

DISCUSSION

L-AmpB was safe and effective in the treatment of systemic fungal infections even failing to respond to conventional AmpB. L-AmpB is easier to administer than conventional AmpB. Because lower infusion volumes of L-AmpB then AmpB, there are can be used shorter infusion periods and usually, no premedication is required. In addition, patients can be treated on an outpatient basis due in part to the lack of acute side effects and ease of administration. Patients with impaired renal function related to the previous administration of conventional AmpB were found to tolerate L-AmpB. During L-AmpB treatment, a gradual improvement in renal function was consistently observed which potentially facilitates the co-administration of other necessary but potentially nephrotoxic drugs such as the aminoglycosides and cyclosporine.

In those patients for whom long-term follow-up was available, no recurrent or new fungal infections were observed. The response to treatment with L-AmpB in spite of profound neutropenia is an encouraging finding in this study, since chemotherapy for the primary disease does not need to be discontinued.

The improved therapeutic index observed with L-AmpB may be related to modifications in the interactions of AmpB with fungal and mammalian cells when presented in the liposomal form. *In vitro* experiments comparing the differential toxicity of L-AmpB to red blood cells and fungal cells support this latter concept.[28] We observed in mice injected intravenously with AmpB or L-AmpB that at 24 hours the liver concentration of free AmpB or L-AmpB was similar. However, high and persistent concentrations of AmpB were observed in mice with systemic candidiasis. This latter finding and the superior activity of L-AmpB to treat experimental candidiasis suggests an enhanced bioavailability to infected tissues. Such a process may be related to capillary leakage or to secondary transport by peripheral phagocytes.

Hepatosplenic candidiasis is becoming recognized as a variant of systemic candidiasis particularly in patients with hematologic malignancies.[24] Christiansen et. al.[30] observed high tissue concentrations of AmpB in patients with aspergillosis or candida infection in the same organs. Of relevance was that AmpB extracted from the infected tissues retained the antifungal potency against the infecting organism, suggesting that it was not resistance but other factors limiting the availability of the drug to the fungus. Our experience with patients who have hepatosplenic candidiasis lends further support to an enhanced availability of the drug to interact with the fungi in the liposomal form.

Further studies in diverse fungal infections will shed light on the spectrum of activity of L-AmpB. Scale-up procedures for the pharmaceutical production are being developed, and several studies are underway with a formulation of similar phospholipid composition. Studies should include treatment and prophylactic studies, both in systemic mycoses and leishmaniasis.

REFERENCES

1. E. M. Hersh, G. P. Bodey, B. A. Nies, and E. J Freireich, Causes of death in acute leukemia. A ten-year study of 414 patients from 1954 to 1963, JAMA 193(2):99 (1965).
2. H. S. Mirsk, and J. Cuttner, Fungal infection in acute leukemia, Cancer 30(2):348 (1972).
3. G. P. Bodey, V Rodriguez, H-Y Chang, and G. Narboni G, Fever and infection leukemic patients. Cancer 41:1610 (1978).
4. M. W. Degregorio, W. M. F. Lee, C. A. Linder, R. A. Jacobs, and C. A. Ries, Fungal infections in patients with acute leukemia, Amer J Med 73:543 (1982).
5. W. M. J. Gold, Opportunistic fungal infections in patients with neoplastic disease, Amer J Med 76:458 (1984).
6. G. P. Bodey, Candidiasis in cancer patients, Am J Med 77(4D):13 (1984).
7. E. R. Stiehm, T. J. Fischer, J. Fischer, and L. S. Young, Severe candidal infection: clinical perspective, immune defense mechanisms, and current concepts of therapy, Ann Intern Med 89:91 (1978).
8. J. M. Wiley, N. Smith, B. G. Leventhal, M. L. Graham, L. C. Strauss, C. A. Hurwitz, J. Modlin, D. Mellits, R. Baumgardner, B. J. Corden, et. al. Invasive fungal disease in pediatric acute leukemia patients with fever and neutropenia during induction chemotherapy: a multivariate analysis of risk factors, J Clin Oncol 8(2):280 (1990).

9. T. J. Walsh, and A. Pizzo, Treatment of systemic fungal infections: Recent progress and current problems, Eur J Clin Microbiol Infect Dis 7(4):460 (1988).
10. P. E. Hermans, and T. K. Keys, Antifungal agents used for deep-seated mycotic infections, Mayo Clin Proc 58:223 (1983).
11. A. M. Maksymiuk, S. Thongpraset, R. Hopfer, M. Luna, V. Fainstein, and G. P. Bodey, Systemic candidiasis in cancer patients, Am J Med 77:20 (1984).
12. J. R. Graybill, The long and the short of antifungal therapy, Infect Dis Clinics NA 2(4):805 (1988).
13. B. D. Fisher, D. Armstrong, B. Yu, and J. W. M. Gold, Invasive aspergillosis. Progress in early diagnosis and treatment, Am J Med 71:571 (1981).
14. J. M. Benson, and M. C. Nahata, Drug Review. Clinical use of systemic antifungal agents, Clin Pharm 7:424 (1988).
15. J. M. T. Hamilton-Miller, Chemistry and biology of the polyene macrolide antibiotics, Bacteriol Rev 37:166 (1973).
16. T. E. Andreoli, The structure and function of amphotericin B-cholesterol pores in lipid bilayer membranes, Ann NY Acad Sci 235:448 (1974).
17. G. Lopez-Berestein, R. Mehta, and R. L. Hopfer, Treatment and prophylaxis of disseminated infection due to *Candida albicans* in mice with liposome-encapsulated amphotericin B, J Infect Dis 147:939 (1983).
18. G. Lopez-Berestein, R. L. Hopfer, R. Mehta, K. Mehta, E. M. Hersh, and R. L. Juliano, Liposome-encapsulated amphotericin B for the treatment of disseminated candidiasis in neutropenic mice, J Infect Dis 150:278 (1984).
19. G. Lopez-Berestein, R. L. Hopfer, R. Mehta, K. Mehta, E. M. Hersh, and R. L. Juliano. Prophylaxis of *C. albicans* infection in neutropenic mice with liposome-encapsulated amphotericin B, Antimicrob Agents Chemother 25:366 (1984).
20. J. R. Graybill, P. C. Craven, R. L. Taylor, D. M. Williams, and W. E. Magee, Treatment of murine cryptococcosis with liposome associated amphotericin B, J Infect Dis 145:740 (1982).
21. R. R. C. New, M. L. Chance, and S. Heath, Antileishmanial activity of amphotericin and other antifungal agents entrapped in liposomes, J Antimicrob Chemother 1:378 (1981).
22. J.-P. Sculier, A. Coune, F. Meunier, C. Brassinne, C. Laduron, C. Hollaert, N. Collette, C. Heymans, and J Klastersky, Pilot study of amphotericin B entrapped in sonicated liposomes in cancer patients with fungal infections, Eur J Cancer Clin Oncol 24(3):527 (1988).
23. J.-P. Sculier, C. Delcroix, C. Brassinne, C. Laduron, C. Hollaert, and A. Coune, Pharmacokinetics of amphotericin B in patients receiving repeated intravenous high doses of amphotericin B entrapped into sonicated liposomes, J Lip Res 1(2):151 (1989).
24. G. Lopez-Berestein, G. P. Bodey, V. Fainstein, M. Keating, L. S. Frankel, B. Zeluff, L. Gentry, and K. Mehta, Treatment of systemic fungal infections with liposomal amphotericin B, Arch Intern Med 149:2533 (1989).
25. G. Lopez-Berestein, M. G. Rosenblum and R. Mehta, Altered tissue distribution of amphotericin B by liposomal encapsulation: comparison of normal mice to mice infected with *Candida albicans*, Cancer Drug Deliv 1:199 (1984).

26. J. M. Benson, and M. C. Nahata, Pharmacokinetics of amphotericin B in children, <u>Antimicrob Agents Chemother</u> 33(11):1989 (1989).
27. G. Koren, A. Lau, J. Klein, C. Golas, M. Bologa-Campeanu, S. Soldin, S. M. MacLeod, and C. Prober, Pharmacokinetics and adverse effects of amphotericin B in infants and children, <u>J Pediatr</u> 113(3):559 (1988).
28. R. Mehta, G. Lopez-Berestein, R. Hopfer, K. Mills, and R. L. Juliano, Liposomal-amphotericin B is toxic to fungal cells but not to mammalian cells, <u>Biochim Biophys Acta</u> 770:230 (1984).
29. L. S. Tashjian, J. S. Abramson, and J. E. Peacock, Jr., Focal hepatic candidiasis: a distinct clinical variant of candidiasis in immunocompromised patients, <u>Rev Infect Dis</u> 6:689 (1984).
30. K. J. Christiansen, E. M. Bernard, J. W. M. Gold, and D. Armstrong, Distribution and activity of amphotericin B in humans, <u>J Inf Dis</u> 152:1037 (1985).

THE POTENTIAL ROLE OF IMMUNOMODULATION IN THE TREATMENT OF HIV-INFECTION AND MALIGNANT DISEASES

Evan M. Hersh, Carole Y. Funk, Eskild A. Petersen

The University of Arizona Health Sciences Center
Tucson, Arizona 85724

INTRODUCTION

The AIDS epidemic continues to worsen worldwide.[1] The incidence of malignant disease is also increasing.[2] Cancer and AIDS can be considered to be related in several ways. In both, immunodeficiency is related to a poor prognosis.[3,4] Also, AIDS may be considered the most important of the clinical states which predisposed to malignancy and up to 20% of HIV seropositive subjects will eventually get malignant diseases.[5] This suggests that immunorestorative therapy may be useful in both AIDS and cancer.

Approaches to the therapy of HIV-infection have concentrated on anti-retroviral chemotherapeutic agents such as zidovudine, anti-retroviral biologics such as interferon α (IFNα) and the development of preventive and therapeutic AIDS vaccines.

Little attention has been paid to immunorestoration or immunomodulation in the treatment of AIDS. However, there have been some leads. Several reports cite either immunological improvement, clinical benefit, or both from the administration of thymic hormones[6], isoprinosine,[7] and diethyldithiocarbamate.[8,9,10,11] Benefits observed have included increased numbers of circulating CD4+ cells, improved cutaneous delayed hypersensitivity, improved mitogen responses, diminished symptoms, reduced lymphadenopathy and splenomegaly, reduced opportunistic infections, and reduced mortality.

The immunomodulatory drugs used in patients with HIV-infection or in relevant animal models are listed in Table 1. They include the thymic hormones, cytokines and chemical immunomodulators of diverse classes including: nucleic acid analogues, imidazoles, thiols and cyanoaziridines.

Of these, we have focused our preclinical and clinical work on the thiol compound diethyldithiocarbamate (ditiocarb, Imuthiol[R]) and the cyanoaziridine compound Imexon.

There are a variety of animal models of human AIDS which have been accepted as relevant models in which to examine putative AIDS therapies.[12] There are murine models including: graft versus host disease, Rauscher leukemia, Duplan MuLV LP-BM5 virus infection, the HIV

Combination Therapies, Edited by A.L. Goldstein and
E. Garaci, Plenum Press, New York, 1992

Table 1. Immunomodulatory Drugs of Potential Value for the
Treatment of HIV-Infection.

Thymic Hormones	Chemical Immunomodulators
Thymosin *a* 1	Nucleic Acid Analogues
Thomopoeitin Pentapeptide	Isoprinosine
Thymic Humoral Factor	inosine monophosphate methylester
Cytokines	Imidazoles
Interferon *a*	Levamisole
Interleukin-2	Thiols
	Ditiocarb
	N-acetylcysteine
	Cyanoaziridines
	Azimexon
	Imexon

transgenic mouse and severe combined Immune Deficiency (SCID) mice
reconstituted with human cells and infected with HIV.[13] In addition,
feline immunodeficiency virus (FIV) infection, simian immunodeficiency
virus infection (SIV) and chimpanzees infected with HIV are useful in
the study of various aspects of HIV prevention and therapy.

We have utilized the LP-BM5 model to investigate immunomodulatory
drugs for HIV-infection. This disease is induced by a mixture of
replication-competent non-pathogenic MuLV and a replication-defective
pathogenic mink-cell focus forming virus.[14] The natural history of the
LP-BM5 retrovirus induced immunodeficiency disease is shown in Figure 1.
Within 2 weeks after virus inoculation the animals develop impaired T-
cell function and hypergammaglobulinemia. There is progressive
lymphadenopathy and splenomegaly. Animals begin to die at 15 weeks and
are all dead by 23-24 weeks after virus inoculation. Similar to AIDS,
there is opportunistic infection, opportunistic malignancy (B-cell
lymphoma) and neurological involvement. The disease responds to
azidothymidine.[15] Different from HIV, LP-BM5 is related to MuLV and not
a Lente virus, the infected cells are B-cells, macrophages and glial
cells rather than T-cells, macrophages and glial cells as in HIV. While
there is complete loss of T-cell function, T-cells are not depleted in
number.

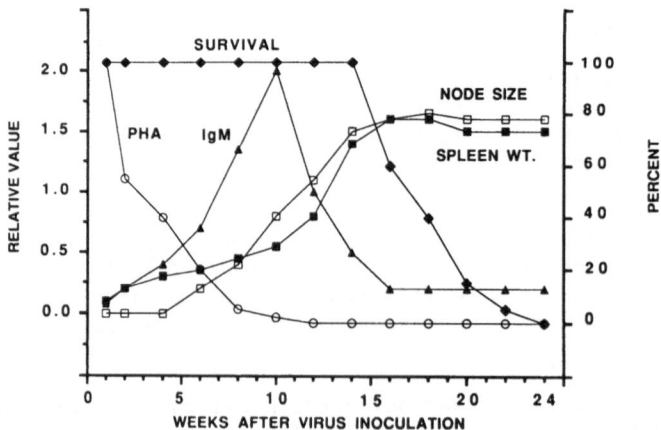

Figure 1.   Natural history of LP-BM5 infection of C57BL6 mice.
Relative value scale for IgM serum level, lymph node
size and splenomegaly is shown on left. Percent scale
of animals with a measurable PHA response and survival
are shown on the right.

METHODS

C57BL/10 mice were maintained in microisolator cages, 5 animals per cage and were manipulated only in a laminar air flow hood. The animals were maintained with conventional water and food. Mice of approximately 6-8 weeks, weight 20 gm were used. There were 5-8 animals per group. Mice were inoculated with a virus dose chosen so there would be an approximate doubling of the serum IgM level at 2 weeks after virus inoculation.

DTC solution was prepared fresh daily and injected IP in a volume of 0.1 ml containing 20, 200, 400, 600 or 800 mg/kg. 5 days per week (Monday-Friday).

Animals were examined weekly for lymphadenopathy and the number of animals with palpable lymph nodes and the approximate lymph node size were measured with calipers and recorded. The day of mortality was also recorded. The animals were bled from the retro-orbital plexus. Serum IgM was measured using the ELISA method. For the measurement of lymphocyte blastogenesis animals were sacrificed by cervical dislocation, their spleens removed, weighed, minced with a single cell suspension resulting. T and B cells were stimulated by the addition of phytohaemagglutin (PHA) 1 μg/ml and lipopolysaccharide from E. Coli 0111:B4 (LPS) 50 μg/ml respectively. Proliferation was measured by [^{3}H] thymidine incorporation.

The methods used in the clinical study of ditiocarb in patients with HIV-infection, which is summarized below, are given in the original manuscript.[16]

RESULTS

We investigated the effects of ditiocarb therapy in the LP-BM5 model. Table 2 shows the effects of 200, 400 and 600 mg/kg intra-peritoneally given 5 days per week starting on the day of virus inoculation. A dose response effect on both lymphadenopathy and survival was noted with the 600 mg/kg dose being most active. This dose was not exceeded since prior studies had shown it to be the maximally tolerated dose.

Table 2. Effect of Diethyldithiocarbamate (Ditiocarb) on the Course of the LP-BM5 Retrovirus-Induced Immunodeficiency Disease.

Dose mg/kg/d[1]	Percent With Lymphadenopathy[2]	Average Node Size[2]	Percent Survival[3]
None	100	204	28
200	100	120	28
400	43	50	57
600	14	14	86

[1] Drug given 5 days per week starting the day of virus inoculation.
[2] Area of cervical lymph nodes measured in mm^2 at 15 weeks.
[3] Percent of mice surviving at 19 weeks.

Of interest, ditiocarb could be administered late in the course of disease with striking effect. Thus, as shown in Figure 2, ditiocarb

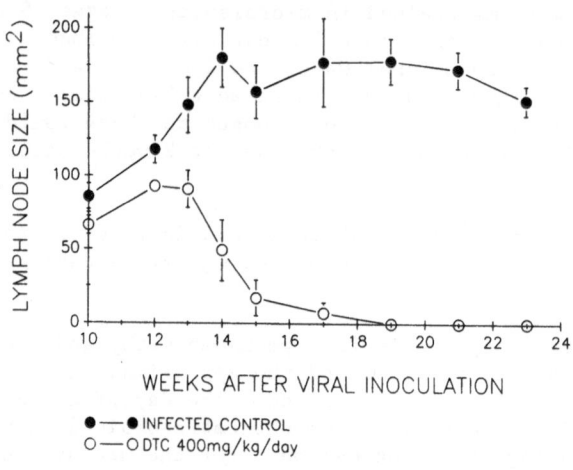

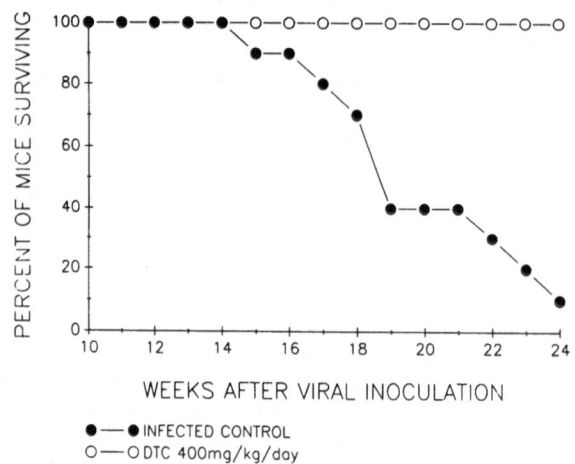

Figure 2.   Effect of ditiocarb on LP-BM5 infection. Treatment with
400 mg/kg 5 days per week intraperitoneally was started
10 weeks after virus inoculation. Top panel - lymph
node size; Bottom panel - survival.

started 10 weeks after virus inoculation abrogated lymphadenopathy and
prevented mortality up to 24 weeks after virus inoculation.

When drug was stopped lymphadenopathy reappeared and mortality occurred
(data not shown).

    We also investigated the effects of Imexon administered at doses of
50-150 mg/kg intraperitoneally 5 days per week. As with ditiocarb, we
noted that the drug could be started as late as 13 weeks after virus
inoculation with striking effects on lymphadenopathy and survival (Table
3). The maximally tolerated dose in the mouse is 150 mg per kg twice
weekly. However, even 50 mg per kg was active.

Table 3. Effect of Imexon on the Course of the LP-BM5
         Retrovirus-Induced Immunodeficiency Disease
         When Started 13 Weeks Post Viral Inoculation.

Dose In mg/kg/d[1]	Average Node Size MM^2 At 21 Week[2]	Survival At 21 Weeks (%)
none	94	0
50	0	62
75	0	75
100	0	75
150	25	62

[1] Drug given daily 5 days per week except twice a
    week in 150 mg group.
[2] Measurement of area of cervical lymph nodes.

We next explored whether Imexon could be combined with anti-
retroviral therapy with zidovudine or azidothymidine (AZT). Selected
results are shown in Figures 3 and 4. Therapy was started with AZT at
0.2 mg/ml in the drinking water and Imexon was given at 50 mg/kg 5 days
per week, both starting 2 weeks after virus inoculation. A synergistic
effect on the prevention of the development of lymphadenopathy and on
survival was noted in the group receiving combination therapy.

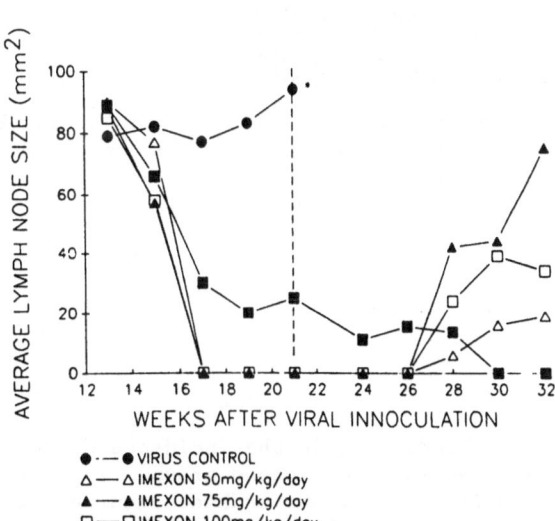

Figure 3. Effect of combined therapy with AZT and Imexon on
          the course of LP-BM5 infection. Average lymph node
          size when animals were treated starting 2 weeks
          after virus infection with 0.2 mg/ml AZT in drinking
          water and 50 mg/kg Imexon 5 days per week is shown.

This combination regimen was also immunorestorative. The response of spleen lymphocytes to the mitogens PHA and LPS were markedly improved by the combination (Figure 5).

Clinically, immunomodulators are being studied for the treatment of patients with HIV-infection. We conducted a randomized, double-blind, placebo-controlled trial of ditiocarb in 387 patients with AIDS related complex (ARC) and AIDS.[16] The results are summarized in Table 4. At entry the drug and placebo groups were well-balanced with regard to the usual clinical parameters as well as for peripheral blood CD4+ cells and CDC AIDS classification groups.

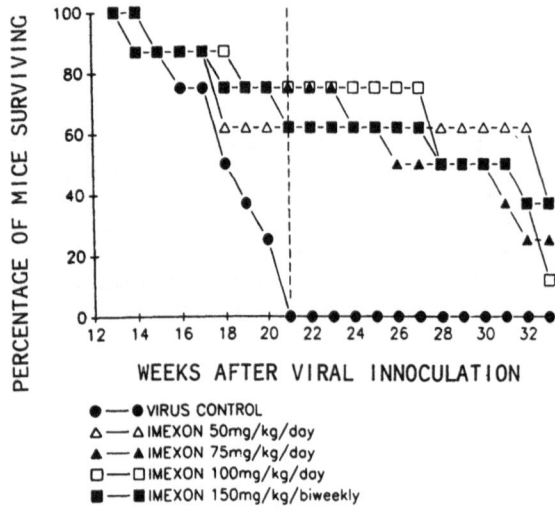

Figure 4.   Effect of combined therapy with AZT and Imexon on the course of LP-BM5 infection on the course of LP-BM5 infection. The survival of animals in the same experiment as Figure 3 is shown.

There was a significant reduction in the incidence of new opportunistic infections in the drug versus the placebo group. There was a significant reduction in other events such as recurrent opportunistic infection, severe fall in CD4+ cell count, other infections in the drug versus the placebo group. There was no difference in the low incidence of Kaposi's sarcoma or mortality. There was no significant toxicity in the drug versus the placebo groups. Thirty-five patients in each group received concurrent zidovudine. There was no adverse effect of the combination and the trend of benefit from the drug was seen in this subset as well.

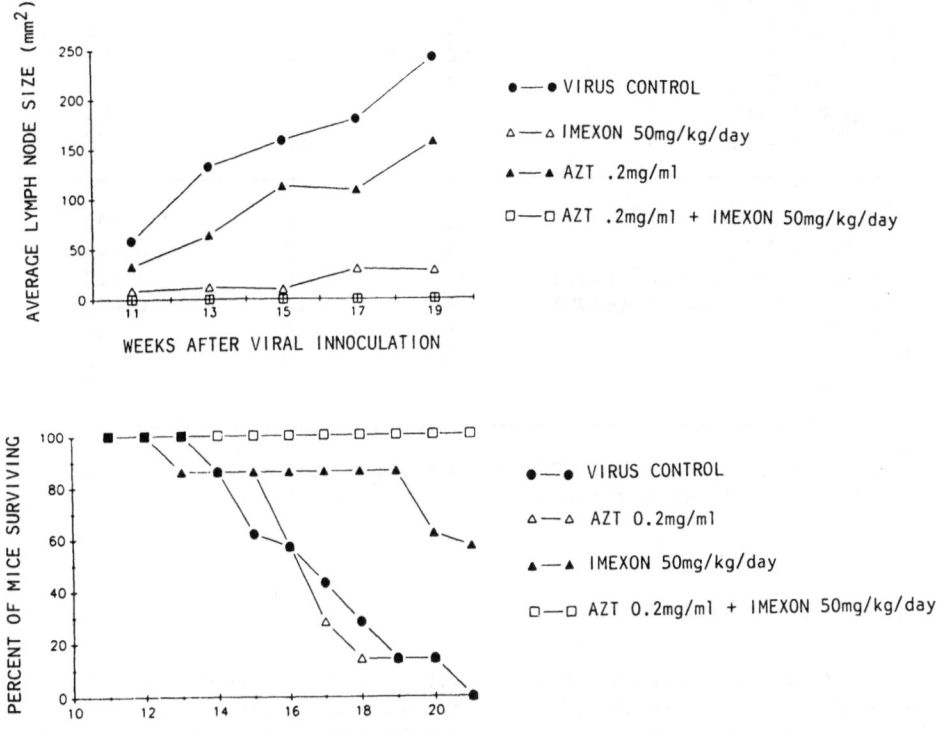

Figure 5.   Effect of combined therapy with AZT and Imexon on the lymphocyte proliferative responses as a percent of the uninfected control are shown for the phytohemagglutinin response (top panel) and the lipopolysaccharride response (bottom panel).

Table 4. Randomized, Double-Blind, Placebo-Controlled Study of Ditiocarb In Patients With HIV-Infection.

Parameter	Ditiocarb	Placebo	P
Number of patients	191	196	NS
age (median years)	35	34	NS
weight (median kg)	73	73	NS
ARC patients	137	140	NS
AIDS patients	53	56	NS
CD4 cells/mm^3	263	213	NS
CDC group II-III	56	58	NS
CDC group IVA	26	28	NS
CDC group IVC2	56	54	NS
CDC group IVC1	43	40	NS
CDC group IVD	10	16	NS
On AZT Therapy	35	37	NS
new OIs (all)	10	21	0.032
new OIs (AIDS)	1	7	0.046
OIs and other events* (all)	17	39	0.002
OIs and other events (AIDS)	6	14	0.079
New KS	4	4	NS
Deaths	8	8	NS
Toxicity	2	5	NS

*Other events: recurrent CDC defined OIs, OIs not CDC defined, progression to an indication for zidovudine therapy.

DISCUSSION

These results suggest that therapy with immunomodulators should be further explored, both alone and in combination with antiviral therapy in HIV-infection and in cancer. Ditiocarb has immunorestorative effects in immunosuppressed animals,[17] is effective in murine autoimmune models[18] and is effective in human HIV-infection. There have been 4 randomized trials in HIV patients showing benefit of this drug.[9,10,11,16] The mechanism of action is not known but probably includes inhibition of polyclonal B-cell activation, inhibition of macrophage release of toxic products such as NO_2, O_3^- and of cytokines such as TNF and IL-1. It may also serve as a glutathione repleter.

Imexon has not been used clinically but a related cyanoaziridine compound, azimexon was shown to have in-vitro immunorestorative activity and some benefit in patients with HIV-infection.[19] The mechanism of action is not known but Imexon is immunorestorative in immunosuppressed animals and is also active in murine models of malignant disease.[20]

Immunomodulatory therapy is of potential benefit for human disease. Plans for future work in this area should include studies of mechanism of action using in-vitro systems, investigation of combination therapy in animal models and systematic investigation in human disease.

ACKNOWLEDGEMENTS

Supported by NIAID Grant AI 25617-04 and a Grant from the Merieux
Institute, Miami, Florida.

REFERENCES

1. Center for Disease Control, HIV Prevalence Estimates and AIDS Case
    Projections for the United States, MMWR, 39:1 (1990).
2. American Cancer Society. Cancer Statistics 1990. CA, 40:9 (1990).
3. J. J. Goedert, C. M. Kessler, L. M. Aledort, R. J. Biggar, W. A.
    Andes, G. C. White II, J. E. Drummond, K. Vaidya, D. L. Mann, M. E.
    Eyster, M. V. Ragni, M. M. Lederman, A. R. Cohen, G. L. Bray, P. S.
    Rosenberg, R. M. Friedman, M. W. Hilgartner, W. A. Blattner, B.
    Kroner, and M. H. Gail. A prospective study of human
    immunodeficiency virus type 1 infection and the development of AIDS
    in subjects with hemophilia, N Engl J Med, 321:1141 (1989).
4. E. M. Hersh, J. U. Gutterman, G. M. Mavligit, C. W. Mountain, C. M.
    McBride, and M. A. Burgess, Immunocompetence and immunodeficiency
    and prognosis in cancer, Ann NY Acad Sci, 276:386 (1976).
5. L. D. Kaplan, D. I. Abrams, E. Feigal, M. McGrath, J Kahn, P. Neville,
    J. Ziegler, and P. A. Volberding. AIDS-associated non-hodgkin's
    lymphoma in san francisco, JAMA, 261:719 (1989).
6. R. S. Schulof, G. L. Simon, M. B. Sztein, D. M. Parenti, R. A.
    DiGioia, J. W. Courtless, J. M. Orenstein, C. M. Kessler, P. D.
    Kind, S. Schlesselman, H. M. Paxton, M. R. Guroff, P. H. Naylor,
    and A. L. Goldstein. Phase I/II trial of thymosin fraction 5 and
    thymosin alpha one in HTLV-III seropositive subjects, J Biol
    Response Mod, 5:429 (1986).
7. C. Pedersen, E. Sandstrom, C. S. Petersen, C. Norkrans, J. Gerstoft,
    A. Karlsson, K. C. Christensen, C. Hakansson, P. O. Phrson, J. O.
    Nielsen, H. J. Jurgensen, and Scandinavian Study Group. The
    efficacy of inosine pranobex in preventing the acquired
    immunodeficiency syndrome in patients with human immunodeficiency
    virus infection, N Engl J Med, 322:1757 (1990).
8. J. M. Lange, F. Oberling, A. Aleksijevic, A. Falkenrodt, and S. Mayer.
    Immunomodulation with diethyldithiocarbamate in patients with AIDS-
    related complex, Lancet, 2:1066 (1985).
9. J. M. Lange, J. L. Touraine, C. Trepo, P. Choutet, M. Kirstetter, A.
    Falkenrodt, L Herviou, J. M. Livrozet, G. Retornaz, F. Touraine, G.
    Renoux, M. Renoux, M. Musset, J. Caraux, and the AIDS-Imuthiol
    French Study Group. Randomized, double-blind, placebo-controlled
    trial of ditiocarb sodium ('imuthiol') in human immunodeficiency
    virus infection, Lancet, 24:702 (1988).
10. G. W. Brewton, E. M. Hersh, A. Rios, P. W. A. Mansell, B. Hollinger,
    and J. M. Reuben. A pilot study of diethyldithiocarbamate in
    patients with acquired immune deficiency syndrome (AIDS) and the
    AIDS-related complex, Life Sciences, 45(26):2509 (1989).
11. E. C. Reisinger, P. Kern, M. Ernst, P. Bock, H. D. Flad, M. Dietrich
    and German DTC Study Group. Inhibition of HIV progression by
    ditiocarb, Lancet, 335:679 (1990).
12. L. A. Salzman. Animal models of retrovirus infection and their
    relationship to AIDS, Academic Press, Inc., New York (1986).
13. R. Namikawa, H. Kaneshima, M. Lieberman, I. L. Weissman, and J. M.
    McCune. Infection of the SCID-hu mouse by HIV-1, Science, 242:684
    (1988).

14. D. E. Mosier, R. A. Yetter, and H. C. Morse, III. Retroviral induction of acute lymphoproliferative disease and profound immunosuppression in adult C57BL/6 mice, J Exp Med, 161:766 (1985).

15. J. A. Bilello, E. Tracey, B. Benjers, R. Yetter, and P. M. Hoffman. Murine retrovirus model systems for evaluating antiviral agents: Efficacy of AZT and DDC in vitro and in vivo. III International Conference on AIDS, 165 (1987).

16. E. M. Hersh, G. Brewton, D. Abrams, J. Bartlett, J. Galpin, P. Gill, R. Gorter, M. Gottlieb, J. Jonikas, S. Landesman, A. Levine, A. Marcel, E. A. Petersen, M. Whiteside, J. Zahradnik, C. Negron, F. Boutitie, J. Caraux, J. M. Dupuy, and L. R. Salmi. Ditiocarb sodium (diethyldithiocarbamate) therapy in patients with symptomatic HIV infection and AIDS. A randomized double-blind, placebo-controlled, multicenter study. JAMA, 265:1538 (1991).

17. G. Renoux and M. Renoux. The effects of sodium diethyldithiocarbamate, azathioprine, cyclophosphamide, or hydrocortisone acetate administered alone or in association for 4 weeks on the immune responses of BALC/c mice, Clin Immunol and Immunopath, 15:23 (1980).

18. M. D. Halpern, E. Hersh, and D. E. Yocum. Diethyldithiocarbamate, a novel immunomodulator, prolongs survival in autoimmune MRL-1pr/1pr mice, Clin Immuno and Immunopath, 55:242 (1990).

19. Y. Z. Patt, P. W. A. Mansell, J. M. Reuben, and E. M. Hersh. Effect of azimexon therapy on host defense parameters and disease associated symptoms in acquired immune deficiency syndrome (AIDS) and AIDS related complex (ARC), AIDS Research, 2:191 (1986).

20. U. F. Bicker. Immunopharmacological properties of 2-cyanaziridine derivatives, in: Immune Modulating Agents and Their Mechanisms, R. L. Fenichel and M. A. Chirigos, eds., Marcel Dekker, New York (1984).

USE OF DRUGS TARGETED TO INHIBIT DIFFERENT STAGES OF THE HIV LIFE CYCLE

IN THE TREATMENT OF AIDS

Prem S. Sarin, Allan Goldstein, S. Agrawal*, and
Paul Zamecnik*

Dept. of Biochemistry and Molecular Biology,
The George Washington University Medical Center,
Washington, D.C.
*Worcester Foundation for Experimental Biology,
Shrewsbury, MA 01545

Acquired immune deficiency syndrome (AIDS) is a global disease which has presented extraordinary challenge to the scientific community in terms of understanding the pathogenesis, treatment and prevention of the disease. With the identification of human immunodeficiency virus (HIV) as the etiological agent (1-3), it is now possible to investigate approaches to develop treatments for the disease and vaccines for the prevention of the disease. With an estimated six to ten million HIV-1 infected individuals worldwide and over 160,000 known cases of AIDS in the United States, it is extremely important and urgent to look for strategies to control the disease by antiviral therapy.

HIV is a cytopathic retrovirus that selectively infects and kills T helper cells resulting in immune suppression (1-4). HIV contains reverse transcriptase like other animal retroviruses and buds from the cell membrane (2). The virus enters the cell by attaching through the CD4 receptor and after entry undergoes uncoating followed by synthesis of DNA copy of the viral RNA which subsequently integrates into the host genome. The viral DNA can also be present in the unintegrated form and can replicate in the cytoplasm. The virus membrane is known to contain very high cholesterol to phospholipid ratio (5,6) thus making it another target for antiviral agents.

Various approaches are currently being pursued in controlling the disease using antiviral agents that interfere with the virus life cycle at different stages of replication. These include: (i) inhibition of reverse transcriptase and RNA directed DNA synthesis by nucleoside analogs, such as AZT, dideoxycytidine (ddC) and dideoxyinosine (ddI) (4,7), phosphonoformic acid or foscarnet (8,9); (ii) binding or removal of cholesterol from viral membrane by agents such as amphotericin methyl ester and AL-721 (10,11); (iii) inhibition of tat gene function by agents such as D-penicillamine (12,13); (iv) inhibition of virus packaging by agents such as avarol and avarone (14); and (v) inhibition of regulatory gene functions or splicing by antisense oligonucleotides (15-20).

Reverse Transcriptase Inhibitors

Inhibition of reverse transcriptase has been a major target to block HIV replication. Several compounds have been identified that

Combination Therapies, Edited by A.L. Goldstein and
E. Garaci, Plenum Press, New York, 1992

block virus replication by inhibiting reverse transcriptase and/or terminate DNA synthesis. One of the first compounds that was identified to block reverse transcriptase was suramin (21) which was later shown to have severe toxic side effects in treatment of AIDS patients. We and others identified foscarnet as the second compound that was found to be an effective inhibitor of HIV-1 reverse transcriptase (8,9). This compound was first used in the treatment of cytomegalovirus (CMV) infections. Foscarnet is currently undergoing clinical trials in several countries. The main disadvantage of this drug is the need to give the drug by intravenous infusions. We have recently prepared palmitoyl analogs of foscarnet that are also effective inhibitors of HIV-1 replication (22). The presence of the lipid group may be useful in the passage of the drug through the blood brain barrier. More recently, we have observed that prolonged treatment of the virus infected cells with foscarnet results in the development of resistant HIV strains. (Sarin et al, unpublished results). Nucleoside analogs form another group of compounds that inhibit HIV replication by blocking DNA synthesis. The most widely known compound is AZT which has been used in clinical trials in adults with AIDS and pneumocystis carinii pneumonia (PCP). (4). Other nucleoside analogs that are currently being evaluated in clinical trials include dideoxycytidine (ddC), dideoxyadenosine (ddA), and ddI (4,7). The terminal plasma half life for these compounds is rather low ranging from 0.5 hr for ddI to approximately 1 hr for AZT and ddC (4). Although, weight gain and immunological improvements have been observed in some patients, a number of patients experience bone marrow suppression, anemia requiring blood transfusion, nausea, insomnia, severe headaches and neutropenia. AZT is also being tried on a limited scale on pediatric patients with AIDS. ddC was the second nucleoside analog that was tried in clinical trials. Despite early evidence of reduction in HIV p24 antigen levels, a number of patients on ddC administration developed fever, oral ulcerations and peripheral neuropathy especially involving feet (4). ddI (7) is currently being evaluated in clinical trials on AIDS patients. To overcome the toxicity problems associated with both AZT and ddC, a combination therapy protocol was designed and preliminary results indicate that the toxicity of the two agents can be reduced to lower levels with this approach (4, 23). Other combinations protocols that have shown efficacy in vitro include combination of AZT with foscarnet (24,25), castanospermine (26) and amphotericin methylester (Sarin et al., unpublished results) await further evaluations in clinical trials. Since glycerophospholipid analogs of anticancer agents such as ara-C diphosphate have shown improved efficacy (27,28), dimyristrin conjugates of nucleotide analogs have been examined by Hostetler et al. (29) with the goal of targeting these analogs to macrophages. We have examined the HIV inhibitory capacity of a monophosphate diglyceride conjugate of AZT containing esterified saturated palmitoyl and unsaturated oleoyl fatty acids (30). The compound AZTMPDG obtained by the condensation of sn-1-palmitoyl-sn-2-oleoyl phosphatidic acid and AZT, and extruded unilamellar vesicles containing AZTMPDG with the molar compositions: 20% AZTMPDG/80%egg phosphatidyl choline (PC); AZTMPDG 80%/20% cholesterol; and 18% AZTMPDG/35% cholesterol / 47% egg PC, when examined for anti HIV activity showed very good inhibition of HIV in cell culture. Relative to free AZT the IC50 of AZTMPDG for inhibition of HIV-1 p17 and p24 differ by a factor of about 3. Similar values were obtained for other mixed liposome preparations (30). The activity of the conjugate does not arise from free AZT, since no free AZT is released upon incubation for 3 days at 37°C in fresh human serum. The lack of toxicity of these AZT derivatives in cell culture and the potential for passage of such compounds through the blood brain barrier suggests that this class of anti HIV dideoxynucleotide conjugates of glycerophospholipids may be useful in the treatment of AIDS.

Antisense Oligodeoxynucleotides as Inhibitors of AIDS Virus

In 1978, Zamecnik and Stephenson used oligonucleotides complementary to Rous sarcoma virus RNA to inhibit viral replication and proposed the possible us of oligonucleotides in chemotherapy (31,32).

Antisense oligonucleotide approach to chemotherapy is based on considerations: (a) that the complementary synthetic oligonucleotide acts by hybridizing with the 'sense' or instructional strand of a sequence genome thereby impairing the replication, transcription, or translation of that strand; and (b) that the length of the synthetic antisense strand, or 'hybridon' (31), should be sufficient to make it unique for the viral or human genomic segment to be blocked or modulated.

It is assumed that oligonucleotides complementary to conserved regions of HIV-RNA should be most effective in inhibiting processes involving single-stranded RNA. In order to evaluate inhibition of HIV replication by oligomers, several targets were selected which are involved in viral recognition step. They include the extreme 5'-end of RNA the AUG initiator codons and sites that are involved in processing RNA such as the splice donor and acceptor sites. Although these sites involved in translation and processing of RNA are likely to have some homology with most sequences, an oligonucleotide, 17-mer or longer should be specific for viral sequences.

Inhibition of reverse transcription is the other target of choice, and should be specific as this is not a normal cellular function. Three other sites initially selected were: (a) binding site for tRNA primer (PBS), (b) immediately upstream of tRNA binding site (nest to PBS) and (c) middle of the 5'-repeated region. Oligonucleotide binding to tRNA primer site, would compete with tRNA and prevent initiation of transcription. An oligonucleotide complementary to the region 5' to PBS may block initiation of transcription by reverse transcriptase with steric interaction or by inability of the enzyme to unwind a DNA-RNA hybrid.

HIV-1 _rev_ gene, which is essential for viral replication and regulates the expression of various proteins, in part by affecting the splicing of the viral mRNA has also been used as a target. Other sites which have been studied for antisense inhibitors are (a) TAR - the portion of transactivator responsive region which is essential for transcription stimulation by the tat protein, (b) nef and vif, start codons of the genes for the regulatory protein nef, and the virus infectivity factor vif respectively.

Several oligonucleotides (20-mers) complementary to HIV have been tested and all showed activity to some extent. An oligonucleotide which is grossly mismatched showed no activity. The most active oligonucleotides were complementary to the poly(A) signal, to 5'end of RNA (cap 5'-untranslated region, next to PBS and the primer binding site) (15,16).

Of the internal sites, only the splice acceptor site for tat (5349-5368) was the most active. Of comparable activity was the oligonucleotide complementary to another splice acceptor site, upstream of env-initiator (7947-7966). The ID50 as assayed by syncytia formation and p24 antigen expression was in the range of 20-100 μg ml-1 (3.5-16 μM). In general, at this concentration range oligonucleotides show no cytotoxicity in the tissue culture system. Unmodified oligonucleotides were not active when they were added to cells which were infected for 24 hours or more, or chronically infected (20).

Oligonucleotide analogs such as, methylphosphonates also form stable duplexes with DNA/RNA (33), but because of their nonionic nature, the binding of the oligomer to its target is an equilibrium process, and excess of oligomer is required to drive the binding equilibrium towards the bound state. In previous studies, methylphosphonate oligomers were found to be effective over a concentration range of 30-150 μM (34).

We have tested several oligonucleotides (20-mers), containing 5 to 18 methylphosphonate residues for their anti-HIV activity and compared them to unmodified oligodeoxynucleotides. The oligomer sequences tested were complementary to splice acceptor site of tat encoded mRNA (18). The effects of these oligomers on HIV-induced syncytia formation, viral antigens (p17 and p24) expression and cell viability showed similar levels of inhibition. Inhibition of HIV replication by an oligonucleotide methylphosphonate complementary to tat gene splice acceptor site showed a strong does dependent inhibition with 80-100% inhibition seen at 5 to 10 μg/ml [approximately 1 μM]. A self complementary 20-mer phosphorothioate oligomer was ineffective even up to 15 μM concentration assayed under the same conditions.

We also observed that phosphorothioate homooligomers of S-dC20, S-dA20, S-dG20, S-T20 and also mismatched oligomers showed some anti-HIV activity, if they were added to cell culture simultaneously with the virus. At low concentration they were less effective than a complementary sequence, but at a higher concentration, showed similar activity. Thus, at a higher concentration of this series of compounds, mechanisms of action other than hybridization arrest' may be operational. Similar results were obtained by Matsukura and coworkers (35). They observed 80% inhibition of p24 at concentration of 25 μM of 28-mer complementary to rev gene, whereas homopolymer of cytidine, S-dC28, was effective at 0.5 μM concentration and protected 100% cells against HIV infection. This effect was both dose and chain length dependent.

In subsequent studies, we added the phosphorothioate oligomers to the cell culture after 24 hours and in a separate experiment 48 hours after infection. Phosphorothioate oligomer which was complementary to tat gene splice acceptor site "antisense oligomer" was effective and sense or random phosphorothioate oligomers failed to protect cells from HIV-induced cytopathic effect (20). The effective dose of antisense oligomer' after 24 hours or 48 hours post infection addition was higher than when added simultaneously with the virus. At 1.5 μM concentration, the inhibition of p17 at 0, 24, and 48 hours post infection was 96%, 88% and 36% respectively.

Sequence specific and non-sequence specific effect of phosphorothioate oligomers was much clearer in a model experiment, where oligomers were added at 0 hour (simultaneously with the virus) and 4,8, 24 and 48 hours after infection. Three oligomers were studied, one complementary to splice donor site, one mismatched and one S-dA20, all 20-mers in length. When added simultaneously, all three oligomers were effective at about the same dose, but as the time of post-infection and addition of oligomer goes from 0 to 48 hours, there is a marked difference in doses of all three oligomers. Antisense oligomers required approximately 3-fold higher amount to inhibit syncytia by 50% whereas the mismatched oligomer and a S-dA20, required 8- and 11-fold excess respectively. These studies suggest that the effect observed with the antisense oligomers is sequence specific in chronically infected cells. Since HIV-1 has been shown to contain a high cholesterol to phospholipid ratio (5,6) compared to the normal lymphocyte membrane, we examined a number of unmodified and thiophosphate oligomers bound to cholesterol for their capacity to inhibit HIV-1 replication (19). The reason being that the cholesterol modified oligomer will be more hydrophobic due to the presence of cholesterol. This may enhance the affinity of the cholesteryl-oligomer to HIV and HIV infected cell membrane and thus increase the chances of oligomer uptake by the cells and subsequent interference with virus replication.

The cholesterol conjugated oligomers are water soluble, show normal thermal dissociation characteristics and form complexes with complementary oligonucleotides. The attachment of cholesterol group enhances the anti HIV-1 activity of both the phosphodiester and phosphorothioate oligomers. The attachment of a cholesterol residue to a oligomer (20 mer) complementary to the splice acceptor site (5349-5368) changes the ID50 from>100 for the unmodified oligomer to a value of 10 for oligomer which contains the cholesterol residue. Similarly, in the phosphorothioate analogs, oligomer without the cholesterol residue has an ID50 of 6 whereas the oligomer with cholesterol residue has an ID50 of 0.8. Similar effect is observed when a comparison is made between oligomers of shorter chain length. For example, a 15 mer oligomer shows an ID50 of 14.5 which after attachment of a cholesteryl residue has a value of 3.2. Similar improvement in activity is observed with a 10 mer from an ID50 value of >100 to a value of 3.5 for the oligomer with a cholesterol residue attached. The TD_{50} values for all these compounds are >100 suggesting that these compounds will be non-toxic at therapeutic doses needed to block HIV replication, and hence these compounds could prove to be very useful as antiviral agents in the treatment of AIDS.

Preliminary studies on the acute toxicity of oligonucleotides in mice and rats were performed with a 20-mer unmodified oligonucleotide (16), as well as its phosphorothioate and phosphoromorpholidate analogues (20). The sequence tested was complementary to the splice acceptor site of HIV tat-gene. The oligonucleotides were injected intraperitoneally in 1 ml volume (in saline) into two male and female animals. In mice, no symptoms of toxicity were observed for up to 14 days at doses up to 100 mg/Kg body weight. Phosphorothioate and phosphoromorpholidate analogues gave identical results. In rats, unmodified oligonucleotide as well as its phosphorothioate analogue of the same sequence and length as in mice, showed no toxicity up to a dose of 150 mg/Kg of body weight (20).

Oligonucleotide phosphorothioates are effective in inhibiting HIV replication in tissue culture at a concentration of 1×10^{-7} M, which translates into a dose of 0.6 mg/Kg body weight. A non-toxic dose of 100 mg/Kg, in acute toxicity experiments above, represents an exploitable therapeutic window for oligonucleotide therapy. Clinical evaluation of these oligomers either alone or in combination with other antiviral agents will determine the efficacy of the antisense compounds in the treatment of AIDS.

The use of antisense oligonucleotides in control of gene regulation and inhibition of virus replication is a unique approach designed to interfere with cell and virus replication machinery at the molecular level. This technique has a wide applicability and has already been used in the inhibition of replication of HIV (36,37), vesicular stomatitis virus (38,39), herpes simplex (40), and influenza (41,42) viruses. Antisense oligonucleotides have also been used in elucidating the functions of certain protoonocogene product in cell differentiation (43,44). In the cell free system, both the rabbit reticulocyte (45) and Krebs-2 (46) have been used to measure inhibition of specific mRNA function, such as globin mRNA translation in rabbit reticulocyte system. Another system that has been successfully utilized to measure the effect of antisense oligomers on mRNA translation is the Xenopus oocytes. This system has been used (47) to study the inhibition of IL-2 expression by antisense oligomers. In other studies the antisense RNA approach has also been used in plants to study segregation and recombination (48, 49), and lymphokine biosynthesis and autocrine growth (50).

Evaluation of the studies carried out thus far with antisense approach suggest the potential for a wider applicability of this technique for understanding mechanisms of gene regulation and for therapeutic control of viral diseases such as AIDS. One of the major hinderance in the use of antisense approach in the treatment of AIDS is

the cost of large scale production of antisense oligomers. Once
techniques become available for production of large quantities of
antisense oligomers, this approach could be very useful in not only
therapeutic control of AIDS and viral diseases but experiments in
correction of genetic defects may also become obvious.

Other Approaches to the Development of Antiviral Agents

A number of other approaches are being investigated to obtain
drugs that could prove to be useful in the treatment of AIDS. These
include blocking of virus attachment by interfering with the CD4
receptor (51, 52), inhibiting virus replication and amplification by
blocking tat gene function by agents such as D-penicillamine (12,13),
blocking virus assembly by agents such as avarol and avarone (14) and
metal chelators such as mono and disulfonic acid derivatives (53,54).
Other approaches that may prove to be useful in the development of
agents for the treatment of AIDS should focus on the need to obtain
compounds that can cross the blood brain barrier. Preparation of
glycerophospholipid analogs of known antiviral agents or liposomal
encapsulation may be useful in crossing the blood brain barrier as well
as decreasing the toxicity of these agents. These approaches need to be
investigated in order to provide agents that could be used either alone
or in combination with other drugs or immunomodulators in the treatment
of patients with AIDS with minimal side effects.

REFERENCES

1.   Gallo, R.C., _Sci. Amer_. 256, 46-56, 1987.
2.   Sarin, P.S., _Ann. Rev. Pharmacol_. 28, 411-428, 1988.
3.   Haseltine, W.A., _J. AIDS_ 2, 311-334, 1989.
4.   Yarchoan, R. _et al_., _New Engl. J. Med_. 321, 726-738, 1989.
5.   Aloia, R.C. _et al_., _Proc. Natl. Acad. Sci. USA_ 85, 900-904, 1988.
6.   Crews, F.T. _et al_., _Drug Dev. Res_. 14, 31-44, 1988.
7.   Yarchoan, R. _et al_, _Science_ 245, 412-415, 1989.
8.   Sarin, P.S. _et al_., _Biochem. Pharmacol_. 34, 4075-4079, 1985.
9.   Sandstrom, E.G. _et al_., _Lancet_ 1, 1480-1482, 1985.
10.   Schafner, C.P. _et al_., _Biochem. Pharmacol_. 35, 4110-4113, 1986.
11.   Sarin, P.S. _et al_., _New Engl. J. Med_. 313, 1289-1290, 1985.
12.   Chandra, P. and Sarin, P.S., _Arznei Forsch (Drug Res)_ 36, 184-186,
      1986.
13.   Chandra, A. _et al_., _J. Natl. Cancer Inst._ 78, 663-666, 1987.
14.   Sarin, P.S. _et al_., _J. Natl. Cancer Inst._ 78, 663-666, 1987.
15.   Zamecnik, P.C. _et al_., _Proc. Natl. Acad. Sci. USA_
16.   Goodchild, J. _et al_., _Proc. Natl. Acad. Sci. USA_ 85, 5507-5511,
      1988.
17.   Agrawal, S. _et al_., _Proc. Natl. Acad. Sci. USA_ 85, 7079-7083,
      1988.
18.   Sarin, P.S. _et al_., _Proc. Natl. Acad. Sci. USA_ 85, 7448-7451,
      1988.
19.   Letsinger, R. L. _et al_., _Proc. Natl. Acad. Sci. USA_ 86, 6553-6556,
      1989.
20.   Agrawal, S. _et al_., _Proc. Natl. Acad. Sci. USA_ 86, 7790-7794,
      1989.
21.   Levine, A.M. _et al_., _Ann. Intern. Med._ 105, 32-37, 1986.
22.   Neto, C.C. _et al_., _Biochem. Biophys. Res. Commun._ 171, 458-464,
      1990.
23.   Spectoe, S.A., Ripley, D., and Hsia, K., _Antimicrob. Agents.
      Chemotherapy_ 33, 920-923, 1989.
24.   Eriksson, B.F.H., and Schinazi, R.F., _Antimicrob. Agents.
      Chemotherapy_ 33, 663-669, 1989.

25. Koshida, R. et al., Antimicrob. Agents. Chemotherapy 33, 778-780, 1989.
26. Johnson, V.A. et al., Antimicrob. Agents. Chemotherapy 33, 53-57, 1989.
27. Raetz, C.H.R. et al., Science 196, 303-305, 1977.
28. Ryn, E.K. et al., J. Med. Chem. 25, 1322-1329, 1982.
29. Hostetler, K.Y. et al., J. Biol. Chem. 265, 6112-6117, 1990.
30. Sterin, J. M. et al., Biochem. Biophys. Res. Commun. 171, 451-457, 1990.
31. Stephenson, M.L., and Zamecnik, P.C., Proc. Natl. Acad. Sci. USA 75, 285-289, 1978.
32. Zamecnik, P.C., and Stephenson, M.L., Proc. Natl. Acad. Sci. USA 75, 280-284, 1978.
33. Quartin, R.S., and Wetmur, J.G., Biochemistry 28, 1040-1044, 1989.
34. Ts'o, P.O.P., et al., Annals of New York Academy of Sciences 507, 220-229, 1987.
35. Matsukura, M. et al., Proc. Natl. Acad. Sci. USA 84, 7706-7710, 1987.
36. Zamecnik, P.C. Agrawal, S., Eds., Annual Review of AIDS Research, New York, Marcel Dekker Press, In press.
37. Agrawal, S., and Sarin, P.S., Eds., Advanced Drug Delivery Rev., Amsterdam, Elsevier, In press.
38. Agris, C.H. et al., Biochemistry 25, 2628-2632, 1986.
39. Lemaitre, M., Bayard, B., and LeBleu, B., Proc. Natl. Acad. Sci. USA 84, 648-653, 1987.
40. Miller, P.S., and Ts'o, P.O.P., Anti-Cancer Drug Design 2, 117-129, 1987.
41. Kabanov, A.V. et al., FEBS Lett 259, 327-331, 1990.
42. Leiter, J.M.E. et al., Proc. Natl. Acad. Sci. USA .87, 3430-3434, 1990.
43. Gewirtz, A.M., and Calabretta, B., Science 242, 1303-1306, 1988.
44. Heikkila, R. et al., Nature (London) 328, 445-447, 1987.
45. Blake, K.R., Murakani, A. and Miller, P.S., Biochemistry 24, 6132-6137, 1990.
46. Miroshniechenko, N.A. et al., FEBS Lett 234, 65-68, 1988.
47. Kawasaki, E.S., Nucleic Acids Res. 13, 4991-4997, 1985.
48. Cheon, C.I., Delaney, A.J. Verma, D.P.S., Plant. Sci. 66, 231-238, 1990.
49. Hiatt, W.R., Kramer, M. and Sheehy, R.E., Genet. Eng. 11, 49-63, 1989.
50. Harel-Bellan, A. et al., Colloq. Inserm. 81, 1989.
51. Traunecker, A., Luke, W., and Kajalainen, K., Nature 331, 84-86, 1988.
52. Capon, J.D. et al., Nature 337, 525-531, 1989.
53. Motran, P. et al., Life Sci. 47, 993-999, 1990.
54. Mohan, P. et al.,, AIDS 4, 821-822, 1990.

ASPIRIN AS A BIOLOGICAL RESPONSE MODIFIER

Judith Hsia   and Ting Tang

Department of Medicine
George Washington University
Washington, DC

BACKGROUND

For some time our laboratory has been interested in the development
and control of cellular immunity, both by the thymosins and other
agents. Thymosins are a family of peptide hormones produced by the
thymus and thymus-derived tissues such as T lymphocytes, which modulate
differentiation of a variety of T cells providing us with immunity
against viruses, mycobacteria, fungi and tumors. About ten years ago,
while studying thymosins, Dr. Allan Goldstein's laboratory looked at
cyclooxygenase inhibitors, among other agents, to determine whether they
might influence or inhibit thymic peptides. These studies demonstrated
that acetyl salicylic acid (aspirin) could enhance immune responses and
synergize with thymosins.

The eicosanoids have been demonstrated to play an important regulatory role in lymphocyte function. Prostaglandins of the E series exert
inhibitory control over immune function[1,2,3]; these prostaglandins are
synthesized and secreted by macrophages and other adherent cells[3].
Aspirin, by inhibiting cyclooxygenase activity[4], reduces prostaglandin
production and is thought to permit immune activation. This observation
is of clinical interest in that it has been suggested that other cells
such as cancer cells, which produce significant quantities of prostaglandins, might be deleterious to the host by secreting prostaglandins,
the end effect of would be down regulation of the very immune system
with which the body tries to fight these cancer cells.

Initial studies conducted in our laboratory focused on aspirin's
effects on cytokine production in vitro.

IN VITRO STUDIES

We have previously reported stimulation by aspirin of interleukin-2
production by mitogen-stimulated peripheral blood mononuclear cells
(PBMC)[5]. Subsequently these studies were extended by evaluating the
effect of aspirin on interferon-γ production by human PBMC in vitro.
For these experiments, PBMC were isolated from heparinized blood samples

Table 1.   Samples of PBMC were incubated with phytohemagglutinin
and serum as described in the absence or presence of
aspirin at the indicated concentrations. After 72
hours, interferon-γ content of the supernatants was
determined by radioimmunoassay.

Aspirin-Stimulated Production of Interferon-γ by PBMC

Aspirin, μM	Interferon-γ, U/ml
0	97 ± 6
150	166 ± 23
300	217 ± 22
600	258 ± 10

obtained from normal volunteers who had abstained from aspirin
consumption for at least two weeks. Blood samples were diluted with Hanks
Balanced Salt Solution, layered on a cushion of lymphocyte separation
medium (Litton Bionetics), centrifuged (600 x g, 30 min) and PBMC collected from the plasma-lymphocyte separation medium interface. PBMC are a
mixed population of cells including lymphocytes and monocytes.

For interferon assays, PBMC were incubated in 96-well plates with
phytohemagglutinin, 1 μg/ml, and 1% human AB serum in the absence or
presence of aspirin for 72 hours. Supernatants were frozen and thawed, and
interferon-γ content determined by solid phase radioimmunoassay (Centacor).
As shown in Table 1, interferon-γ production was doubled in the presence of
aspirin. Monocytes are thought to play a central role in regulating
production of cytokines, such as interleukin-2 and interferon-γ, by
secreting interleukin-1 and prostaglandins. To assess the role of monocytes in aspirin-induced stimulation of cytokine release, interferon-γ
production in the absence or presence of aspirin was assessed in PBMC
depleted of monocytes and in samples to which the monocytes had been
restored. It was apparent that monocytes were absolutely required for
interferon-γ production, whether or not aspirin was included in the cultures[6]. Further, no effect of aspirin was demonstrable in the absence of
mitogen.

Following this in vitro evidence of aspirin's value as a biological
response modifier, we moved on to conduct in vivo dose ranging studies.

IN VIVO STUDIES

To evaluate aspirin's efficacy in humans, a series of dose ranging and
time course studies were conducted. In the current model of immune
regulation, interferon-γ production is induced by interleukin-2, so we
first looked at interleukin-2 production following aspirin ingestion. For
these studies volunteers who had abstained from aspirin and other non-
steroidal anti-inflammatory agents for 2 weeks took oral aspirin and had
blood samples drawn at various times thereafter. PBMC were isolated and
incubated with phytohemagglutinin and serum in the presence or absence of
aspirin for 24 hours. Interleukin-2 content of the supernatants was
determined in a bioassay using IL-2-dependent CT6 or CTLL cells[6] .

Initially the time course of cytokine production following single dose
aspirin was assessed. Following 325 mg of aspirin, interleukin-2 production was unchanged at 2, 4, and 8 hours. At 10 hours after ingestion,
however, interleukin-2 production was almost twice baseline. Levels fell to
normal during the subsequent 14 hours (Table 2).

Table 2.   Samples of PBMC were isolated from blood samples collected at the indicated times after ingestion of 325 mg of aspirin. PBMC were incubated with phytohemagglutinin and serum as described for 24 hours (for interleukin-2) or 72 hours (for interferon-γ) and cytokine content of the supernatants determined.

Interleukin-2 and Interferon-γ Production After Aspirin Ingestion

Time After Ingestion (hours)	Interleukin-2 U/ml	Interferon-γ U/ml
0	100	183
2	120	148
4	82	170
8	94	164
10	206	ND
24	62	426
48	ND	364
72	ND	202

Interferon-γ levels were similarly unchanged for the first 8 hours. At 24 hours after ingestion, however, production was approximately twice baseline; interferon-γ production reverted to normal over the next 48 hours.

To determine whether a sustained increase in interferon-γ production could be achieved by multiple dose aspirin, a volunteer received a 650mg loading dose or aspirin, followed by 325 mg each day for 7 days. There was an initial increase in phytohemagglutinin-stimulated interferon-γ production by PBMC collected 24 hours after the loading dose, but rapid tachyphylaxis was apparent thereafter, with interferon-γ production unchanged from baseline[7]. It was subsequently determined that alternate day aspirin led to a sustained increase in interleukin-2 and interferon-γ production for at least 6 days[7].

Two years ago we began to apply this new information about aspirin in a clinical setting to determine whether 1) the immunomodulatory effects could be confirmed in a randomized, placebo-controlled trial of aspirin, and 2) it was possible to intervene with aspirin to prevent the common cold.

A PLACEBO-CONTROLLED TRIAL OF ASPIRIN

As part of a placebo-controlled trial of aspirin in experimental rhinovirus infection, twenty normal volunteers were randomized to receive aspirin, 325 mg every other day for three doses, or identical appearing placebo. PBMC were isolated from blood samples collected before and 24 hours after aspirin ingestion (but before rhinovirus infection) and phytohemagglutinin-stimulated interferon-γ production determined. There was a significant increase ($p<.05$) in both interleukin-2 and interferon-γ production among aspirin recipients; no such increase was apparent in placebo recipients[7].

Subsequently, both groups were nasally inoculated with rhinovirus to determine whether aspirin could prevent experimental rhinovirus infection. There was no difference between the treatment groups when symptoms, days of virus shedding in nasal secretions, or serologic evidence of infection were evaluated. Thus, aspirin was not able to protect these individuals against experimental rhinovirus colds. One possible explanation for this observation may be that the administration of a large number of virions directly into the nose may be an overwhelming challenge, not comparable to infectious exposure in the community. No community trial has been conducted, however, to evaluate aspirin's efficacy in a more typical clinical setting.

Thus, although aspirin did not alter the incidence or clinical course of experimental rhinovirus infection, production of interleukin-2 and interferon-γ by PBMC was stimulated by oral aspirin in this randomized trial. Our next step in seeking a clinical setting in which aspirin's immunostimulatory activity would be efficacious was to evaluate aspirin's effect on influenza vaccination.

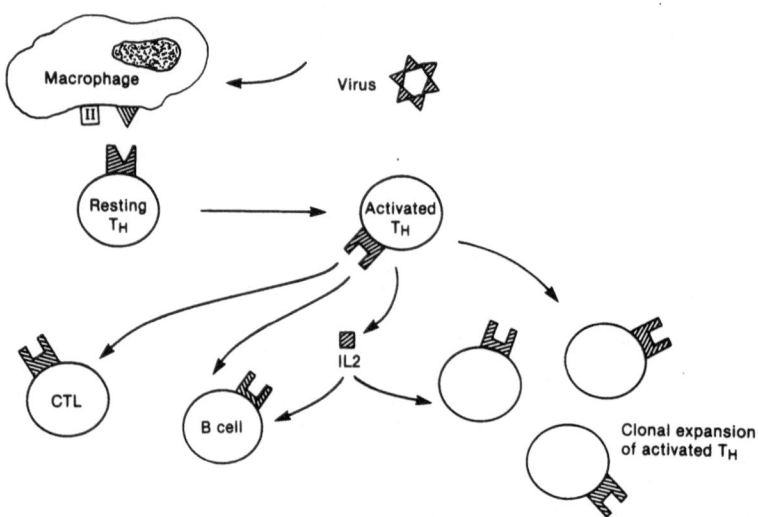

Figure 1.   Schematic of Immune Response to Virus. Viral antigens and major histocompatibility complex, class II antigens are presented jointly to helper T lymphocytes (CD4-bearing cells) by macrophages. The activated CD4$^+$ cell secretes interleukin-2 inducing a three-pronged immune response: cytotoxic lymphocyte induction, B lymphocyte activation and clonal expansion of activated CD4$^+$ cells.

ASPIRIN AS AN ADJUVANT TO INFLUENZA VACCINATION IN MICE

The objective of this study was to determine whether aspirin was an effective adjuvant, increasing the immune response to influenza vaccination in mice[8]. In deciding on endpoints to evaluate, we took into account the considerable body of knowledge on immune responses to viruses which has been established by a number of investigators. Viral antigen and major histocompatibility complex type II antigens are jointly presented by the monocyte to a CD4-bearing lymphocyte, that is, a helper cell (Figure 1). The lymphocyte is thereby activated and secretes interleukin-2. Proliferation of CD4-bearing lymphocytes, B lymphocytes and cytotoxic lymphocytes is then induced by the interleukin-2.

On the basis of this model we chose to evaluate the following immunologic endpoints: antigen-stimulated interleukin-2 production as a marker of the first step of immune activation, and antigen-stimulated blastogenesis as a measure of CD4 activity. Cytotoxicity, which is a CD8 cell function, was not evaluated in this trial, but probably should be in future studies. To determine the extent of immune protection afforded by aspirin as an adjuvant during vaccination, a viral challenge was conducted using mouse-adapted influenza virus of the same strain from which the vaccine was derived.

Three hundred Balb/c mice were randomized into 6 treatment groups. The randomization scheme is summarized in Table 3. Mice in groups 1,2,3 and 4 received initial aspirin/placebo injections on day 1. Mice in all 6 treatment groups were inoculated intramuscularly with real or sham vaccine on day 2. Subsequent intraperitoneal aspirin/placebo injections were administered as indicated in Table 3. On day 28, half the mice in each treatment group received an intranasal challenge with mouse-adapted influenza virus of the same strain used in the vaccine. Five days later all mice were sacrificed (Figure 2).

Spleens were collected from uninfected mice. Spleen cells were isolated, washed and rate frozen for subsequent use in interleukin-2 and blastogenesis assays. Lungs from infected mice were crushed and extracted for determination of pulmonary virus content by hemagglutination.

For antigen-stimulated interleukin-2 studies, spleen cells were incubated with various concentrations of influenza antigen, ranging from 4 to 34 ng/ml, in 5% fetal calf serum for 48 hours, then interleukin-2 content of the supernatants was determined by bioassay. Interleukin-2 production is generally induced to a much smaller extent by antigen than by mitogen, and in fact, values for five of the six treatment groups were below the usual limit of the assay, 25 U/ml. Interleukin-2 production was, however, increased by aspirin treatment.

For antigen-stimulated blastogenesis assays, spleen cells were incubated with various concentrations of influenza antigen ranging from 4 to 34 ng/ml, with 5% fetal calf serum for 5 days. Cells were pulsed

Table 3.   Balb/c mice were randomized into six
            treatment groups, which received either
            sham vaccine or influenza vaccine on
            day 2, and aspirin or placebo as indicated.

Mouse Influenza Trial: Treatment Groups

#1 - sham vaccine (day 2), placebo (days 1,2,3,5,7)
#2 - vaccine, placebo (days 1,2,3,5,7)
#3 - vaccine, aspirin 4.7mg/kg (days 1,2,3,5,7)
#4 - vaccine, aspirin 2.5mg/kg (days 1,2,3,5,7)
#5 - vaccine, aspirin 4.7mg/kg (days 5,6,7,9,11)
#6 - vaccine, aspirin 2.5mg/kg (days 5,6,7,9,11)

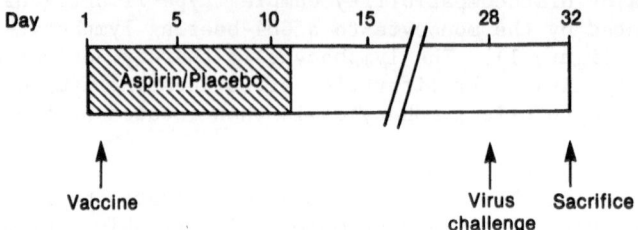

Figure 2.   Protocol for Mouse Influenza Vaccination Study.
Mice received intraperitoneal aspirin or placebo on day 1 or
as indicated in Table 3, then sham vaccine or influenza
vaccine on day 2. Half the mice in each group underwent
viral challenge on day 28 and all mice were sacrificed on
day 32.

with ^{3}H-thymidine for 16 hours, then harvested onto glass fiber filters
using a multiple automated sample harvester. Thymidine incorporation
was determined by radioassay. Specific thymidine incorporation, defined
as cpm in samples containing antigen minus cpm in samples containing
medium alone, was determined for each mouse.

The mice not receiving vaccine, group 1, did not recognize the
influenza antigen and had essentially no blastogenic response. In
contrast, Group 2, the mice receiving real vaccine but no aspirin, had
significantly greater antigen-stimulated thymidine incorporation. Mice
in Groups 3 and 4, the mice receiving early aspirin, had greater blastogenic responses than group 2. The late aspirin regimens, in groups 5
and 6, seemed less effective.

Following viral challenge, hemagglutination titers of pulmonary
extracts were determined as a measure of virus replication in the lungs.
Pulmonary extracts were serially diluted and incubated with rooster
erythrocytes at room temperature. Hemagglutination titer was the
greatest dilution at which hemagglutination was detected. More mice
were protected against infection, that has had absent titers, in treatment group 3, the early, higher dose aspirin recipients, than in group 2
(5 mice vs. 1 mouse), however, the difference was not statistically
significant.

We concluded from this trial that aspirin appeared to increase
cellular immune responses to the vaccine in mice. A clinical trial will
be necessary to confirm aspirin's efficacy as a vaccine adjuvant in
humans.

FUTURE APPLICATIONS

Many other avenues for future research remain:

1-   Does aspirin augment immune function in the elderly and in other
      immunosuppressed populations?

      There is no question that aspirin is an effective immune modula-
      tor, at least in young healthy adults, but how effective is it in
      elderly populations whose immune systems are suppressed? A clini-
      cal trial is planned to evaluate aspirin's effectiveness as an
      adjuvant to influenza vaccination in the elderly, a group which
      develops mediocre levels of protection following vaccination
      because of the immunosuppression of aging.

2-   Can aspirin speed recovery from immunosuppressive treatment for
      cancer or inflammatory illnesses?

      One of the side effects of conventional anti-tumor treatment,
      whether chemotherapy, radiation or surgery, is suppression of host
      immunity. A great potential value of biological response modifi-
      ers such as aspirin, may be to restore some of that systemic host
      immunity, particularly if given in combination with conventional
      anti-tumor treatment.

3-   Will aspirin have a future role as an adjuvant to conventional
      anti-tumor treatment?

      Recent evidence suggests that combination treatment of chronic
      active hepatitis with interferon and thymosin α_1 is more effective
      than interferon alone. The low toxicity of biological response
      modifiers such as thymosin and aspirin increases the feasibility
      of jointly administering these agents with more toxic conventional
      chemo- or immuno-therapeutic agents.

Aspirin, a relatively inexpensive, widely available and comparatively
safe drug, appears to have potential as a biological response modifier
in man. Future studies, both in animals and in well-controlled clinical
studies, will demonstrate whether or not the modulation of cytokine
responses can be translated into clinical efficacy, particularly in
populations characterized by immune imbalance or suppression.

REFERENCES

1.   R.S. Rappaport and G. R. Dodge, Prostaglandin E inhibits the
      production of human interleukin 2, _J. Exp. Med._ 155:943 (1982).

2.   S. Chouaib, L. Chatenould, D. Klatzmann, et al., The mechanisms of
      inhibition of human IL 2 production. II. PGE_2 induction of suppres-
      sor T lymphocytes, _J Immunol_. 133:1851 (1984).

3.   J.S. Goodwin and D. R. Webb, Regulation of the immune response by
      prostaglandins, _Clin. Immunol. Immunopath._ 15:106 (1980).

4.   J. R. Vane, Inhibition of prostaglandin synthesis as a mechanism of
      action of aspirin-like drugs, _Nature New Biol._ 231:232 (1971).

5.   M. M. Zatz, A. Skotnicki, J. M. Bailey, J. H. Oliver, and A. L.
      Goldstein, Mechanism of action of thymosin. II. Effects of aspirin
      and thymosin on enhancement of IL-2 production, _Immunopharmacol._
      9:1989 (1985).

6.   J. Hsia, N. Sarin, J. H. Oliver, and A. L. Goldstein, Aspirin and
      thymosin increase interleukin-2 and interferon-γ production by human
      peripheral blood lymphocytes, _Immunopharmacol._ 17:167 (1989).

7.   J. Hsia, G. L. Simon, N. Higgins, A. L. Goldstein, and F. G. Hayden,
      Immune Modulation by Aspirin during Experimental Rhinovirus Colds,
      Bull. N. Y. Acad. Med. 65:47 (1989).

8.   J. Hsia and T. Tang, Augmentation of Influenza Vaccine Response by
      Aspirin, _Clin. Res._ in press.

BIOLOGICAL THERAPIES IN GERIATRIC POPULATIONS

William B. Ershler and Stefan Gravenstein

Department of Medicine
Institute on Aging and Adult Life
University of Wisconsin
Madison, Wisconsin 53706

INTRODUCTION

There is an age-associated decline in immune capacity that involves primarily thymus-related (T cell) functions, including the production of certain T cell-produced lymphokines such as gamma interferon and interleukin-2 (IL-2). The reduction of these factors may relate to an age-associated mild to moderate clinical immune deficiency. Although this immune deficiency has been well characterized (as below), the clinical consequences have not been established. Nonetheless, it is commonly believed that the increased prevalence and severity of infections in older people relates to this decline in immune function. Furthermore, the incidence and severity of neoplastic disease may similarly be related.

Efforts to reconstitute age-associated immune deficiency have been clinically tested, particularly in association with vaccine trials. Furthermore, elderly cancer patients have received various immune modulating therapies, such as interferon, thymosin and interleukin-2 and their effects have not been completely assessed, especially with reference to patient age.

In this manuscript we shall review our experience with certain immune modulating therapies in older hosts. We have examined the effects of Thymosin Alpha 1 (TA1) in conjunction with tetanus toxoid and influenza hemagglutinin vaccines in experimental animals and in clinical trials. We have also explored the influence of age upon the efficacy of exogenous interleukin-2 (IL-2) in a murine fibrosarcoma model. Our results indicate that these therapies can be administered safely in older hosts, and that beneficial response can be expected.

Combination Therapies, Edited by A.L. Goldstein and
E. Garaci, Plenum Press, New York, 1992

IMMUNESENESCENCE

In all mammalian species studied to date, there is an age-related decline in immune function which begins before sexual maturation and develops progressively thereafter. Extensive reports have described a wide variety of age-related abnormalities and these have been nicely reviewed by Thoman and Weigle (1989). It is generally believed that age-related immune deficiency develops coincident with the gradual involution of the thymus gland and thymic-related (or T-cell) functions are most profoundly affected (Price and Makinodan, 1972; Stutman, 1974; Weksler et al., 1976). Humoral immunity is less affected, but age-associated alterations have been reported (Serge and Serge, 1976; Callard and Basten, 1977). Although less well studied, changes in monocyte/macrophage function have been observed with age but these are less in magnitude than those described for T-cell function (Antonaci et al., 1984; Rabatic et al., 1988). Age-related change in the production of cytokines have been reported, most notably for interleukin-2 (IL-2) (Thoman and Weigle, 1981; ibid., 1982; Gillis et al., 1981; Chang et al., 1983; Ershler et al., 1986a), but also for others, including the monokines IL-1 (Inamizu et al., 1985; Bruley-Rosset and Vergnon, 1984) and tumor necrosis factor (Bradley et al., 1989). The defect in IL-2 production appears at the level of gene expression, as reduced levels of IL-2 mRNA are observed in mitogen-stimulated lymphocytes from old individuals (Fong and Makinodan, 1989; Wu et al., 1986).

THYMOSIN AND AGING

There have been a number of peptides originally derived from thymic tissue that have been collectively termed Thymosins. One such peptide, Thymosin Alpha 1 (TA1) has been a focus of research in our laboratory for several years. This 28 amino acid peptide was initially purified from a calf thymus preparation (Thymosin Fraction 5) (Low and Goldstein, 1979) and was demonstrated to have both *in vitro* and *in vivo* immunomodulatory activity (Goldstein, 1983). The peptide was shown to be present in thymic epithelial cells and its role in intra-thymic lymphocyte maturation has been proposed (Low and Goldstein., 1984). With the well characterized age-associated decline in thymic tissue mass, it was proposed that TA1 level and function decline with age (Ershler, 1984a). Accordingly, we and others have investigated the role of TA1 in enhancing certain immune functions in elderly people (as mentioned below).

However, recently, work from Horecker and colleagues has demonstrated that TA1 is actually the N-terminal sequence of a much larger protein (termed Prothymosin) (Panneerselvam et al., 1988; Frangou-Lazaridis et al., 1988). What this group has demonstrated is that the larger molecule is widely found throughout many tissues and that it appears to be an important regulator of cellular proliferation. The mechanism of cleavage of TA1 and its secretion have not been established.

Despite the uncertainty about the physiologic role of this peptide the rationale for its use to reconstitute certain specific age-reduced responses was strengthened by the observation that *in vitro* specific antibody synthesis was enhanced in a dose-response fashion by incubation with thymic peptides (Ershler et al., 1984b; *ibid* 1984c). Furthermore, young and old mice treated with TA1 immediately after inoculation with tetanus toxoid produced greater levels of specific antitetanus antibody than vaccinated mice without the TA1 (Ershler et al., 1985). In subhuman primates we found that TA1 could be safely administered and that certain measures of immune competence could be influenced (Ershler et al., 1988).

As mentioned above, certain infections are more prevalent and severe in geriatric populations. The most prominent of these is influenza. A vaccine comprised of purified viral hemagglutinin is available and its administration is recommended for people over 65 years of age (Centers for Disease Control, 1986). However, antibody response to the vaccine has been demonstrably low in a large per centage of this population, particularly the frail elderly, those with underlying medical illnesses and those residing in nursing homes (Ershler et al., 1984c; Gravenstein et al., 1990). Influenza in these patients can be life threatening. We chose, therefore, to determine if a short course of TA1 could enhance vaccine response in frail nursing home patients.

From the three clinical trials that we have conducted we now confidently conclude:

1)   Thymic hormone can be administered safely in elderly people, including those that are frail, and institutionalized (Gravenstein et al., 1989);

2)   Treated volunteers (900 milligrams per meter squared subcutaneously twice weekly for four weeks), especially those older than 80 years, had high specific influenza antibody as measured by ELISA, hemagglutination inhibition and serum neutralization activity (Gravenstein et al., 1989);

3)   Treated volunteers had less laboratory confirmed influenza, and those that did get influenza had less respiratory symptoms when compared to placebo-treated controls (Gravenstein et al., manuscript in preparation).

It is apparent, therefore, that TA1 maybe useful as an adjunct to influenza vaccine for elderly patients and current research strategies are to determine the minimal effective dose, route of administration, and schedule.

BIOLOGICAL THERAPIES IN EXPERIMENTAL CANCER/AGING MODELS

Interleukin-2 (IL-2) also declines with age. This lymphokine, under active clinical investigation as a cancer treatment, has been administered alone, with autologous lymphocytes, or with lymphocytes that had been co-incubated with tumor and/or IL-2. These latter therapies have proven to be successful especially for patients with malignant melanoma and renal cell cancer (Rosenberg et al., 1987). In light of the encountered toxicities, especially the capillary leak syndrome (which has clinically resulted in pulmonary edema), there has been some reluctance to treat older patients with this agent, and no systematic evaluation of IL-2 use in the elderly has been reported. In addressing this question in a murine fibrosarcoma model involving young and old mice, we found that lymphokine activated killer (LAK) cell generation and antitumor response were equivalent with regard to age. Furthermore, there was no evidence for increased toxicity in the old mice.

Splenocytes from old mice were less effective at killing YAC cells (commonly-used natural killer cell targets) than young. However when freshly prepared fibrosarcoma cells (MV2) were used as targets, there was no age difference (figure 1). For this assay freshly-prepared MV2 cells were labeled with 51-chromium and served as targets. Freshly-prepared splenocytes were cultured for three days in the presence of IL-2 (500 units/ml) and were then cocultured with the radiolabelled tumor cell targets.

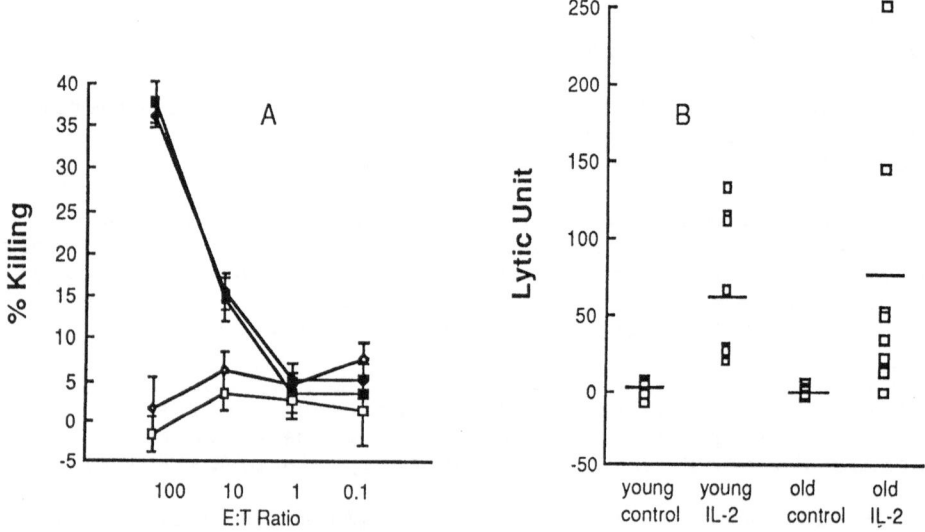

Figure 1. LAK activity in young and old mice. Splenocytes from individual mice were cultured at 1-2 x10^6/ml with 500 U /ml of IL-2 for 3 days and cytotoxicity was determined with MV2 cells as the target. (Adapted from Ho et al., 1990, with permission).

(A). Open diamonds: Control young mouse splenocytes; Open squares: Control old mouse splenocytes; Closed diamonds: IL-2-stimulated young mouse splenocytes; Closed squares: IL-2-stimulated old mouse splenocytes.

(B). Activity expressed in lytic unit (LU) at 20% lysis per 10 million cells as described by Pross et al. (1981). Mean activity is depicted by the horizontal bar.

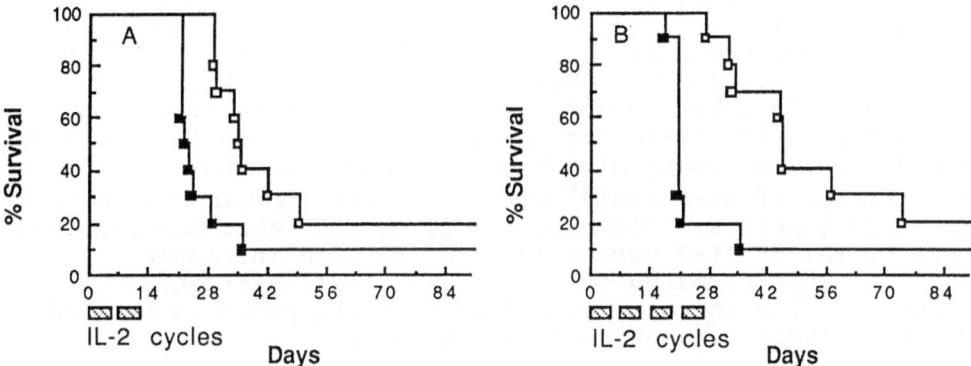

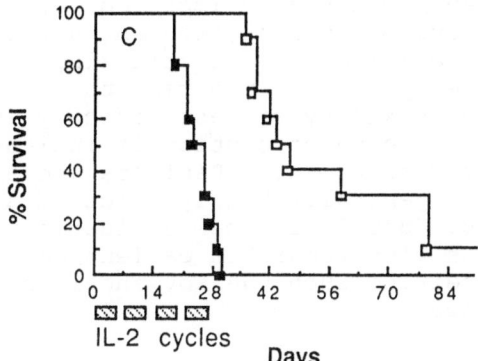

Figure 2. Survival curve of mice inoculated with 10^3 MV2 cells intraperitoneally on day 0, and treated with 5×10^4 U of IL-2 i.p. bid, for 5 days treatment cycles. Ten mice were used in each group. Closed square, control; Open square, IL-2 treated. (Adapted from Ho et al., 1990 with permission).

(A). Young mice treated with 2 cycles, separated by two days.

(B). Young mice treated with 4 cycles, each cycle separated by two days.

(C). Old mice treated with 4 cycles each cycle separated by two days.

In vivo **IL-2 Effects.** Preliminary experiments had indicated that an i.p. inoculation of 10^3 MV2 cells would result in lethal tumor in 90% of young (3 months) C57BL/6 mice. When inoculated with tumor cells under identical conditions, old mice developed a lethal tumor at a greater incidence than young, and survival was greater for young tumor bearing animals, a finding typical for antigenic murine tumors (Flood et al., 1982; Urban et al., 1982; Urban and Schrieber, 1984; Ershler et al., 1986b). For the IL-2 experiments, tumor cells were injected (day 0) and IL-2 was administered i.p. beginning on the following day (day 1). As seen in figure 2, the survival of young mice that had received either two or four cycles of IL-2 (5×10^4 units bid) was greater than saline injected controls. Old mice (23-24 months) that had received four cycles of IL-2 were also shown to have increased survival when compared to age-matched, saline-treated controls. The increase in median survival produced by IL-2 was comparable in young and old animals.

CONCLUSIONS

There may prove to be a distinct rationale for the use of certain biologic such as TA1 for specific immune enhancement in elderly people. Indeed, influenza vaccine responses have been demonstrably improved, and this improvement has resulted in less frequent and less severe influenza. In the clinical trials utilizing biologic therapies for cancer patients, the results to date have not indicated increased toxicity or less efficacy in older patients. However, a note of caution is indicated with regard to the latter statement. Patients who are enrolled in clinical trials are generally highly selected and of good performance status. Until critical evaluation of these biologic approaches with regard to patient age are reported, older patients receiving such therapy should be subjected to special surveillance.

REFERENCES

Antonaci S., Jirillo E., Ventura M.T., Garofolo A.R., and Bonomo L., 1984, Non-specific immunity in aging: Deficiency of monocyte and polymorphonuclear cell-mediated functions, _Mechanisms of Ageing and Development_, 24:367.

Bradley, S.F., Vibhagool, A., Kunkel, S.L., and Kauffman, C.A., 1989, Monokine secretion in aging and protein malnutrition, _J. Leukocyte Biology_, 45:510.

Bruley-Rosset, M.and Vergnon, I., 1984, Interleukin-1 synthesis and activity in aged mice. _Mechanisms of Ageing and Development_, 24:247.

Callard, R.E.and Basten, A., 1977, Immune function in aged mice. II. B-cell function, _Cellular Immunol._,31:26.

Centers for Disease Control, Department of Health and Human Services, 1986, Recommendation for prevention and

control of influenza: Recommendation of the
Immunizations Practices Advisory Committee. <u>Ann.
Internal Med.</u>, 105:399.

Chang, M.P., Makinodan, T., Peterson, W.J. and, Strehler,
B.L., 1983, Role of T-cells and adherent cells in age-
related decline in murine interleukin-2 production, <u>J.
Immunol.</u>, 129:2426.

Ershler, W.B., 1984a, Augmentation of antibody synthesis *in
vitro* by Thymosin Fraction 5: The influence of age, in:
<u>Thymic Hormones and Lymphokines: Basic Chemistry and
Clinical Applications</u> (A.L. Goldstein, ed.), pp. 297-306,
Plenum Press, New York.

Ershler, W.B., Moore, A.L., Hacker, M.P., Ninomiya, J.,
Naylor, P.B., Goldstein, A.L., 1984b, Specific antibody
synthesis in vitro. II. Age associated thymosin
enhancement of antitetanus antibody synthesis.
<u>Immunopharmacol.</u>, 8:69.

Ershler, W.B., Moore, A.L., Socinski, M.A., 1984c, Influenza
and aging: Age related changes and the effects of
thymosin on the antibody response to influenza vaccine.
<u>J. Clin. Immunol.</u>, 4:445.

Ershler, W.B., Hebert, J.C., Blow, A.J., Granter, S.R.,
Lynch, J, 1985,. Effect of thymosin alpha one on
specific antibody response and susceptibility to
infection in young and aged mice, <u>International J.
Immunopharmacol.</u>, 7:465.

Ershler, W.B., Moore, A.L., Roessner, K., and Ranges, G.E.,
1986a, Interleukin-2 and aging: Decreased IL-2
production in healthy older people does not correlate
with reduced helper cell numbers or antibody response to
influenza vaccine and is not corrected <u>in</u> <u>vitro</u> by
Thymosin Alpha One, <u>Immunopharmacol.</u>, 10:11.

Ershler, W. B., 1986b, Why tumors grow more slowly in older
people, <u>J. Natl. Cancer Inst.</u>, 77: 837.

Ershler, W.B., Coe, C.L., Laughlin, N., Klopp, R.G.,
Gravenstein, S., Schultz, K.T., Roecker, E, 1988, Aging
and immunity in nonhuman primates: II. Lymphocyte
response in Thymosin treated middle aged monkeys, <u>J.
Gerontol.</u>, 43:B142.

Flood, P.M., Urban, J.L., and Kripke, M.L., and Schreiber,
H., 1980, Loss of tumor-specific and idiotype-specific
immunity with age, <u>J. Exp. Med.</u>, 154:275.

Fong, T.C., and Makinodan T., 1989, In situ hybridization
analysis of the age-associated decline in IL-2 messenger
RNA expressing murine T-cells, <u>Cellular Immunology</u>,
118:199.

Frangou-Lazaridis, M., Clinton, M., Goodall, G.J., Horecker,

B.L., 1988, Prothymosin alpha and parathymosin: Amino acid sequences deduced from the cloned rat spleen cDNAs, Arch. Biochem. Biophys.,263:305.

Gillis, S., Kozak, R., Durante, M., and Weksler, M.E., 1981 Immunologic studies of aging: Decreased production and response to T-cell growth factor by lymphocytes from aged humans, J. Clin. Invest., 67:942.

Goldstein, A. L., Low, T.L.K., Zatz, M.M, Hall, N.R., and Naylor, P.H., 1983, Thymosins. Clinics in Immunology and Allergy, 3:119.

Gravenstein, S., Miller, B.A., Duthie, E., Drinka, P., Prathipati, K., and Ershler, W.B., 1989, Augmentation of influenza antibody response in elderly men by Thymosin alpha one: A double-blind placebo-controlled trial. J Am. Geriatr. Soc., 37:1.

Gravenstein, S., Drinka, P.J., Duthie, E.H., Miller, B.A., Langer, E., Bliefuss, G., Holdridge, N., Beck, C., Jacobs, L., Tomczak, J., Boettcher, C., Brown, C.S., Hensley, M., Circo, R., and Ershler, W.B., 1990, Risks for influenza and respiratory illness in vaccinated elderly. Aging: Immunology and Infectious Diseases, 2:185.

Ho, S.-P., Kramer, K.E., Ershler, W.B., 1990, Effect of host age upon interleukin-2-mediated antitumor responses in a murine fibrosarcoma model. Cancer Immunol. Immunother., 31:146.

Inamizu, T., Chang, M.P., and Makinodan, T., 1985, Influence of age on the production and regulation of interleukin-1 in mice, Immunology, 55:447.

Low, T.L.K., and Goldstein, A.L., 1979, The chemistry and biology of thymosin. II. Amino acid sequence analysis of thymosin $\alpha 1$ and ploypeptide $\beta 1$, J.Biol.Chem., 254:981.

Low, T.L.K., and Goldstein, A.L., 1984, Thymosins: Isolation, structural studies, and biological activities, in: Thymic Hormones and Lymphokines: Basic Chemistry and Clinical Applications (A.L. Goldstein, ed.), pp. 21-35, Plenum Press, New York.

Panneerselvam, C., Wellner, D., Horecker, B.L., The amino acid sequence of bovine thymus prothymosin alpha. Arch. Biochem. Biophys., 265:454.

Price, G.B.and Makinodan, T., 1972, Immunologic deficiencies in senescence. I. Characterization of intrinsic deficiencies, J. Immunol.,108:403.

Pross, H. F., Baines, M. G., Rubin, P., Shragge, P., and Patterson, M. S., 1981, Spontaneous human lymphocyte-mediated cytotoxicity against tumor target cells. IX: The quantitation of natural killer cell activity. J. Clin. Immunol., 1:51.

Rabatic, S., Sabioncello, A., Dekaris, D., and Kardum, I., 1988, Age-related changes in functions of peripheral blood phagocytes, Mechanisms of Ageing and Development, 45:223.

Rosenberg, S.A., Lotz, M.T., and Muul, L.M., 1987, A progress report on the treatment of 157 patients with advanced cancer using lymphokine-activated killer cells and interleukin-2 or high-dose interleukin-2 alone. N. Engl. J. Med., 316:889.

Serge, M. and Serge, D., 1976, Humoral immunity in aged mice. I. Age-related decline in the secondary responses to DNP of spleen cells propagated in diffusion chambers, J. Immunol., 116:731.

Stutman, O., 1974, Cell-mediated immunity and aging, Fed. Proc., 33:2028.

Thoman, M.and Weigle, W.O., 1982, Cell mediated immunity in aged mice: An underlying lesion in IL-2 synthesis, J. Immunol.,128:2358.

Thoman, M.and Weigle, W.O., 1981, Lymphokines and aging: Interleukin-2 production and activity in aged animals, J. Immunol., 127:2102.

Thoman, M.L. and Weigle, W.O., 1989, The cellular and subcellular bases of Immunosenescence, Advances in Immunology, 46:221.

Urban, J.L., Burton, R.C., Holland, J.M., Kripke M.L., and Schreiber H., 1982, Mechanisms of syngeneic tumor rejection: susceptibility of host selected progressor variants to various immunologic effector cells, J. Exp. Med.,155:557.

Urban, J.L., Schreiber, H., 1984, Rescue of the tumor-specific immune response of aged mice in vitro, J. Immunol., 133:527.

Weksler, M.E., Innes, J.B., and Goldstein, G., 1976, Immunological studies of aging IV. The contribution of thymic involution to the immune deficiencies of aging mice, and reversal with thymopoietin, J. Exp. Med., 148:996.

Wu, W., Pahlavani, M., Cheung, H.T., and Richardson, A., 1986, The effect of aging on the expression of Interleukin-2 messenger ribonucleic acid, Cellular Immunology, 100:224.

THYMOSIN: AN INNOVATIVE APPROACH TO THE TREATMENT OF

CHRONIC HEPATITIS B

Milton G. Mutchnick,[1] Glen D. Cummings,[1]
Jay H. Hoofnagle[2] and David A. Shafritz[3]

[1]Department of Medicine, Wayne State University School
of Medicine, Detroit, MI 48201; [2]Liver Disease Section,
Digestive Diseases Branch, National Institute of
Diabetes and Digestive and Kidney Diseases, National
Institutes of Health, Bethesda, MD 20892; [3]Liver
Research Center, Albert Einstein College of Medicine,
New York, NY 10461

INTRODUCTION

Chronic hepatitis B virus infection is a common disease afflicting
300 million people worldwide, including approximately one million
Americans who are carriers of the hepatitis B surface antigen (HB_sAg).
Many such carriers have concomitant chronic liver disease and are at
risk for developing cirrhosis, liver failure and hepatocellular
carcinoma (1, 2). Impaired effectiveness of the host cellular immune
mechanisms in clearing hepatitis B virus (HBV) infected hepatocytes has
been proposed to explain development of chronic HBV infection (3, 4).

Recent therapeutic trials in patients with chronic hepatitis B
(CH-B) have been directed towards utilization of antiviral agents,
immunomodulators, immunosuppressives or combinations thereof (Reviewed
in 3, 5-8). At present, α-interferon (IFN-α) is the most extensively
evaluated therapeutic agent for HBV (9-11). However, in these studies
a response to IFN-α was induced in less than 50% of patients with CH-B
and was associated with significant side effects that sometimes led to
early cessation of therapy (9-12).

Another class of immune modifiers, thymosin fraction 5 (TF5) and
thymosin α_1 ($T\alpha_1$), has been shown to trigger maturational events in
lymphocytes, to augment T cell function and to promote reconstitution
of immune defects (13). These thymosins may, thus provide an alternate
approach to the treatment of chronic HBV infection.

TF5, originally described by Goldstein et al (14), is a partially
purified extract of bovine thymus containing at least 40 peptide
components, 20 of which have been purified to homogeneity or near
homogeneity (13). $T\alpha_1$, initially isolated from TF5, has been sequenced
and chemically synthesized (15). $T\alpha_1$ is an acidic peptide 3108 m.w.
that has shown activity similar to TF5 in modulating the maturation of
T cells (16). TF5 and $T\alpha_1$ can influence immunoregulatory T cell
function, promote IFN-α, IFN-γ and IL2 production by normal human

lymphocytes and increase lymphocyte IL2 receptor expression (17-23).

Clinical trials of $T\alpha_1$ as primary or adjunctive therapy indicate that it enhances immune responsiveness and augments specific lymphocyte function in patients with immunodeficiency or cancer (24). Furthermore, $T\alpha_1$ appears to reconstitute immune defects rather than nonspecifically augmenting relatively normal immune parameters to higher levels.

We have previously reported that TF5 decreases spontaneous cell mediated lysis of hepatocytes, using peripheral blood mononuclear cells (PBM) from patients with CH-B. No effect on cytotoxicity was seen with TF5 treated PBM obtained from healthy volunteers (25). Additional studies showed that TF5 increased Con A induced suppressor cell function in PBM from patients with CH-B (26). $T\alpha_1$ has also been shown to enhance in vivo production of anti-HB_s following Heptavax-B vaccination in previously non-responsive hemodialysis patients (27).

Previously, we reported on the initial results of a randomized, double-blind and placebo-controlled Phase II study designed to assess the efficacy and safety of a single dose concentration of TF5 and $T\alpha_1$ in the treatment of CH-B (28). We describe here the results of the completed Phase II study which utilized two doses of TF5 and $T\alpha_1$ in the treatment of CH-B.

PATIENTS AND METHODS

Study Population

Patients between the ages of 18 and 70 years with CH-B were included based on the following criteria: Presence of hepatitis B surface antigen (HB_sAg) and elevated serum alanine aminotransferase (ALT) levels for at least 6 months; positive serum test for hepatitis B virus DNA (HBV DNA); histologic confirmation of chronic hepatitis (29) within 3 months of randomization and evidence of mild or moderately decompensated liver disease (prolongation of prothrombin time less than 4 seconds over control values, serum albumin $\geq$ 3 gm/dl, and serum total bilirubin $\leq$ 4 mg/dl). Additional requirements included a hemoglobin $\geq$ 10 gm, a platelet count $\geq$ 70,000/mm^3, a white cell count (WBC) $\geq$ 3000/mm^3, a polymorphonuclear count (PMN) $\geq$ 1500/mm^3 and serum creatinine $\leq$ 1.4 mg/dl. Patients with a history of hepatic encephalopathy, bleeding esophageal or gastric varices, previous antiviral or immunosuppressive therapy were excluded. Additional causes for exclusion included a history of intravenous drug abuse, presence of hepatitis D antibody, malignancy, pregnancy, homosexuality and a positive test for antibody to human immunodeficiency virus. Women agreed to practice birth control for the duration of the study (1 year) and to avoid use of contraceptive medications.

Study Protocol

In this 3 arm study, the first 12 patients (Group I) were randomly assigned by a computer generated program to receive TF5 (90 mg/M^2 body surface area), $T\alpha_1$ (900 µg/M^2) or placebo (1.4% sodium bicarbonate) by subcutaneous injection twice weekly for 6 months. The remaining 8 patients (Group II) were randomized to receive higher dosages of TF5 (1200 mg/M^2), $T\alpha_1$ (1200 µg/M^2)or placebo. TF5, synthetic $T\alpha_1$ and placebo were supplied by Alpha 1 Biomedicals, Inc., Foster City, CA. Patients were instructed on self administration of the TF5, $T\alpha_1$ or placebo injections. Compliance was monitored weekly by nurse clinicians who maintained a record of the injection schedule.

Side effects were specifically sought from all patients by the nurse clinicians who, in turn, transmitted the information to a physician monitor not directly involved in the clinical trial. If patients experienced local discomfort at the injection site, the monitor would make the determination to continue treatment or, if the patient was receiving TF5, to change the treatment to $T\alpha_1$. The clinicians remained blinded to problems associated with the injections and any change in treatment. Patients were seen at 2 week intervals for 6 months and then monthly for an additional 6 months. Clinical and laboratory assessments were obtained at each visit and included serum analysis for HB_sAg, antibody to HB_sAg (anti-HB_s), hepatitis B e antigen and antibody (HB_eAg and anti-HB_e, respectively), HBV DNA, ALT, aspartate aminotransferase (AST), total bilirubin, alkaline phosphatase, blood urea nitrogen (BUN), creatinine, cholesterol, uric acid and total protein. Monthly determinations of serum albumin, prothrombin time, hemoglobin, WBC, PMN, lymphocytes and platelet counts and urine analyses were made.

Immunological analyses were conducted prior to treatment and monthly thereafter for the study period (1 year). Analysis of peripheral blood lymphocytes included absolute numbers for CD3, CD4, CD8, CD11 and NK subsets by indirect immunofluorescence staining using a modification of a previously described method (30) and PBM production of IFN-γ using solid-phase radioimmunoassay (IMRX Interferon-γ RIA, Centocor Inc., Malvern, PA; 30). Blood samples obtained from healthy adult volunteers were included for each of the above assays and constituted a panel of normal values used in statistical analyses. Percutaneous liver biopsy was repeated in all Group I patients at 1 year and in most at 6 months. Only 4 of 8 patients in Group II had repeat liver biopsy at 1 year. A positive response to treatment was defined as loss of serum HBV DNA, HB_eAg (if present initially), and normalization or near normalization of ALT and AST levels at 1 year. When possible, portions of liver biopsy tissue were frozen in liquid nitrogen and analyzed by hybridization for the presence of HBV DNA molecular forms, as previously reported (31).

Statistics

Group means were compared by Student's 2-tailed t test. Changes in the measurements between the inclusion values and subsequent time points were compared by Student's 2-tailed paired t test.

RESULTS

Twenty patients (Group I=12, Group II=8) were assessed in this study. The number of patients entered into each arm for the two doses of TF5 and $T\alpha_1$ and placebo are shown in Table 1.

Group I results have been reported elsewhere (28) and we present the combined findings of Group I and II here. The biological effects of TF5 and $T\alpha_1$ are similar (24). Since analysis of the pretreatment characteristics and response to treatment were similar for the TF5 and $T\alpha_1$ treatment arms using both dosages, all patients given thymosin were combined. The final study groups consisted of 12 patients receiving TF5, $T\alpha_1$ or TF5/$T\alpha_1$ (thymosin group) and 8 patients given placebo.

Table 1. Treatment Groups

Treatment	Number
Group I	
TF5	2
$T\alpha_1$	3
$TF5/T\alpha_1$ [a]	2
Placebo	5
Group II	
TF5	1
$T\alpha_1$	2
$TF5/T\alpha_1$ [a]	2
Placebo	3

[a] Patients were first treated with TF5 for 1 or 2 weeks, followed by $T\alpha_1$ for 24 or 25 weeks.

At inclusion, the thymosin and placebo groups were comparable with respect to sex, age, biochemical and serological parameters (Table 2).

None of the patients tested positive for antibody to hepatitis delta virus and only one patient, who responded to $T\alpha_1$, was positive for antibody to hepatitis C virus. Clearance rates for HBV DNA, HB_eAg and HB_sAg at completion of the trial (12 months) are shown in Table 3 and indicate a significantly higher HBV DNA clearance rate in the thymosin group as compared to the placebo group. Serum HBV DNA levels decreased in all 9 patients responding to thymosin during the 6 month treatment period. Serum HBV DNA disappeared in 6 patients during treatment and in the remaining 3 patients at 2, 5 and 6 months, respectively, after completing treatment.

Table 2. Characteristics of Study Groups at Inclusion

Characteristic	Thymosin Group	Placebo
Number	12	8
Male:Female	10:2	6:2
Age	48 (26-67)	49 (23-64)
Duration of HB_sAg (yr)	3.5 (0.8-13.0)	1.8 (0.6-6.0)
ALT (IU/L)	203 ± 124[a]	148 ± 83
AST (IU/L)	151 ± 118	198 ± 98
Bilirubin (mg/dl)	0.8 ± 0.2	1.2 ± 1.0
Albumin (g/dl)	4.0 ± 0.5	3.5 ± 0.4
Prothrombin time (sec)	12.9 ± 0.7	13.1 ± 1.3
HBV DNA (0-5+)	2.3 (0.5-4.5)	2.9 (0.5-10.0)

Normal values: ALT<40 IU/L, AST<45 IU/L, Bilirubin <1.5mg/dl

[a] Means ± S.D.

The thymosin group had normal or near normal ALT (59±17, SEM) and AST (54±12) levels at 1 year compared to the placebo group (135±48 and 143±38, respectively). In the 9 thymosin treated responders, the ALT levels at 1 year were 45±6. Transient ALT elevations (2-6 fold over pre-inclusion values) were observed in 6 of the 9 responders to thymosin and preceded clearance of HBV DNA in each case. By 27 ± 4 months of follow up, 4 of the 9 responders to thymosin cleared serum HB_sAg.

Table 3. HBV Marker Seropositivity at Inclusion and at 12 Months

HBV Marker		Thymosin-Treated (12)	Placebo (8)	p value
DNA	Initial	12 (100%)	8 (100%)	NS
	12 Months	3 (25%)	6 (75%)	<0.04[a]
HB_eAg	Initial	11 (92%)	5 (63%)	NS
	12 Months	5 (42%)	4 (50%)	NS
HB_sAg	Initial	12 (100%)	8 (100%)	NS
	12 Months	10 (83%)	8 (100%)	NS

[a] Fisher's exact test

Liver biopsy samples obtained prior to inclusion and at 1 year were available for patients in Group I which included 7 patients treated with thymosin (6 of whom were responders) and for 5 patients given placebo (including 1 patient who had a spontaneous remission). Replicative forms of HBV DNA were present in the liver tissue of all 12 patients at inclusion. HBV molecular forms observed at 1 year are shown in Table 4. The single placebo treated patient with absent HBV molecular forms at 1 year had spontaneous remission of disease and the single patient with replicative forms in the thymosin group did not respond to treatment. Histologic improvement was observed in the 12 month liver biopsy specimens of the 7 thymosin treated patients which was significant (p<0.01) when compared to the 12 month biopsy specimens of the 5 placebo treated patients (28).

Prior to randomization, the 20 patients with CH-B had significantly lower peripheral blood lymphocyte (p<0.001), CD3 (p<0.001), CD4 (p<001), CD8 (p<0.02), and CD11 (p<0.001) counts when compared to healthy volunteers. No significant differences were noted in these parameters between the thymosin and placebo groups. Within one month of initiating treatment, the thymosin group exhibited higher lymphocyte, CD3, CD4 and CD11 counts when compared to the initial values. No change was seen in the placebo group. At 12 months the lymphocyte count was significantly higher in the thymosin group than in the placebo group (1962 ± 475 cells/mm^3 vs 1407 ± 618, p<0.05).

Table 4. HBV Molecular Forms in Liver Tissue at 12 Months

Group	HBV Molecular Forms		
	Replicative	Free Genome	Absent
Thymosin (7)	1	2	4
Placebo (5)	4	0	1

At inclusion, no differences were found in _in vitro_ IFN-γ production between study groups or between either treatment group and healthy volunteer controls (144 ± 89 U/ml/10^3 PBM, thymosin group; 165 ± 85, placebo group; 149 ± 103, controls). After inclusion, PBM synthesis of IFN-γ in the thymosin group rose to levels above those seen with the healthy volunteers and was significantly higher than in the placebo group (233 ± 132 vs 99 ± 70, $p < 0.05$).

Therapy with TF5 and $T\alpha_1$ was not associated with significant side effects. Six patients reported local discomfort at the sites of the TF5 injections during the first 2 weeks. Four of these patients were changed to $T\alpha_1$ without further difficulty and the remaining 2 patients continued with TF5 with disappearance of the local discomfort. No local, systemic or constitutional symptoms were observed with $T\alpha_1$ administration. No significant changes from normal values were observed in hematologic status, biochemical parameters or in renal function, including creatinine clearance, throughout the treatment and follow up periods in the thymosin and placebo groups.

DISCUSSION

The results of this Phase II trial suggest that TF5 and $T\alpha_1$ are safe and effective in the treatment of CH-B. Moreover, the improvement in clinical, biochemical and immunologic parameters is associated with cessation of HBV replication and either elimination of HBV DNA from liver tissue or conversion from replicative forms to free genomes with transition to a latent form of infection.

It is not yet possible to define the mechanism by which thymosin mediates its effects in patients with CH-B. TF5 and $T\alpha_1$ are not believed to possess antiviral properties (32). The results of the Phase II study suggest that the salutary responses to these agents may be derived from the modulation of immune responses by these peptides. There is evidence to suggest that $T\alpha_1$ may function in a manner similar to IFN-α. The C-terminal sequence of IFN-α shares homology (36%) with prothymosin α, the precursor form of $T\alpha_1$ (32). Unlike the N-terminal domain of IFN-α, which may direct antiviral activity, the C-terminal domain may be responsible for IFN-α immunomodulatory activity. Furthermore, the octapeptide corresponding to the region of highest homology between IFN-α2 and $T\alpha_1$ competes for the same receptor on thymocytes responsible for induction of proliferation in the presence of Con A (32).

Based on the findings of the Phase II study, a controlled investigation was initiated wherein 6 chronic woodchuck hepatitis virus (WHV) carrier woodchucks were given twice weekly subcutaneous injections of Tα_1 (10µg/Kg) for 28 weeks (33). At the conclusion of treatment, WHV DNA levels were undetectable in 4 of the treated animals and were depressed 100-fold in the remaining 2 animals. Liver biopsy specimens obtained at the conclusion of treatment revealed a 50 to 300-fold decrease in the levels of WHV DNA replication intermediates in the 4 animals in whom serum WHV DNA was undetectable - but no change from pretreatment levels in the other 2 animals. No changes were identified in serum WHV DNA levels or in tissue WHV DNA replication intermediates during the 28 week period in any of the 6 untreated control animals

A prospective, double-blind and placebo controlled, Phase III multicenter study is currently in progress to establish the efficacy of thymosin α_1 in the treatment of CH-B.

REFERENCES

1. Seeff LB, Koff RS: Evolving concepts of the clinical and serologic consequences of hepatitis B virus infection. Sem Liver Dis 6:11-22, 1986
2. Hoofnagle JH, Alter HJ. Chronic viral hepatitis. In: Vyas GN, Dienstag JL, Hoofnagle JH, eds. Viral hepatitis and liver disease. New York: Grune & Stratton, 97-113, 1984
3. Thomas HC, Lever AML, Scully LJ, Pignatelli M: Approaches to the treatment of hepatitis B virus and Delta-related liver disease. Sem Liver Dis 6:34-41, 1986
4. Dienstag JL: Immunologic mechanisms in chronic viral hepatitis. In: Vyas GN, Dienstag JL, Hoofnagle JH, eds. Viral hepatitis and liver disease. New York: Grune & Stratton, 135-66, 1984
5. Alexander GJM, Williams R: Natural history and therapy of chronic hepatitis B virus infection. Am J Med 85:143-146, 1988
6. DiBisceglie AM, Hoofnagle JH: Antiviral therapy of chronic viral hepatitis. Am J Gastro 85:650-654, 1990
7. Lever AML: Treatment of the chronic hepatitis B virus carrier state. J Infect 16:221-229, 1988
8. Aach, RD: The treatment of chronic type B viral hepatitis. Ann Int Med 109:89-91, 1988
9. Perrillo RP, Regenstein FG, Peters MG, et al: Prednisone withdrawal followed by recombinant alpha interferon in the treatment of chronic type B hepatitis. Ann Int Med 109:95-100, 1988
10. Hoofnagle JH, Peters M, Mullen KD, et al: Randomized, controlled trial of recombinant human α-interferon in patients with chronic hepatitis B. Gastroenterology 95:1318-1325, 1988
11. Perrillo RP, Schiff ER, Davis GL, et al: A randomized controlled trial of interferon alfa-2b alone and after prednisone withdrawal for the treatment of chronic hepatitis B. N Eng J Med 323:295-301, 1990
12. Renault PF, Hoofnagle JH, Park Y, et al: Psychiatric complications of long-term interferon alfa (sic) therapy. Arch Intern Med 147:1577-1580, 1987
13. Low TLK, Goldstein AL: Thymosins: structure, function and therapeutic applications. Thymus 6:27-42, 1984
14. Goldstein AL, Guha A, Zatz MM, et al: Purification and biological activity of thymosin, a hormone of the thymus gland. Proc Natl Acad Sci USA 69:1800-1803, 1972

15. Wetzel R, Heyneker HL, Goeddel DV, et al: Production of biologically active N^α-desacetyl thymosin α_1 in E. coli through expression of a chemically synthesized gene. Biochem 19:6096-6104, 1980

16. Low TLK, Thurman GB, McAdoo M, et al: I. Isolation, characterization and biological activities of thymosin α_1 and polypeptide β_1 from calf thymus. J Biol Chem 254:981-86, 1979

17. Marshall GD, Thurman GB, Rossio JL, Goldstein AL: In vivo generation of suppressor T-cells by thymosin in congenitally athymic nude mice. J Immunol 126:741-44, 1981

18. Mutchnick MG, Prieto JA, Schaffner JA, Weller FE. Thymosin modulation of regulatory T cell function. Clin Immunol Immuno 23:626-33, 1982

19. Sztein MB, Serrate SA, Goldstein AL: Modulation of interleukin 2 receptor expression on normal human lymphocytes by thymic hormones. Proc Natl Acad Sci USA 83:6107-6111, 1986

20. Serrate SA, Schulof RS, Leondaridis L, et al: Modulation of human natural killer cell cytotoxic activity, lymphokine production, and interleukin 2 receptor expression by thymic hormones. J Immunol 139:2338-2343, 1987

21. Favalli C, Jezzi T, Mastino A, et al: Modulation of natural killer activity by thymosin alpha 1 and interferon. Cancer Immunol Immunother 20:189-192, 1985

22. Baxevanis CN, Reclos GJ, Perez S, et al: Immunoregulatory effects of fraction 5 thymus peptides. I. Thymosin enhances while thymosin B4 suppresses the human autologous and allogeneic mixed lymphocyte reaction. Immunopharm 13:133-141, 1987

23. Svedersky LP, Hui A, May L, et al: Induction and augmentation of mitogen-induced immune interferon production in human peripheral blood lymphocytes by N alpha - desacetylthmosin α_1. J Immunol 12:244-247, 1982

24. Sztein MB, Goldstein AL: Thymic hormones-a clinical update. Springer Sem Immunopathol 9:1-18, 1986

25. Mutchnick MG, Missirian A, Johnson AG: Lymphocyte cytotoxicity in human liver disease using rat hepatocyte monolayer cultures. Clin Immunol Immunopathol 16:423-437, 1980

26. Mutchnick MG, Schaffner JA, Prieto JA, et al: Increased thymic hormone responsive suppressor T lymphocyte function in chronic active hepatitis. Dig Dis Sci 28:328-334, 1983

27. Shen S, Josselson J, McRoy C, et al: Effects of thymosin alpha-1 (TA-1) on peripheral T-cell and Heptavax-B vaccination (V) in previously non-responsive hemodialysis (HD) patients (Pts). Hepatology 7:1120, 1987

28. Mutchnick MG, Appelman HD, Chung HT, et al: Thymosin treatment of chronic hepatitis B: A placebo-controlled pilot trial. Hepatology (in press).

29. Knodell RG, Ishak KG, Black WC, et al: Formulation and application of a numerical scoring system for assessing histological activity in asymptomatic chronic active hepatitis. Hepatology 1:431-35, 1981

30. Mutchnick MG, Lee HH, Hollander DI, et al: Defective in vitro gamma interferon production and elevated serum immunoreactive thymosin β_4 levels in patients with inflammatory bowel disease. Clin Immunol Immunopathol 47:84-92, 1988

31. Shafritz DA, Shouval D, Sherman HI, et al: Integration of hepatitis B virus DNA into the genome of liver cells in chronic liver disease and hepatocellular carcinoma. N Engl J Med 305:1067-1073, 1981

32. Zav'yalov VP, Denesyuk AI, Zav'yalova GA: Theoretical analysis of
     conformation and active sites of interferons. Immunol Lett
     22:173-181, 1989
33. Korba BE, Tennant BC, Cote PJ, Mutchnick M, Gerin JL: Treatment
     of chronic woodchuck hepatitis virus infection with thymosin
     alpha-1. Hepatology 12:880, 1990

CELL WALL CONSTITUENTS OF *CANDIDA ALBICANS* AS BIOLOGICAL RESPONSE MODIFIERS

Antonio Cassone,[a] Antonella Torosantucci,[a]
Carla Palma,[a,b] Maria J. Gomez,[a]
Clara M. Ausiello,[a] and Julie Y. Djeu[b]

a) Department of Bacteriology and Medical Mycology
Istituto Superiore di Sanità, Rome, Italy
b) Department of Microbiology and Immunology
University of South Florida, Tampa, FL

INTRODUCTION

Candida albicans is an opportunistic fungal agent which has become a highly prevalent and incident cause of disease, especially life-threatening in neutropenic, bone-marrow transplanted subjects with underlying malignant hemopathy[1,2]. An extensive experimental evidence demonstrates that this fungus, and materials extracted from it, can also be used to influence or modify multiple biologic functions[3,4]. A particular point of interest in the "Biological Response Modifier" (BRM)-activities of *Candida*, that make this microorganism quite particular in comparison to other more popular microbial immunomodulators (for instance, BCG), is that *Candida* is a human commensal. Thus, almost every normal subject is primed for immune response to candidal antigens, as shown by the presence in its serum of measurable, sometimes elevated, levels of specific antibodies, and positive cell-mediated response to *Candida antigens*[5,6]. While generating restrictions to the use of certain fungal materials as immunomodulators (mostly concerning undesired hypersensitivity reactions) the human commensalism also tells us that *Candida*-induced immunomodulation may take place under natural conditions and can be easily amplified. A rather dramatic example of this amplification is the generation of LAK- like effectors following *Candida* vaccination of normal mice[7] or exposure of peripheral blood mononuclear cells (PBMC) from normal human donors to a mannoprotein extract of *C. albicans*[8]. Moreover, certain fungal products are potent recall antigens to probe the efficiency of the immune system, both in normal and pathological conditions[9,10]. Most of the BRM-effects of *C. albicans* are mediated by the glucan and the mannoprotein constituents of the fungal cell wall[4]. In this note, we will mostly address the latter components (hereafter referred to as MP), and will attempt to summarize some of our recent results on the immunogenic and immunomodulatory effects of a purified and chemically-characterized mannoprotein fraction (F2). Localization of this constituent throughout the fungal cell wall, and its differential antigenic ex-pression in yeast and mycelial forms of *C. albicans* have recently been

Table 1. Main reasons for attempting purification and separation of mannoproteins from *C. albicans*

---

1 - Only purified constituents may allow to study the interaction between antigens/immunomodulators and receptors on immune cells, then the resolution of the specific mechanisms involved in the biologic response modification.

2-Most of bulky "mannan" preparations used in immunological work are based on extraction steps involving strong alkali or acid treatment which degrade significantly the native structure of mannoproteins and probably generate inhibitory "mannan" fragments[a].

3 -A bulk preparation of mannoprotein may contain constituents endowed with opposing biological effects, for instance immunostimulatory and immunosuppressive[b]. Moreover, it containsantigenic molecules which are distinct from other molecules which exert lectin-like actions[c] or possibly interact with cells of thenatural immunity (natural killer/professional phagocytes)[d].

---

a) see Ref. 17
b) see Ref. 13, 14
c) see Ref. 18
d) see Ref. 21

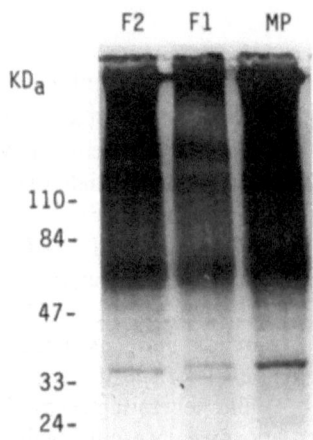

Figure 1. Concanavalin A-peroxidase stain of F2 fraction run in SDS-PAGE 5-10% gel gradient and transblotted onto nitrocellulose filter. F1 in an antigenic, but lymphoproliferation-induction inactive fraction from the MP extract. The bars indicate M.W. standards. For technical details, see Ref. 12.

demonstrated[11]. The general structure of MP molecules and their polydisperse, heterogeneous constitution have been discussed elsewhere[4,12].

RESULTS AND DISCUSSION

A main problem that has strongly limited the validity of past studies with MP constituents as immunomodulators, is that bulk preparations of cell wall materials have generally been used. Apart from the obvious notation that only purified and well characterized constituents may allow to study how precisely the mannoprotein immunomodulators interact with cells and/or soluble factors of the immune system, there are several other compelling reasons for the purification of the distinct mannoprotein constituents, as outlined in Table 1. In particular, lectin-like and immunosuppressive mannan components have been described, including inhibitors of phagocyte function[13-18]. Thus, several efforts have been made to separation and molecular characterization of the distinct immunologically active mannoproteins from *Candida*. We addressed extraction and purification schemes preserving as much as possible the biological attributes of MP from *C. albicans*, as exemplified in the preparation of GMP and its active F2 fraction. This latter proved to possess most if not all of the BRM-properties of candidal MP: it contains the antigenic activator of human T cell proliferation and LAK-like cytotoxicity generation,[12] a major adjuvant for primary antibody response in vitro to Candida- unrelated antigen[19], and a strong stimulatory constituent of murine macrophages[20] and human neutrophils (Palma et al., submitted).

Molecular composition and activity of MP-F2 fraction

Although F2 is a substantially pure and characteristic "mannoprotein" material (mannan was > 95% of the whole polysaccharide, as detected by Fehling reagent, and mannose was essentially the only detectable sugar in HPLC analysis, *unpublished data*) recent experimental approaches with gradient gel SDS-PAGE, transblotting and Concanavalin A- peroxidase-or immuno-detection with anti-Candida sera or monoclonal anti-MP antibodies, revealed the molecular complexity of this fraction. At least five polydisperse but sharply distinct molecular bands were detected by Con A-peroxidase staining. These molecules shared common oligomannoside epitopes,[11] and their M.W. ranged from > 200 to 34-36 Kda (Figure 1).

The most representative molecular constituents were eluted from the gel and tested for their ability to mimic the F2 fraction in stimulating the proliferation of PBMC from normal human subjects. Although being still preliminary, the results have shown that the PBMC- stimulatory activity is not possessed by all constituents but mainly associated with a molecular complex of 60-64 Kda. Interestingly, the M.W. of this complex ranges close to, or within, that of other glycoprotein constituents which bind C3 and other immunologically relevant host proteins.[22]

MP as probes to detect an efficient immune response

The antigenic, T cell response to candidal MP with associated lymphokine cascade and generation of MHC-unrestricted cell cytotoxicity is so widespread in normal individuals, that these purified constituents can be exploited as probes to detect to efficiency of particular T-cell mediated responses, or specific cytokine production in abnormal subjects. Particular examples are those concerning AIDS and gliomatous patients. The PBMC from HIV-infected subjects at CDC stages III and IV were found to have substantially lost their ability to proliferate and produce IFN- in response to MP,

Table 2. Interferon-γ production in cultures of PBMC from glioma-bearing subjects and controls[a].

Subjects group	N°	IFN-γ production (I.U./ml) after:				
		F2		PHA		
		mean ± SEM	R/T	mean ± SEM	R/T	
Normal	21	410.7±181[c]	20/21[d]	680±208[c]	21/21[f]	
Glioma	20	9.3±6.7[c]	2/20[d]	175±85[e]	13/21[f]	

a   For technical details on culture, stimulation and measurement of
    IFN-γ production, see Refs 8, 9.
b   R = responder (>10 I.U./ml); T = total.
c   P < 0.001 (Student's t test).
d   P < 0.001 (χ2 test).
e   P < 0.01 (Student's t test).
f   P < 0.01 (χ2 test).

and this loss could be detected at least as efficiently and precociously as the one to tetanus toxoid, a widely used test antigen[10]. On the other band, the PBMC from glioma-bearing subjects, while efficiently responding to *Candida* antigen stimulation for lymphoproliferation had a rather dramatic loss of capacity to produce IFN-γ, an immunodeficiency that is also present, although less marked, after stimulation with PHA (Table 2). This lack of IFN-γ production is rather characteristic, is inevitably followed by lack of MP-stimulated generation of LAK-like activity, and suggests that IFN-γ, possibly in association with other cytokines, could be useful in the immunomodulatory treatment of gliomatous subjects.

The Stimulatory Effect of F2 Fraction on the Antimicrobial Activity of, and Cytokine Production by, Human Neutrophils

We have recently discovered that the F2-MP fraction is also capable of strongly stimulating various activities of highly purified (> 99%) PMN from normal human subjects. In particular, it primes the antimicrobial activity, both intra-and extracellularly expressed, of these essential phagocytic and inflammatory cells. This priming effect is seen in a range of 1 to 10 μg/ml of F2, was greater at lower effector: target (E:T) ratio, and as intense as to be formally equivalent to a twofold increase in the E:T ratio. In particular, the mannoprotein stimulation of PMN anticandidal activity was studied with a large number of separate subjects, and in comparison with well known exogenous (LPS) or endogenous (GM-CSF) stimulators of PMN activity. As summarized in Table 3, the F2 stimulatory activity was of the same order of magnitude as that of LPS and GM-CSF, and relied upon the integrity of the mannan portion of the molecule. In a typical experiment, the F2 fraction was treated with pronase or-D-mannosidase, and these enzyme-treated preparations were used in comparison to untreated F2 in the same subject, simultaneously for PBMC proliferation (the antigenic response) and PMN activation (the phagocytic response). The experiment (results summarized in Table 4)

Table 3. The PMN-stimulatory ability of F2 versus LPS and GM-CSF for growth inhibition of *Candida albicans*.

Experimental Group	N° of experiments	Inhibition Units[a]			
		mean ± SEM	Range	P_1	P_2
F2 vs LPS					
unstimulated		450±55.1	288– 767	–	–
F2-stimulated	11	1244±196.5	608–2684	<0.005	NS
LPS-stimulated		1142±171.6	564–2402	<0.005	NS
F2 vs GM-CSF					
unstimulated		416±33.3	281– 767	–	–
F2-stimulated	16	1411±160	596±2967	<0.005	NS
LPS-stimulated		1521±149	741–2626	<0.005	NS

[a] Defined as PMN number causing the reduction of 20% of *Candida* growth in a standard 3H-glucose uptake assay (see Ref. 21).

[b] P_1 is the probability of a difference between unstimulated and stimulated PMN.

[c] P_2 is the probability of a difference between the two stimuli given to PMN.

Both P_1 and P_2 were calculated by the Student't test (pooled data, one tail).

Table 4. The effects of proteolytic or saccharidic degradation of F2 moieties on lymphocyte versus PMN activation in the same donor.

Material[a]	PBMC proliferation[b]	PMN activation[c]
F2	27,350 ± 1,9	647
F2-pronase	3,580 ± 1,4	702
F2-mannosidase	24,890 ± 3,5	85
F2-heated	26,305 ± 2,7	692

[a] For enzyme treatments, see Ref. 6, 12

[b] Measured as ^{3}H-Thymidine incorporation (cpm) (see Ref. 6).

[c] *Candida-growth* Inhibition Units (see Table 3).

gave a clear-cut indication that the proteolytic treatment, causing the reduction or loss of protein moiety but leaving almost unaltered the mannan moiety, abolished the lymphocyte multiplication,whereas the treatment with an enzyme degrading the mannan moiety abolished the neutrophil activation but not the lymphoproliferation. These experiments also suggest that mannan receptors may exist on PMN surface, as they do on monocyte surface. These findings should also be considered in the light of previous reports on the inhibitory effects of crude mannan preparations from Saccharomyces cerevisiae on PMN phagocytosis and mieloperoxidase activity[16].

F2 also proved as effective as LPS in the induction of message for cytokines. However, the kinetics of both IL-1 and TNF- production by F2-stimulated PMN indicated a long-lasting effect (characteristic of monocyte cytokine production) (Djeu et al., manuscript in preparation). The production of pro-inflammatory and immunomodulatory cytokines by PMN, following mannoprotein stimulation, points to a more general, previously unsuspected, immunoregulatory role of these cells, and suggests that PMN could have a part in the potent antitumour or anti- infections effects elicited by Candidal materials in murine models. Considering that activators of PMN are widespread and largely shared microbial products like LPS, MP and, probably, peptidoglycan fragments, it could be speculated that this activation represents for the antimicrobial activity of neutrophils an efficient alternative to Fc- dependent mechanisms, requiring previous specific immunization.

CONCLUSION

A remarkable body of evidence has been accumulated that *C. albicans* is endowed with powerful properties of a human-indigenous BRM, that both antigenic and non-antigenic immunomodulatory properties are expressed in particular by candidal mannoproteins, with apparently different molecular moieties coming into play in different activation processes. The enhanced PMN activity and the synthesis/secretion by these cells of important pro-inflammatory and immunomodulatory cytokines raises the problem of considering these professional phagocytes as efficient, though short-lived cells participating in the general immunomodulations triggered by *Candida*.

ACKNOWLEDGEMENTS

The experimental work described in this note was supported by grants from the National AIDS Project 1989-1990 (Istituto Superiore di Sanità, Ministero della Sanità, Unit A. Cassone). The authors are indebted to Mrs Anna M. Marella for assistance in manuscript preparation. The technical assistance of Miss Carla Bromuro is also gratefully acknowledged.

REFERENCES

1.   F. C. Odds, Candida infections: an overview, *CRC Crit. Rev. Microbiol.* 15:1 (1987).
2.   R. Horn, B. Wong, T. E. Kiehn, and D. Armstrong, Fungemia in a cancer hospital: changing frequency, earlier onset, and results of therapy, *Rev. Infect. Dis.* 7:646 (1985).
3.   A. Cassone, P. Marconi, F. Bistoni, E. Mattia, G. Sbaraglia, E. Garaci, and E. Bonmassar, Immunoadjuvant effects of *Candida albicans* andits cell wall fractions in a mouse lymphoma model, *Cancer Immunol. Immunother.* 10:181 (1981).

4. A. Cassone, Cell wall of *Candida albicans*, its functions and impact on the host, *Current Topics Med. Mycol.*, 3:249 (1989).

5. F. C. Odds, "Candida and candidosis", Baillière Tindall, London (1988).

6. C. M. Ausiello, G. C. Spagnoli, M. Boccanera, I. Casalinuovo, F. Malavasi, C. U. Casciani, and A. Cassone, Proliferation of human peripheral blood mononuclear cells induced by *Candida albicans* and its cell wall fractions, *J. Med. Microbiol.* 22:195 (1986).

7. L. Scaringi, P. Cornacchione, E. Rosati, M. Boccanera, A. Cassone, F. Bistoni, and P. Marconi, Induction of LAK-like cells in the peritoneal cavity of mice by inactivated *Candida albicans*, *Cell. Immunol.* 129:271 (1990).

8. C. M. Ausiello, C. Palma, G. C. Spagnoli, A. Piazza, C. U. Casciani, and A. Cassone, Cytotoxic effectors in human peripheral blood mononuclear cells induced by a mannoprotein complex of *Candida albicans*: a comparison with interleukin- 2 activate killer cells, *Cell. Immunol.* 121:349 (1989).

9. C. M. Ausiello, C. Palma, A. Maleci, G. C. Spagnoli, C. Amici, G. Antonelli, C. U. Casciani, and A. Cassone. Cell-mediated cytotoxicity and cytokine production in peripheral blood mononuclear cells of glioma patients. *Eur. J. Cancer*, in press (1991).

10. I. Quinti, C. Palma, E. C. Guerra, M. J. Gomez, I. Mezzaroma, F. Aiuti and A. Cassone. Proliferative and cytotoxic responses to mannoproteins of *Candida albicans* by peripheral blood lymphocytes of HIV-infected subjects. *Exptl. Clin. Immunol.*, in press (1991).

11. A. Torosantucci, M. Boccanera, I. Casalinuovo, G. Pellegrini and A. Cassone. Differences in the antigenic expression of immunomodulatory mannoprotein constituents on yeast and mycelial forms of *Candida albicans*. J. Gen. Microbiol. 136:1421 (1990).

12. A. Torosantucci, C. Palma, M. Boccanera, C. M. Ausiello, G. C. Spagnoli and A. Cassone. Lymphoproliferative and cytotoxic responses of human peripheral blood mononuclear cells to mannoprotein constituents of *Candida albicans*. *J. Gen. Microbiol.* 136:2155 (1990).

13. E. W. Carrow, and J. Domer. Immunoregulation in experimental murine candidiasis: specific suppression induced by *Candida albicans* cell wall glycoprotein. *Infect. Immun.* 49:172 (1985).

14. J. Domer, K. Elkins, D. Ennist and P. Baker. Modulation of immune responses by surface polysaccharides of *Candida albicans*. Rev. *Infect. Dis.* 10:419 (1988).

15. C. F. Cuff, C. M. Rogers, B. J. Lamb, and T. J. Rogers. Induction of suppressor cells in vitro by *Candida albicans*. *Cell. Immunol.* 100:47 (1986).

16. C. D. Wright, M. J. Herron, G. R. Gray, B. Holmes, and R. D. Nelson. Influence of yeast mannan on human neutrophil functions: inhibition of release of mieloperoxidase related to carbohydrate-binding properties of the enzyme. *Infect. Immun.* 32:731 (1981).

17. R. Podzorski, G. R. Gray and R. D. Nelson. Different effects of native *Candida albicans* mannan and mannan-derived oligosaccharides on antigen-stimulated lymphoproliferation in in vitro. *J. Immunol.* 144:707 (1990).

18. J. Tollemar, O. Ringdèn, and K.Holmberg *Candida albicans*: mannan and protein activation of cells from various human lymphoid organs. *Scand. J. Immunol.* 30:473 (1989).

19. A. L. Luzzati, E. Giacomini, A. Torosantucci, L. Giordani and A. Cassone. A mannoprotein constituent of *Candida albicans* cooperates with antigenic in the induction of a specific primary antibody response in cultures of human lymphocytes. *J. Biol. Regul. Hom. Agents.* 4:142 (1990).

20.   A. Vecchiarelli, M. Puliti, A. Torosantucci, A. Cassone and F.Bistoni. In vitro production of tumor necrosis factor by murine splenic macrophages stimulated with mannoprotein constituents of *Candida albicans* cell wall. *Cell. Immunol.* 134:65 (1991).

21.   J. Y. Djeu and D. Kay-Blanchard. Regulation of human polymorphonuclear neutrophil (PMN) activity against *Candida albicans* by large granular lymphocytes via release of a PMN-activating factor. *J. Immunol.* 139:2761 (1987).

22.   A. Saxena and R. Calderone. Purification and characterization of the extracellular C3d-binding protein of *Candida albicans*. *Infect. Immun.* 58:309 (1990).

CYTOKINES MODULATE HIV REPLICATION AND THE ACTIVITY OF ANTIVIRAL DRUGS IN CELLS OF MONOCYTE/MACROPHAGE LINEAGE

C.F. Perno*, A. Bergamini**, G. Milanese**,
M. Capozzi**, G. Zon §, R. Calio*, and G. Rocchi**

* Dept. Experimental Medicine, and ** Chair of
Infectious Diseases, II University of Rome, Tor
Vergata, Italy.
§ Applied Biosystems, Foster City, CA, USA

SUMMARY

The role of cytokines in modulating either replication of HIV, the cause of acquired immunodeficiency syndrome (AIDS), or the activity of antiviral drugs, is not yet fully understood. We then undertook an investigation to evaluate viral replication in cells of monocyte/macrophage lineage (M/M) exposed to granulocyte-macrophage colony stimulating factor (GM-CSF) or macrophage-colony stimulating factor (M-CSF) in combination with various anti-HIV drugs. We found that GM-CSF and M-CSF potently enhance HIV replication in M/M. Moreover, the antiviral activity of 2',3'-dideoxyadenosine (ddA), a prototype drug working as reverse transcriptase inhibitor, is decreased by GM-CSF. By contrast, neither GM-CSF nor M-CSF interfere with the antiviral activity of soluble CD4, and antisense phosphorothioate oligonucleotides against rev gene of the virus; these two molecules inhibit viral binding on CD4 molecule and viral translation respectively. Cytokines such as GM-CSF and M-CSF are able to modulate some immune functions impaired by HIV in AIDS patients. Moreover, even in the case of reduction of antiviral activity of ddA by GM-CSF, complete inhibition of viral replication can be obtained by 10 uM ddA, a concentration similar to that achieved in patients treated with 2',3'-dideoxyinosine (ddI, the active moiety of ddA).
These results suggest that combination of cytokines and antiviral drugs should be used with caution and only after careful evaluation of their activity in _in vitro_ and _in vivo_ models. Nevertheless, association of immunomodulators and anti-HIV drugs can be of great advantage for AIDS patients, and their study is worth to be pursued in advanced preclinical and clinical trials.

INTRODUCTION

Cell of monocyte-macrophage lineage (M/M) are widely

Combination Therapies, Edited by A.L. Goldstein and
E. Garaci, Plenum Press, New York, 1992

recognized as a major target of human immunodeficiency virus (HIV), the causative agent of acquired immunodeficiency syndrome (AIDS) (1,2). M/M infected by HIV have been found in brain, spinal cord, lung, liver, skin, lymph nodes and blood of seropositive patients (3). Recent reports suggest that only a minority of blood-monocytes are infected by HIV (4). However, other studies show that viral production could be sometimes obtained from blood M/M, but not from stimulated lymphocytes of seropositive patients (5). Finally, mature M/M account for the large majority of cell infected by HIV in the central nervous system: their infection and consequent functional impairment is believed to play a major role in the AIDS-related dementia (6).

Viral production by infected M/M is abundant and lasts long time, because such cells are poorly sensitive to the cytophatic effect of HIV (7). Moreover, infected M/M can easily transfer the virus to other cells like T4-lymphocytes, thus contributing to their progressive reduction found in HIV-infected patients.

The role that M/M play in the pathogenesis and progression of HIV-related disease strongly suggests the importance of developing drugs able to suppress viral replication both in M/M and lymphocytes. Previous reports from our group show that the antiviral activity of 2'-azido-2',3'-dideoxythimidine (AZT, zidovudine) and other dideoxynucleosides inhibitor of viral reverse transcriptase, is substantially different in T-lymphocytes and M/M (7). It should also be noted that viral replication is quite marginal in resting lymphocytes, and stimulation with interleukin-2 or other mitogens is indispensable to induce a substantial viral production. In contrast, M/M do produce large amount of virus under resting conditions, thus their activation is not a necessary prerequisite for viral replication (7).

Nevertheless, M/M are major or unique target of several cytokines and growth factors able to induce cell activation and replication (8-10). Such modulation of M/M functions suggests that cytokines can also affect the replication of HIV in these cells, as well as potentially modulate the activity of anti-HIV drugs. Indeed, preliminary studies undertaken by us and other point that granulocyte-macrophage colony stimulating factor (GM-CSF) enhances viral replication in M/M, yet increases the antiviral of AZT and related thymidine congeners (10). In order to expand these observations, we undertook an investigation, to evaluate the potential role of cytokines in modulating either viral replication or the antiviral activity of some anti-HIV drugs already in clinical trials or at the stage of preclinical development.

MATERIALS AND METHODS

CELLS. M/M were obtained from peripheral blood mononuclear cells of normal, seronegative subjects by countercurrent centrifugal elutriation or by short term adherence (2 hours) on plastic dishes. M/M populations obtained with these two methods are substantially similar in term of purity (>95% non specific esterase positive), except that 2-hour adherent M/M are slightly more mature than elutriated cells. After separation, $2*10^5$ M/M were plated in 48-well plates in 1 ml of RPMI 1640 supplemented with 50 U/ml penicillin, 50 ug/ml streptomycin, 2 mM L-glutamine, and 20% fetal calf serum (complete medium). Details of culture conditions used in these experiments are described elsewhere (7).

VIRUS. HTLV-III$_{Ba-L}$, a monocytotropic strain of HIV-1 obtained from pleural effusion of an AIDS pediatric patient (hereafter called HIV$_{Ba-L}$) was used in these experiments. The characteristics of this strain have been previously described (1,7). HIV$_{Ba-L}$ was expanded and titrated in normal M/M, as previously described (11).

CYTOKINES AND DRUGS. Human recombinant granulocyte-macrophage colony stimulating factor (GM-CSF) and human recombinant macrophage colony stimulating factor (M-CSF) were kindly provided by Genetics Institute (Cambridge, MA, USA). The antiviral drugs used in these experiments were: 2',3'-dideoxyadenosine (ddA) (Pharmacia Fine Chemicals, Piscataway, NJ, USA), recombinant soluble CD4 (sCD4) and a phosphorothioate 28 mer DNA antisense oligonucleotide directed against the first exon of the rev regulatory gene of HIV.

ANTIVIRAL DRUG ASSAY. Purified M/M were cultured in 1 ml of 48-well plates for five days with/without 100 U/ml GM-CSF or 1,000 U/ml M-CSF, and then challenged with 300 minimum infectious doses (MID$_{50}$) of HIV$_{Ba-L}$, in the presence or absence of various concentrations of anti-HIV drugs. Cell were then cultivated at 37°C in a humidified atmosphere supplemented with 5% CO_2 for 2 days, washed to remove the excess virus, and maintained in the same culture conditions as before, in the presence of cytokines and drugs. Virus production was evaluated starting from day 10 in the supernatants, using a commercially available ELISA (Abbott Diagnostics, Italy). Syncytia formation was assessed by visual inspection. Drug toxicity was evaluated by trypan blue exclusion method in mock-infected cultures. Results reported in the figures represent the average of at least three experiments. Further details of the techniques used to assess viral production are described elsewhere (7,10,11).

RESULTS

In a preliminary set of experiments, we evaluated the levels of viral replication in M/M exposed to GM-CSF and/or M-CSF. As shown in Fig. 1, M-CSF and GM-CSF similarly enhance the replication of HIV in 2-hour adherent M/M. Such enhancement is consistently achieved from day 7 after infection, and lasts at least up to day 30.

Syncytia formations were present from day 10 after viral challenge: multinucleated giant cells were alive and producing large quantity of cells at least up to day 40 after viral challenge (data not shown). HIV-antigen expression in M/M could also be easily detected by immunofluorescence. Cell fluorescence is evident not only on the membrane, but also within the cytoplasm, thus suggesting that M/M are loaded with viral particles ready to be shed both within intracytoplasmic vacuoles as well as outside the cell (data not shown).

The number of cells infected by HIV varied from culture to culture, but was always greater than 25% (assessed by immunofluorescence). This is in agreement with the variation of the number of CD4-positive M/M found in different donors, as previously described (11). No substantial difference was detected between GM-CSF and M-CSF-exposed M/M in term of number of syncytia or number of HIV-positive cells. It should also be noted that most of M/M staining positive for HIV-p24 antigen were mononuclear and normal shaped even after more than 25 days of culture.

The association of GM-CSF did not increase viral production more than with each cytokine used alone. Similarly, no substantial increase of p24 antigen levels in the supernatants of either control or cytokine-exposed M/M was obtained by disrupting the cells with 0.5% triton X (data not shown).

Based on these data, we assessed the efficacy of some antiviral drugs in inhibiting HIV replication in M/M exposed or not exposed to GM-CSF or M-CSF. We selected one drug active against each of the following stages of HIV replication: viral binding on cell surface, reverse transcriptase activity, and viral transcription.

Figure 2 summarizes the results obtained with soluble CD4, a recombinant molecule that selectively inhibits the binding of HIV-gp120 glycoprotein with CD4 epitope on the cell membrane. About 85% inhibition of HIV replication was achieved with 1 ug/ml sCD4 in M/M not exposed to cytokines, and >98% inhibition was achieved with 5 ug/ml sCD4. GM-CSF did not substantially affect the activity of CD4, since 72% and >98% inhibition of HIV replication was obtained with 1 and 5 ug/ml sCD4 respectively. Results obtained by evaluation of syncytia formation substantially paralleled those achieved by p24-antigen assay (data not shown).

The antiviral effect of ddA, a reverse transcriptase inhibitor, was affected by GM-CSF (Fig.3). Inhibitory dose 50% (ID_{50}) of ddA in control M/M was about 0.01 uM, while the ID_{50} in the presence of GM-CSF increased up to 0.08 uM. The activity of ddA is then about 10 fold reduced in the presence of a cytokine enhancer of viral replication. However, even in this case, >98% viral inhibition was achieved, in the presence of GM-CSF, by 10 uM ddA, a concentration highly effective against viral replication in T-lymphocytes, and more important, clinically achievable in patients with HIV-related disease treated with ddI (the product of conversion of ddA by the ubiquitous enzyme adenosine deaminase). Preliminary results also suggest that M-CSF modulates anti-HIV activity of ddA in a fashion similar to GM-CSF.

In the case of antisense phosphorothioate oligonucleotides directed against the I exon of the rev regulatory gene of HIV, the following results were obtained. Such antisense acts by inhibiting the translation (and probably transcription) of the rev gene, that normally encodes for a regulatory protein that stabilizes viral RNA and regulates the ratio between high and low molecular weight viral RNA. Rev function is indispensable for HIV replication.

Antisense anti-rev thus acts mainly in late (post-

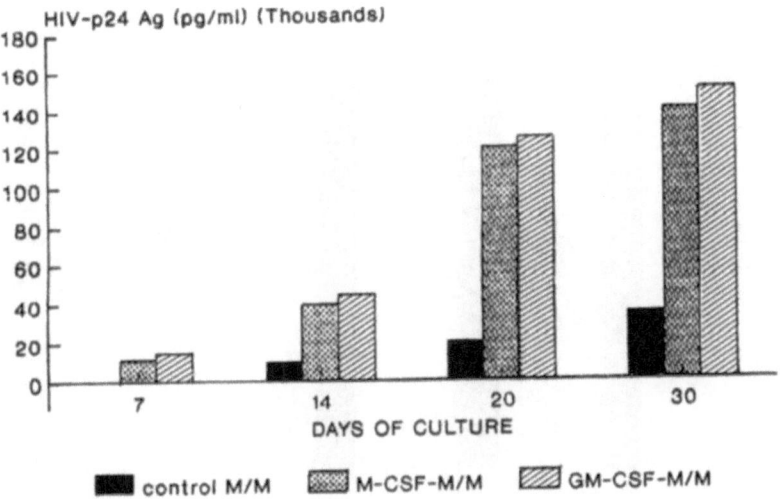

Fig. 1 Enhancement of HIV replication in macrophages exposed to GM-CSF and M-CSF.

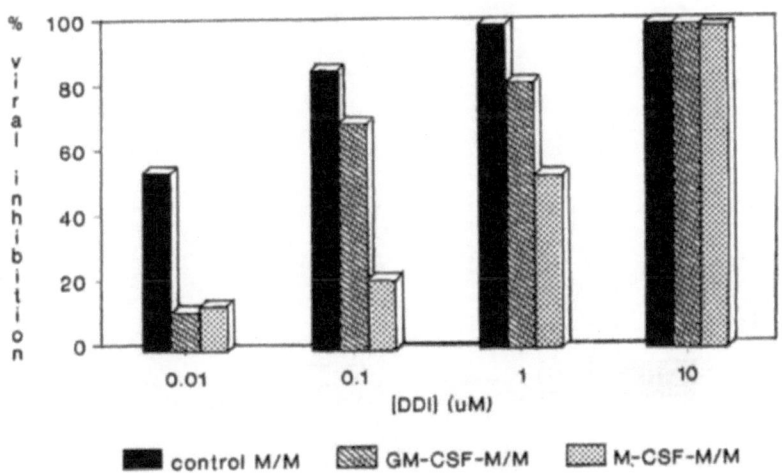

Fig. 2 Anti-HIV Activity of DDI in GM-CSF- or M-CSF- exposed macrophages.

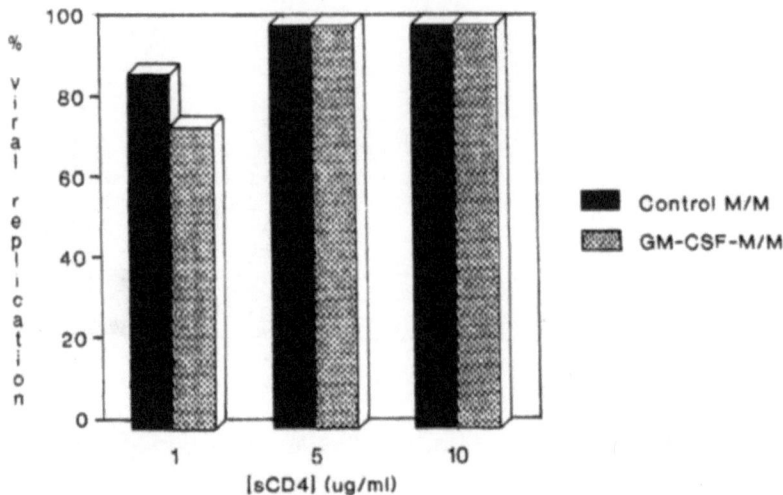

Fig. 3 Inhibition of HIV replication by soluble-CD4 in macrophages.

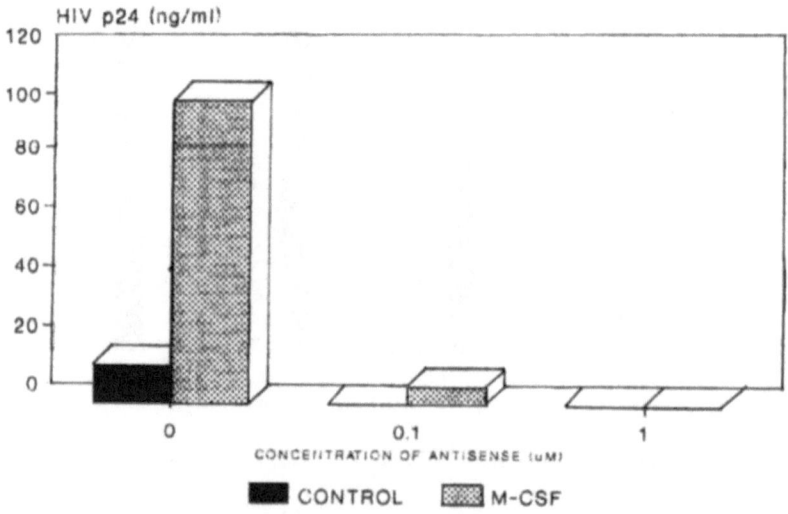

Fig. 4 Inhibition of HIV replication by phosphorothioate antisense to rev in cytokine-exsposed monocytes.

integrational) stages of viral replication. Our data, summarized in the Fig.4, show that the antiviral activity of non toxic concentrations (in animal models) of such antisense are not substantially affected by cytokines like M-CSF. Indeed, potent enhancement of viral replication has been obtained by M-CSF also in this set of experiments: however, either in the presence or absence of M-CSF, >95% viral inhibition was achieved by 0.1 uM antisense, and >99% inhibition was obtained by 1 uM. In a T-lymphocyte model, ID_{50} of the same antisense molecule is between 1 and 5 uM (data not shown); thus, antisense molecules such this are more active in M/M than in T-cells, even when M/M are exposed to cytokines enhancer of viral replication.

DISCUSSION

In this paper we studied, in cells of M/M lineage, the ability of GM-CSF or M-CSF to modulate the replication of HIV and the activity of some anti-HIV drugs acting at different stages of virus replication. We found that the antiviral activity of ddA, a prototype drug acting on viral reverse transcriptase, is more affected than prototype drugs acting at levels of viral binding on cell surface, or at the posttranscriptional level.

There is a large cohort of studies that investigates the role of cytokines on the replication of HIV, either in vivo or in vitro systems (8-10). Among other cytokines, GM-CSF and M-CSF are widely studied in view of their clinical use in patients with HIV-related disease. Immunological disorders correlated with both lymphocyte and M/M disfunctions are the main feature of such patients (12). Moreover, most patients with AIDS experience bone marrow disfunctions, such as anemia, granulocytopenia and thrombocytopenia, either caused by a direct (or indirect) effect of HIV, or by a toxic effect of AZT, an antiviral drug currently used by thousands of patients infected by HIV (13,14). Cytokines such as GM-CSF (and, in part, M-CSF) are able to improve most M/M functions (phagocytosis, antigen presentation, cell killing, superoxide production, etc.), and increase the maturation and dismissal of mature cells from bone marrow compartment (14,15). For this reason, GM-CSF is currently studied in clinical trials in patients with AIDS and neutropenia, in association with AZT.

Nevertheless, it has been demonstrated by us and others that both GM-CSF and M-CSF enhance viral replication in M/M (8-10). The mechanism(s) related to such phenomenon is still poorly understood: it has been hypothesized that cytokines may activate (directly or through a DNA binding protein) enhancer sequences within HIV-long terminal repeat, thus acting at a postintegrational step of viral replication (16). The clinical implications of this phenomenon are still unclear. Indeed, Pluda et al reported that 6/6 patients experienced a substantial increase of HIV-p24 antigemia during treatment with GM-CSF (17). Viral antigenemia immediately returned to the baseline when AZT was administered. Other clinical trials did not show any significant modulation of HIV replication in GM-CSF-treated patients. Nevertheless, this suggests that the use of cytokines should be considered with great caution, and always in association with selected drugs potently active against HIV also in the presence of cytokines. Drugs like sCD4 are able to completely inhibit viral entry and then viral integration, as shown by the absence of proviral genome (by polymerase chain reaction) in sCD4-exposed cells (18). It is then conceivable that inhibition of viral entry induced by such drugs can prevent the modulation of HIV replication induced by cytokines that usually act at postintegrational stages of the replication of the virus. By contrast, proviral DNA has been detected in cells exposed to inhibitors of reverse transcriptase, such as AZT, even in the absence of detectable virus production from these cells. Thus, this suggests that cytokines like GM-CSF or M-CSF are unable to activate viral replication when are present antiviral drugs able to prevent the integration of provirus into cellular DNA. This may at least in part explain the results shown in this paper, that suggest a partial loss of activity of ddA (but not of sCD4) in the presence of GM-CSF or M-CSF. Similarly, viral activation induced by GM-CSF and M-CSF might be balanced (and then almost nullified) by a drug, such as antisense anti-rev, that decreases viral production by inhibiting a postintegrational step of HIV replication later than that activated by cytokines.

It should be mentioned that, even in the case of ddA (and even more of sCD4 and antisense), complete inhibition of HIV replication in cytokine-exposed M/M was achieved with drug concentrations similar or even lower than those active against HIV in lymphocytes, and (in the case of sCD4 and ddA) close to those potentially achievable in patients. Moreover, GM-CSF potently enhances the antiviral activity of AZT in in vitro systems, by increasing both drug entry within the cell and phosphorylation (i.e. activation) of AZT to its triphosphate (active) moiety (10). Thus, association of cytokines and antiviral drugs could be of advantage even in the case of limited cytokine-induced viral enhancement. These results again stress that the development of immunomodulators able to improve the functions of immune system is an important goal in the treatment of AIDS, that parallels the search of good antiviral drugs able to inhibit HIV replication. This suggests that the research of associations of cytokines and antiviral drugs should be further pursued and the results carefully eveluated in preclinical studies before the use in patients with HIV-related disease.

ACKNOWLEDGEMENT

This work has been supported by the Italian Istituto Superiore di Sanità, IV Progetto di Ricerche AIDS 1990, and by two grants of the Italian Consiglio Nazionale delle Ricerche, Project FATMA.

REFERENCES

1) Gartner S., Markovits P., Markovitz D.M., Kaplan M.H., Gallo R.C., Popovic M.,: The role of mononuclear phagocytes in HTLV-III/LAV infection. Science 1986; 233:215.
2) Ho D.D., Rota T.R., Hirsch M.S.: Infection of monocyte/macrophages by human T lymphotropic virus type III. J. Clin. Invest. 1986; 77:1712.

3) Meltzer M.S., Nakamura M., Hansen B.D., Turpin J.A., Kalter D.C., Gendelman H.E.: Macrophages as susceptible targets for HIV infection, persistant viral reservoirs in tissue, and key immunoregulatory cells that control levels of virus replication and extent of disease. AIDS Research and Human Retroviruses 1990; 6:967.

4) Schnittman S.M., Psallidopulos M.C., Lane H.C., Thompson L., Baseler M., Massari F., Fox C.H., Salzman N.P., Fauci A.S.: The reservoir of HIV-1 in human peripheral blood is a T cell that mantains expression of CD4. Science 1989; 245:305.

5) Popovic M., Gartner S.: Isolation of HIV-1 from monocytes but not T-lymphocytes. Lancet 1987; 2:916.

6) Koenig S., Gendelman H.E., Orenstein J.M., Dal Canto M.C., Pezeskhpour G.H., Yungbluth M., Janotta F., Aksamit A., Martin M.A., Fauci A.S.: Detection of AIDS virus in macrophages in brain tissue from AIDS patients with encephalopathy. Science 1986; 233:1089.

7) Perno C.F., Yarchoan R., Cooney D.A., Hartman N.R., Gartner S., Popovic M., Hao Z., Gerrard T.L., Wilson Y.A., Johns D.G., Broder S.: Inhibition of human immunodeficiency virus (HIV-1/HIV-III$_{Ba-L}$) replication in fresh and cultured human peripheral blood monocyte/macrophages by azidothymidine and related 2',3'-dideoxynucleosides. J. Exp. Med. 1988; 168:1111.

8) Koyanagi Y., O'Brien W.A., Zhao J.Q., Golde D.W., Gasson J.C., Chen I.S.Y.: Cytokines alter production of HIV-1 from primary mononuclear phagocytes. Science 1988; 241:1673.

9) Gendelman H.E., Orenstein J.M., Martin M.A., Ferrua C., Mitra R., Phipps T., Wahl L.A., Lane H.C., Fauci A.S., Burke D.S., Skillman D., Meltzer M.S.: Efficient isolation and propagation of human immunodeficiency virus on recombinant colony-stimulating factor 1-treated monocytes. J. Exp. Med. 1988; 167:1428.

10) Perno C.F., Yarchoan R., Cooney A.D., Hartman N.R., Webb D.S.A., Hao Z., Mitsuya H., Johns D.G., Broder S.: Replication of human immunodeficiency virus in monocytes: granulocyte/macrophage colony stimulating factor (GM-CSF) potentiates viral production yet enhances the antiviral effect mediated by 3'-azido-2',3'-dideoxythymidine (AZT) and other dideoxynucleoside congeners of thymidine. J. Exp. Med. 1989; 169:933.

11) Perno C.F. Baseler M.W., Broder S., Yarchoan R.: Infection of monocytes by human immunodeficiency virus type 1 is blocked by inhibitors of CD4-gp120 binding even in the presence of enhancing antibodies. J. Exp. Med. 1990; 171:1043.

12) Yarchoan R., Broder S.: Immunology of HIV Infection. In W. Paul: Fundamental Immunology. Raven Press, 1989, p.1059.

13) Richman D.D., Fischl M.A., Grieco M.H., Gottlieb M.S., Volberding P., Laskin O.L., Leedom J.M., Groopman J.E., Mildvan D., Hirsch M.S., Jackson G.G., Durack D.T., Nusinoff-Lehrman S. and the AZT collaborative working group: The toxicity of azidothymidine (AZT) in the treatment of AIDS and AIDS related complexes (ARC). A double-blind, placebo-controlled trial. N. Engl. J. Med. 1987; 317:192.

14) Weiser W.Y., Van Niel A., Clark C., David J.R., Remold H.G.: Recombinant human granulocyte/macrophage colony-stimulating factor activates intracellular killing of

Leishmania donovani by human monocyte-derived macrophages. J. Exp. Med. 1987; 166:1436.

15) Grabstein K.H., Urdal D.L., Tushinski R.J., Mochizuki D.Y., Price V.L., Cantrell M.A., Gillis S., Conlon P.J.: Induction of macrophage tumoricidal activity by granulocyte-macrophage colony stimulating factor. Science 1986; 232:506.

16) Osborn L., Kunkel S., Nabel G.J.: Tumor necrosis factor alfa and interleukin-1 stimulate the human immunodeficiency virus enhancer by activation of the nuclear factor kB. Proc. Natl. Acad. Sci., Usa 1989; 86:2336.

17) Pluda J.M., Yarchoan R., Smith P.D., McAtee N., Shay L.E., Oette D., Maha M., Wahl S.M., Myers C.E., Broder S.: Subcutaneous recombinant granulocyte-macrophage colony stimulating factor used as a single agent and in an alternative regimen with azidothymidine in leukopenic patients with severe human immunodeficiency virus infection. Blood 1990; 76:463.

18) Ashorn P., Moss B., Weinstein J.N., Chaudhary V.K., Fitzgerald D.J., Pastan I., Berger E.A.: Elimination of infectious human immunodeficiency virus from human T-cell cultures by synergistic action of CD4-pseudomonas exotoxin and reverse transcriptase inhibitors. Proc. Natl. Acad. Sci. USA 1990; 87:8889.

THE CASE FOR SYNERGY OF THYMIC HORMONES AND INTERLEUKINS

IN IMMUNE RECONSTITUTION

J.W. Hadden, P.H. Malec, M. Sosa and E.M. Hadden

Division of Immunopharmacology
University of South Florida Medical College
Tampa, Florida 33612, USA

SUMMARY

The regulation of T cell development can be viewed as a process requiring the thymus and influenced by endocrine and interleukin-type hormonal influences. Thymic hormones are produced by thymic epithelial cells and regulate the differentiation and function of pre and post-thymic T cells but they do not alone induce intrathymic maturation. Interleukins I and II are produced by activated leukocytes (macrophages and T lymphocytes) and, in addition to regulating mature T cell proliferation, promote in a synergistic manner the proliferation and differentiation of pre T cells (prothymocytes and intrathymic precursors) and of immature thymocytes. Thymic epithelial cells produce thymic hormones and IL1, IL6 and GM-CSF which will, with IL2, promote the responses of immature and mature T lymphocytes. Mixed interleukins, but not thymosin fraction V, promote the development of T cells in neonatal mice and their renewal in aged hydrocortisone-treated mice. Combination treatment with mixed interleukins and thymosin fraction V are synergistic in restoring T cell number and function in secondary T cell immunodeficiency associated with aged hydrocortisone-treated mice.

INTRODUCTION

The thymus gland is considered the central lymphoid organ of the cellular immune or T lymphocyte system. It is credited with the guided development of the pre-committed prothymocyte into a fully mature, functional T cell capable of expressing many regulatory and effector functions. Despite this central role for the thymus in T cell development, only recently have we been able to visualize the complexities of this process. Cellular immunologists have delved deeply into defining the many surface markers and functional changes which characterize the stepwise ontogeny of the T cell. This search has developed a static view of the sequence of developmental events and it is difficult to see clearly what regulatory events dictate the initial development of the system, the possible expansion of the system based upon demands placed by intense expression of cellular immunity and, finally, the replenishment of the T cell system following profound depletion as with multidrug chemotherapy or total body irradiation.

Combination Therapies, Edited by A.L. Goldstein and
E. Garaci, Plenum Press, New York, 1992

It will be the purpose of this short review to focus on several recent developments which begin to clarify the molecular and humoral events involved in the development of the cellular immune system. These developments make it clear that immunopharmacologic strategies to promote T lymphocyte development and function should employ combinations of interleukins and thymic hormones.

Humoral Factors on T Cell Development

Thymic Hormones

A number of substances have been extracted from the thymus gland and termed thymic hormones (Goldstein, 1984). These substances are thought to be derived from the hormone-producing cells of the thymus, the thymic epithelial cells. Three thymic hormone preparations have been purified to homogeneity and synthesized either by chemical synthesis or genetic engineering. These are: thymopoietin, thymosin α 1, and thymulin (previously FTS). All of these thymic hormones have been shown to induce prothymocyte differentiation and to modulate T cell function in one or another assay; however, few direct comparisons have been made to allow a proper assessment of differences in their actions. Their capacity to modulate T cell development is generally consistent with events which are known to occur in the presence of a thymus; however, evidence of their intrathymic actions are notably lacking. We have been unable to show that they induce the maturation of immature thymocytes by surface markers or functional criteria (Chen, et al., 1982, 1983; Hadden, et al., 1986a). Others have reached similar conclusions with thymic epithelial cell (TEC) products (Andrews, et al., 1985). It is useful then to consider thymic hormones as being central to thymic chemotactic influences (Champion et al., 1986) which commit prothymocytes to the first step of development (Thy 1 aquisition in the mouse) and, thereafter, sustain T cell commitment and make possible subsequent developmental steps. They cannot be considered to induce these subsequent steps. They modulate IL2 production and receptor display and other responses of mature T cells (Zatz et al., 1984; Sztein et al., 1986); in this sense they operate as humoral regulators maintaining T cell commitment.

Thus, thymic hormones can be visualized to operate as true hormones (i.e., being blood born and acting on target cells at a distance).

The thymic hormones never have qualified as inducing or determining the growth of any cell in the T cell lineage; they are not growth factors. With the knowledge that most cell types have one or more growth factors thought to be critical for their development, it was appropriate to search for alternative regulators of intrathymic development, particularly those which would relate to growth like interleukins I and II (IL1 and IL2).

Interleukins I and II

IL2 is a product of mature T cells and immature large granular lymphocytes (probably pre-T cells). The production of IL2 by mature T cells results from the action of a monocyte/macrophage product called interleukin I (IL1). IL2 acts to allow antigen-primed, mature T cells (triggered to synthesize RNA and protein) to enter DNA synthesis and to replicate clonally. It was previously thought that only mature T cells respond to IL1 to make IL2; however, immature T cells have recently been described to respond to both IL1 and IL2.

We initially showed that IL2 induces immature thymocytes to undergo changes in surface markers characteristics of the transition from the immature to the mature phenotype (Chen, et al., 1982, 1983). We and others (Chen, et al., 1982, 1983; Conlon, et al., 1982; Hadden, et al., 1986a) subsequently showed that recombinant (r)IL2 will induce these cells to mature to the point of acquiring mitogen responsiveness including the ability to make IL2 as well as to respond to it. The responsive cells have been more recently localized in the double negative intrathymic precursor population of mouse thymus and these cells have been further shown to have IL2 receptors (Ceredig, et al., 1985; Raulet, 1985). We further found that these immature thymocytes respond to recombinant IL1 ß to a small degree and show a marked synergy with IL2 to enhance their proliferation (Hadden, et al., 1990). Independently, Falk, et al. (1987) showed that the double negative intrathymic precursor had this synergistic responsiveness to IL1 and IL2. IL1 induces the high affinity IL2 receptor by inducing the beta receptor component so it seems likely that the synergy of IL2 observed with IL1 results from the induction of high affinity IL2 receptors on these cells.

It seemed reasonable to question how early in the ontogeny of T cells this synergistic responsiveness to IL2 and IL1 is expressed. The first step of T cell development was determined initially by the method of Komuro and Boyse (1973). The Komuro-Boyse assay employs prothymocytes obtained from athymic nude mice and the induction of Thy 1 as a measure of one of the earliest steps of T cell differentiation.

A number of thymic hormone preparations are active in the induction of T cell differentiation in this assay. These include, thymosin fraction V, thymosin α 1, thymulin, and thymopoietin (Hadden, et al., 1986a). We (Hadden, et al., 1986b) found that both natural and recombinant IL2 are also active to induce maturation in this assay and that IL2 regulates the basal proliferation of this cell population. These represent the first observations delineating a functional role for IL2 on prothymocytes and indicate that these cells must have IL2 receptors.

We (Hadden, et al., 1989) showed that IL1 alone has a small effect to induce proliferation and acts synergistically with IL2. The effect of the combination of recombinant IL1 and IL2 is somewhat greater than one-half the effect of the natural mixed lymphokine preparation suggesting that other lymphokines are involved.

The degree of maturation in the prothymocyte induction assay is small in terms of the degree of receptor expression found on thymocytes and we found that the additional presence, in coculture, of thymic epithelial cells was necesarry to bring out surface marker induction and IL2-dependent proliferation manifested by the intrathymic immature T cell (Wiranowska, et al., 1987). Mixed thymic hormones (as thymosin fraction V) were not active with IL2 in this regard, implying that unique induction processes (e.g., cell contact) are involved. Thymic epithelial cells (TEC) bind to intrathymic T cells by LFA3-CD2 receptor ligands (Vollger, et al., 1987) and this process leads to IL1 production by the TEC (Le et al, 1990) and to IL2 receptor expression on the T cells (Denning, et al., 1988).

The foregoing observations provide the basis for suggesting that IL1 and IL2 responsiveness can no longer be considered an exclusive trait of mature T lymphocytes; in fact, the responsiveness precedes the first identifiable T cell marker. It seems likely that local sources of IL1 and IL2 in bone marrow and thymus would be important complementary influences to thymic hormones in early T cell development.

The induction of maturation of Thy 1- negative cells to Thy -1 positive functions characteristic of mature T lymphocytes; furthermore, none of the aforementioned substances alone can induce function of Thy 1-positive prothymocytes. The appropriate inducers of intrathymic maturation must, therefore, be provided by the thymic epithelial cells.

Historically, many investigators have probed thymic epithelial cells for active factors. Thymulin, thymopoietin and thymosin α 1 have been confirmed to be present (Dardenne, et al., 1986; Fabien et al., 1988). A host of growth or development promoting factors have been described (Beardsley et al., 1983; Glimcher et al, 1983; Henson et al, 1978; Kruisbeck, 1979; Miyazawa et al 1983; Mizutani et al, 1978; Nieburgs et al, 1987; Ogata et al, 1987; Pfeifer et al, 1981) and a number of lymphokine entities were thought to have been excluded (e.g. IL1, 2,3,4, and IFN). In contrast, recent work (Le, et al., 1987, 1988, 1990; Galy et al, 1989) indicate that TEC produce IL1, IL6, CSF-GM and CSF1. It remains to be determined which other factors are produced by TEC. To our thinking, the production of IL1 by TEC and IA+ dendritic cells is a central event in their contribution to T cell development for the reasons outlined above.

In addition, a variety of other interleukins (IL3, IL4, IL6 and GM-CSF) may be capable of modulating T cell development at different stages. These observations imply that many substances act collectively in promoting T cell development and function. They provide the basis for speculating that interleukins, particularly IL1 and IL2, act as "signals from the periphery" circulating via blood to the thymus to promote a series of maturational steps of immature T cells leading to replenishment of peripheral pool with new, functionally mature T cells.

In order to test the prediction that these substances could promote T cell development in vivo we employed three T cell-deficient animal models; athymic nude mice, neonatal mice and aged, hydrocortisone treated mice. The athymic mouse has few T cells which bear Thy 1.2 surface markers and respond to Con A. It is not clear whether the few T cells which develop in these mice do so extrathymically or via interaction with thymic epithelial remnants known to exist in them (Ikehara, et al., 1984, 1987). Previous experiments suggested that thymic hormones could reconstitute functional T cells in these mice (Ikehara, et al., 1975). Our own experience (Hadden, et al, 1989b) is that prolonged treatment of these mice with thymosin fraction V, mixed natural lymphokines and recombinant IL2 (rIL2) yields no significant effect to induce T cells. After 12 weeks of treatment, only a thymus graft restored functional T cells. While interleukins enhanced immature T cell proliferative responses, we have concluded that interleukins cannot bypass the thymus to yield T cell development.

Neonatal mice (< 10 days) have less than 5% Thy 1-positive T cells in their spleens and these cells have a low level of Thy 1 expression. Responses to Concanavalin A (+ IL2) are less than 10% of the adult response. We (Hadden et al, 1989) found that 5 day treatment of these mice with mixed lymphokine preparation (but not rIL2 or thymic hormones as thymosin fraction V) doubles the number of Thy 1.2+ cells and the Con A (+ IL2) proliferative responses of their spleen cells.

Using a similar protocol (Hadden, et al., 1991), we treated aged mice (12+ months) with 5mg hydrocortisone to further reduce the age-dependent decline of thymus and spleen size. Treatment for 5 days with mixed interleukins (BCIL), but not rIL2 or thymosin fraction V, restored the spleen and thymus weights and cellularity to somewhat greater than pre-treatment levels (Figure 1) BCIL (but not rIL2 or thymosin fraction V) augmented significantly thymocyte proliferative responses to rIL1, rIL2, and BCIL in vitro (Figure

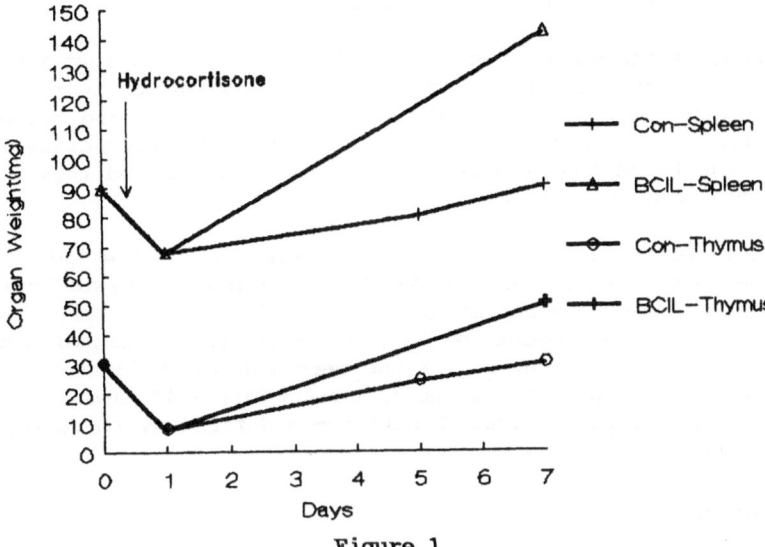

Figure 1

Aged breeder mice (approximately 12 months) were treated at day 0 with hydrocortisone to induce a "chemical thymectomy" and reduction of spleen weight.   Controls (Con) were treated daily with saline i.p. day 2-6 and treated mice (BCIL) received mixed interleukins (50 units IL2 equivalence) daily i.p. day 2-6.   Spleen and thymus weights are expressed in mg.

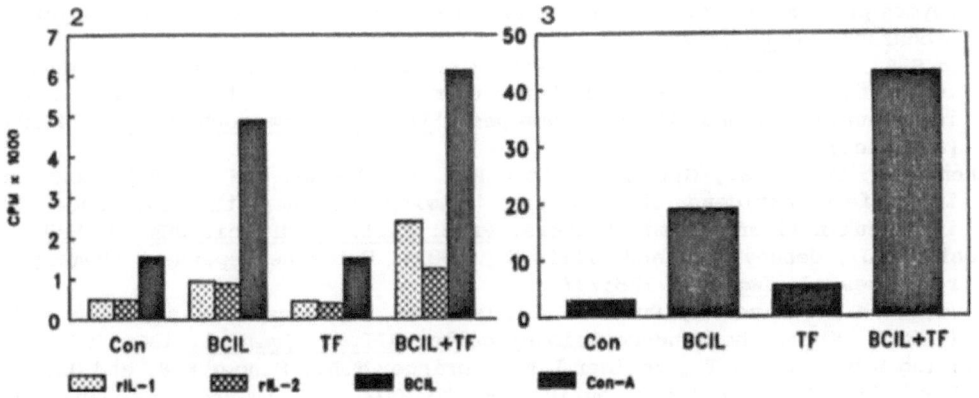

Figure 2 and 3

In the same protocol as Figure 1, mice were treated day 2-6 with saline (Con), BC-IL; thymosin fraction V (TF)(100 ug day i.p.) or the combination of BC-IL and TF.   In vitro proliferative responses of thymocytes to rIL1 (1ng/ml), rIL2 (2 units/ml), or BC-IL (2 units IL2 equivalence/ml) (Figure 2) or to Con-A (1.5 ug/ml) (Figure 3) were measured in vitro by thymidine incorporation (CPM).

2) and to Con A (Figure 3). Thymosin fraction V, while inactive alone, significantly potentiated the effects of BC-IL on thymocyte responses to interleukins (Figure 2) and Con A (Figure 3).

The results of these models are supportive of the notion that interleukins (particularly IL1 and IL2 in synergy) can act in an endocrine manner (i.e., they can be injected in one site and they will circulate and act distally) to enhance the evolution of T cells by marker and functional criteria when a thymus is present and that the presence of interleukins and thymic hormones potentiate T lymphocyte evolution.

The tentative conclusions from this review are that while the thymus provides the endocrine milieu through its secretion of thymic hormones and the informational microenvironmental through cellular contacts, the primary signals for T cell development derive from interleukin hormonal messages to repopulate the periphery based upon the need for replenishment. It seems logical to employ mixed interleukins in conjunction with thymic hormones in those with thymic involution and T cell immunodeficiency to restore T cell number and function.

ACKOWLEDGEMENTS

This work was supported in part by a grant from Cel-Sci, Inc.

REFERENCES

Andrews P., Shortman K., Scollay R., Potworowski E.F., Kruisbeek A.M., Goldstein G., Trainin N. and Bach J-F. (1985). Thymus hormones do not induce proliferative ability or cytolytic function in PNA+ cortical thymocytes. Cell. Immunol. 91:455.

Beardsley T.R., Pierschbacher M., Wetzel G.D. and Hays E.F. (1983). Induction of T cell maturation by a cloned line of thymic epithelial (TEP1). Proc. Natl. Acad. Sci. USA 80:6005.

Ceredig R., Lowenthal J.W., Nahholz M. and MacDonald H.R. (1985). Expression of interleukin-2 receptors as a differentiation marker on intrathymic stem cells. Nature 314:98.

Champion S., Imhof B.A., Savanger P. and Thiery J.P. (1986). The embryonic thymus produces chemotactic peptides involved in the homing of hemopoietic precursors. Cell 44:781.

Chen S.S., Tung J.S., Gillis S., Good R.A. and Hadden J.W. (1982). Changes in surface antigens of immature thymocytes under the influence of interleukin II and thymic hormones. Int. J. Immunopharmacol. 4:381 (abstract).

Chen S.S., Tung J.S., Gillis S., Good R.A. and Hadden J.W. (1983). Changes in surface antigens of immature thymocytes under the influence of interleukin II and thymic factors. Proc. Natl. Acad. Sci. USA 80:5980.

Conlon P.J., Henney C.S. and Gillis S. (1982). Cytokine-dependent thymocyte responses. J. Immunol. 128:797.

Dardenne M., Savino W., Duval D., Kaiserlian D., Hassid J. and Bach J-F. (1986). Thymic hormone-containing cells. VII. J. Immunol. 136:1303.

Denning S.M., Tuck D.T., Vollger L.W., Springer T.A., Singer K.H. and Haynes B.F. (1987). Monoclonal antibodies to CD2 and lymphocytes function associated antigen 3 inhibit human thymic epithelial cell-dependent mature thymocyte activation. J. of Immunology 139:2573.

Denning S.M., Kurtzberg J., Le P.T., Tuck D.T., Singer K.H. and Haynes B.F. (1988). Human thymic epithelial cells directly induce activation of autologous immature thymocytes. Proc. Natl. Acad. Sci. 85:3125.

Fabien N., Auger C. and Monier J-C. (1988). Immunolocalization of thymosin alpha 1, thymopoietin and thymulin in mouse thymic epithelial cells at different stages of culture: a light and electron microscopic study. Immunology 63:721.

Falk W., Kyewski B., Mannel D. and Kramer P.H. (1987). Growth of double negative mouse thymocytes is initiated by the combined action of interleukin I and interleukin 2. Lymph. Res. 6:75 (abstract).

Galy A., Dinarello C., Kupper T., Kameda A. and Hadden J.W. (1990). Effects of cytokines on human thymic epithelial cells in culture. Cell. Immunol. 129:161.

Glimcher L. H., Kruisbeek A.M., Paul W.E. and Green I. (1983). Functional activity of a transformed thymic epithelial cell line. Scand. J. Immunol. 17:1.

Goldstein A. (Ed.)(1984). Thymic Hormones and Lymphokines. New York, Plenum Press.

Hadden J.W., Specter S., Galy A., Touraine J.L. and Hadden E.M. (1986a). Thymic hormones, interleukins, endotoxin and thymomimetic drugs. In: Immunopharmacology III (Chedid L., Hadden J., Spreafico F., Dukor P. and Willoughby D., Eds.) Oxford, Pergamon Press, pp. 487.

Hadden J.W., Chen H., Wang Y., Galy A. and Hadden E.M. (1989a). Strategies of immune reconstitution: Effects of lymphokines on murine T cell development in vitro and in vivo. Life Sciences 44:v-xii.

Hadden J.W., Caspritz G., Zheng Q.Y., Chen H., Wolstencroft, R. and Hadden E.M. (1989). Thymosin, interleukins, isoprinosine and imuthiol do not reconstitute T cells in athymic nude mice. Int. J. Immunopharmacol. 11:13.

Hadden E.M., Malec P. and Hadden J.W. (1991) Int. J. Immunopharmacol. (in press).

Hensen E.J., Hoefsmit E.C.M. and Van Den Tweel J.G. (1978). Augmentation of mitogen responsiveness in human lymphocytes by a humoral factor obtained from thymic epithelial cultures. Clin. Exp. Immunol. 32:309.

Ikehara S., Hamashima Y. and Masuda T. (1975). Immunological restoration of both thymectomised and athymic nude mice by a thymus factor. Nature 258:335.

Ikehara S., Pahwa R., Fernandez G., Hansen C. and Good R.A. (1984). Functional T cells in athymic nude mice. Proc. Natl. Acad. Sci. USA 81:886.

Ikehara S., Shimuzu Y., Yasumizu R., Nakamura T., Inaba M., Inoues S., Oyaizu N., Sugiura K., Oo M.M., Hamashima Y. and Good. R.A. (1987). Thymic rudiments are responsible for induction of functional T cells in nu/nu mice. Thymus 10:93.

Komuro K. and Boyse E.A. (1973). Induction of T lymphocytes from precursor cells in vitro by a product of the thymus. J. Exp. Med. 138:479.

Kruisbeek A.M. (1979). Thymic factors and T cell maturation in vitro: A comparison of the effects of thymic cultures with thymic extracts and thymus dependent serum factors. Thymus 1:163.

Le P.T., Tuck D.T., Dinarello C., Haynes B.F. and Singer K.H. (1987). Human thymic epithelial cell produce interleukin I. J. Immunol. 138:2520.

Le P.T., Kurtzberg J., Brandt S.T., Niedel J.E., Haynes B.F. and Singer K.H. (1988). Human thymic epithelial cells produce granulocyte and macrophage colony-stimulating factors. J. of Immunology 141:1211.

Le P.T., Vollger L.W., Haynes B.F. and Singer K.H. (1990). Ligand binding to the LFA-3 cell adhesion molecule induces IL-1 production by human thymic epithelial cells. J. of Immunology 144:4541.

Miyazawa T., Nakamura H., Sato C. and Suzuki R. (1983). Growth of a cultured leukemia subline was promoted by conditioned medium of thymic reticuloepithelial-like cells (B6TE). Leuk. Res. 7:637.

Mizutani S., Watt S.M., Robertson D., Hussein S., Healy L.E., Furley A.J.W.

and Greaves M.F. (1978). Cloning of human thymic subcapsular cortex epithelial cells with T lymphocyte binding sites and hemopoietic growth factor activity. Proc. Natl. Acad. Sci. USA 84:4999.

Nieburgs A.C., Picciano P., Korn J.H. and Cohen S. (1987). Thymic epithelium in vitro. Cell. Immunol. 104:182.

Ogata M., Sato S., Sano H., Hamgoka T., Doi H., Nakanishi K., Asano Y., Itoh T. and Fujiwara H. (1987). Thymic strom-derived T cell growth factor (TSTGF).   J. Immunol. 139:2675.

Pfeifer J.D., Wetzel G.D. and Dutton R.W. (1986). Partial purification and characterization of a factor from a cloned thymic epithelium cell line. J. Immunol. 136:555.

Raulet D.H. (1985). Expression and function of interleukin-2 receptors on immature thymocytes. Nature 314:101.

Sztein M.B., Serrate S.A. and Goldstein A.L. (1986) Modulation of interleukin 2 receptor expression on normal human lymphoctyes by thymic hormones. Proc. Natl. Acad. Sci. 83:6107.

Wiranowska M., Kaido T., Caspritz G., Cook J. and Hadden J.W. (1987). Interleukins 2 and co-culture with thymic epithelial cells synergistically induce prothymocyte differentiation and proliferation.   Thymus 10:231.

Zatz M.M., Oliver J., Samuels C., Skotnicki, Sztein M.B. and Goldstein A.L. (1984). Thymosin increases production of T-cell growth factor by normal human peripheral blood lymphocytes. Proc. Natl. Acad. Sci. 81:2882.

INDUCING IMMUNITY TO HUMAN MELANOMA CELLS: OPENING THE BAG

OF IMMUNOLOGICAL TRICKS

David Berd

Thomas Jefferson University
Philadelphia, PA

Successful immunotherapy of human cancer requires the induction of a cell-mediated immune response to weakly immunogenic tumor-associated antigens. To accomplish that aim, we have used two immunological strategies, each of which is based on well-established findings in experimental animals.

First, we tested the cytotoxic drug, cyclophosphamide (CY), which augments immunity by inhibiting suppressor T cell function (Maguire and Ettore, 1967). We treated 64 patients with metastatic melanoma using a melanoma vaccine preceded by low dose CY and monitored immunological effects and anti-tumor activity (Berd et al, 1991). On day 0, the patients were given CY 300 mg/M^2 IV. Three days later, they were injected intradermally with vaccine consisting of $10\text{-}25\text{x}10^6$ autologous, enzymatically-dissociated, cryopreserved, irradiated (2500 R) tumor cells mixed with BCG. This treatment sequence was repeated every 28 days. Prior to receiving vaccine, and at various times afterward, they were tested for DTH to autologous melanoma cells and to control materials. Patients were continued on the study until there was clear evidence of progression of metastatic disease or until the supply of vaccine was exhausted. The number of vaccine treatments administered per patient ranged from 2 to 16, with a median of 5.

The vaccine was prepared by a modification of the method of Peters et al (1979). Freshly excised tumor masses were trimmed of skin, fat, and necrotic tissue and minced in cold HBSS (M.A. Bioproducts, Bethesda, MD). Cells that were released into the medium by mechanical dissociation were put aside, stored separately, and used for skin-testing. The minced tumor pieces were placed in an enzyme solution, consisting of collagenase (from *Clostridium* sp.) and deoxyribonuclease (DNAse; bovine) (Sigma Chemical Co., St. Louis, MO), and dissociated as described previously (Berd et al, 1986). Tumor cells were suspended in freezing medium, consisting of RPMI 1640 with 10% dimethylsulfoxide and either 10% pooled human AB+ serum or 1% human albumen without antibiotics, and frozen in a controlled rate freezer (Union Carbide, Indianapolis, IN) and stored in the liquid phase of liquid nitrogen until needed. Fetal bovine serum was not used. On the day that a patient was to be skin-tested or treated, the cells were thawed, irradiated to a dose of 2500 R, washed, and resuspended in HBSS at an appropriate concentration. The vaccine consisted of $10\text{-}25\text{x}10^6$ enzyme-dissociated, trypan blue-excluding tumor cells suspended in 0.2 ml HBSS to which were added BCG, 0.1 ml (approximately $0.8\text{-}2.6\text{x}10^6$ viable organisms) (Glaxo, Research Triangle Park, NC). The mixture was injected intradermally in three adjacent sites on the upper arms or legs; limbs ipsilateral to a lymph node resection were not used.

Combination Therapies, Edited by A.L. Goldstein and
E. Garaci, Plenum Press, New York, 1992

The patients were skin-tested with each of the following materials: 1)1×10^6 melanoma cells dissociated mechanically, *i.e.*, not exposed to enzymes; 2)3×10^6 autologous peripheral blood mononuclear cells, that had been separated on Ficoll-metrizoate (Histopaque; Sigma Chemical Co., St. Louis, MO) and cryopreserved as described for the melanoma cells; 3)PPD (Connaught Laboratories, Willowdale, Ontario, Canada); 4)microbial recall antigens, trichophyton, candida (Hollister-Stier, Spokane, WA) and mumps (Connaught Laboratories); and 5)collagenase and DNAse, separately or mixed, each at a concentration of 1 ug/ml (the highest concentration that did not produce a skin reaction in untreated patients). In the beginning of the study, we suspended the cells in HBSS containing the pH indicator, phenol red. After finding evidence in one patient that the phenol red was itself immunogenic, we used only HBSS without phenol red for the duration of the study. At no time were cells used for skin testing exposed to fetal bovine serum. DTH reactions were determined at 48 hours by measuring the largest diameter and right-angles diameter of the area of induration and calculating the mean.

Standard criteria for determining anti-tumor responses were used: 1)complete response = complete regression of all clinically evident metastases for at least 3 months; 2)partial response = at least 50% reduction in the mean diameter of a metastatic lesion without growth of other tumors or development of new metastases for at least 3 months; 3)delayed response = partial or complete response of metastases that did not appear until after immunotherapy had been started. Patients with stable metastases or tumor regression that did not meet these criteria were categorized as non-responders.

Of 40 evaluable patients with measurable metastases, 5 had responses - 4 complete and 1 partial - with a median duration of 10 months (7-84+ months). In 6 additional patients we observed an anti-tumor response that seems to be peculiar to this vaccine therapy - the regression of metastatic lesions that appeared after the immunotherapy was begun. This type of regression was observed only in subcutaneous and lymph node metastases and in 3/6 patients it occurred in two or more tumors. In one case, the regression of two tumors was preceded by the development of intense erythema and swelling in the subcutaneous tissue around them. Resolution of the inflammatory response and disappearance of the tumor mass (one tumor was excised) occurred over 2-3 weeks. Tumors that regressed completely never recurred, although all these patients eventually died of metastatic disease.

The toxicity of this immunotherapy was mild. A local inflammatory response developed at the vaccine injection site. This consisted of a papule that became ulcerated and drained small amounts of clear fluid with healing by 3-4 weeks after the injection. About 25% of the patients had mild nausea or vomiting following the first dose of CY, and that proportion increased to about 50% with subsequent doses. In most cases, oral prochlorperazine was sufficient to control emesis. No patients developed fever, chills, or malaise, nor did any develop clinical symptoms, such as arthralgias, suggesting auto-immunity. There were no significant changes in blood counts, routine serum chemistries or anti-nuclear antibody titers.

Delayed-type hypersensitivity (DTH) to autologous, mechanically-dissociated melanoma cells that had not been exposed to extraneous antigens, such as enzymes or fetal calf serum, increased significantly following immunotherapy (day 0 vs. day 49, $p < .001$; day 0 vs. day 161, $p < .001$; day 0 vs. day 217, $p = .021$). Overall, 26/43 patients (61%) exhibited a 5 mm or greater DTH response to autologous melanoma cells at some time point.

In our initial vaccine study (Berd et al, 1986), we found that CY-pretreated patients who were immunized with enzymatically-dissociated tumor cells developed strong DTH responses to those enzymes, *i.e.*, collagenase and DNAse; this rendered difficult the interpretation of DTH responses to enzymatically-dissociated cells and necessitated our use of mechanically-dissociated cells for skin-testing. We have confirmed that finding: Of 24 patients tested for DTH with a mixture of collagenase and DNAse (each at 1 ug/ml) after two vaccine treatments (day 49), 21 (88%) had responses >5mm. In seven patients who were skin-tested with each enzyme separately, DTH responses to collagenase were greater than to DNAse (mean difference $\pm$ SE: 6.7 mm $\pm$ 2.3; $p<.05$); this difference was expected since collagenase is of bacterial origin and DNAse is bovine.

Anti-tumor responses to the vaccine were strongly associated with DTH, as indicated by three observations: 1)8/10 patients who exhibited tumor regression had positive DTH. 2)In post-surgical adjuvant patients, there was a highly significant linear relationship ($p < .001$) between the intensity of DTH to autologous melanoma cells and the time to recurrence of tumor. 3)Nine patients who developed DTH to the autologous melanoma cells in their original vaccine developed new metastases that failed to elicit DTH or elicited a much smaller response.

In three cases we were able to excise regressing tumors for histological examination; regressing tumors were characterized by an intense infiltration of lymphocytes with, in some cases, focal tumor cell necrosis. Metastatic tumors excised from these patients before immunotherapy consisted of homogeneous masses of malignant cells without significant lymphocytic infiltration.

To increase the efficiency of the immunization process, we have more recently added a second manipulation: conjugation of the tumor cells to the hapten, dinitrophenyl (DNP). This approach is based on the idea that presentation of tumor antigens in the context of a strongly immunogenic hapten augments the development of immunity to those antigens (Mitchison, 1970; Fujiwara et al, 1984). After being sensitized to DNP by topical application of DNFB (dinitrofluorobenzene), patients were injected with DNP-vaccine every 28 days following pretreatment with low dose CY. The vaccine induced a striking inflammatory response in superficial metastases in 14/24 patients, consisting of erythema, swelling, warmth, and tenderness over tumor masses. Immunohistochemistry and flow cytometric analysis of biopsy specimens showed marked infiltration with lymphocytes, the majority of which were CD8+,HLA-DR+ T cells. Preliminary data suggest that these T cells are cytotoxic for autologous melanoma cells.

These studies indicate that an immune response to melanoma-associated antigens can be elicited in cancer-bearing patients and provide some basis for optimism about the prospects for developing active immunotherapy that has practical therapeutic value.

REFERENCES

Berd, D., Maguire, H.C., McCue, P., and Mastrangelo, M.J., 1990, Treatment of metastatic melanoma with an autologous tumor cell vaccine: Clinical and immunological results in 64 patients. J. Clin. Oncol., 8: 1858-1867.

Berd, D., Maguire, H.C. Jr., Mastrangelo, M.J., 1986, Induction of cell-mediated immunity to autologous melanoma cells and regression of metastases after treatment with a melanoma cell vaccine preceded by cyclophosphamide. Cancer Res. 46:2572-2577.

Fujiwara, H., Aoki, H., Yoshioka, T., Tomita, S., Ikegami, R., and Hamaoka, T., 1984, Establishment of a tumor-specific immunotherapy model utilizing TNP- reactive helper cell activity and its application to the autochthonous tumor system, J. Immunol., 133: 509-514.

Maguire, H.C. and Ettore, V.L., 1967, Enhancement of dinitrochlorobenzene (DNCB) contact sensitization by cyclophosphamide in the guinea pig. J. Invest. Dermatol., 48:39-42.

Mitchison, N.A., 1970, Immunologic approach to cancer. Transplant. Proc., 11: 92-103.

Peters, L.C., Brandhorst, J.S., Hanna, M.G. Jr., 1979, Preparation of
immunotherapeutic autologous tumor cell vaccines from solid tumors.
Cancer Res. 39:1353-1360.

IMMUNE MEDIATED TUMOR DESTRUCTION: CHALLENGES FOR THE 1990's

Paul M. Sondel

Departments of Pediatrics, Human Oncology and Genetics
The University of Wisconsin
Madison, Wisconsin

INTRODUCTION

Numerous experimentally induced tumor models, studied in murine systems, have indicated that successful approaches towards the immune eradication of neoplasms should be a clinical possibility. Central to many of these therapeutic approaches in mice are distinct roles for T lymphocytes, able to mediate antigen specific "major histo-compatibility complex (MHC)-restricted" recognition of tumor cells, as well as natural killer (NK) cells, able to destroy certain tumors in a less specific way, and without requiring the recognition of MHC molecules. Despite the myriad of algorithms enabling effective tumor destruction *in vitro* or in mice utilizing these immune cell popula-tions, successful application of these principles in patients has been possible only in the past few years. Immune mediated destruc-tion of tumors directly in patients, apparently by activated lympho-cytes, has now been reproducibly documented utilizing a number of clinical regimens. Even so, the majority of patients receiving these approaches do not show measurable clinical benefit. Thus, substan-tial improvement is required to enable practical and effective wide-spread application of these immunologic principles to patients with otherwise refractory cancers.

Current innovations involve combining distinct components of these treatments together into regimens hoped to be more effective. The many excellent presentations at this important symposium on combination therapies are reviewing numerous innovative approaches being pursued internationally in preclinical and clinical models. Thus, the purpose of this report is to focus on those preclinical and clinical findings from our own research team rather than comprehen-sively reviewing the vast accumulating information in this important and growing field.

CLINICAL EVIDENCE FOR LYMPHOCYTE INDUCED TUMOR CONTROL-THE "GRAFT VS. LEUKEMIA" EFFECT

Following extensive analyses of murine allogeneic bone marrow transplant (BMT) results, a clear clinical association between graft vs. host disease and prevention of leukemic relapse has been noted.[1] Analyses of International Bone Marrow Transplant Registry data indi-cate that graft vs. host disease (GVHD) itself is associated with a measurable "anti-leukemic" effect. Even without any clinically detectable GVHD, recipients of allogeneic BMT have less leukemic relapse than recipients of syngeneic BMT, indicating a role for some allorecognition event. Furthermore, individuals receiving

Combination Therapies, Edited by A.L. Goldstein and
E. Garaci, Plenum Press, New York, 1992

"unmanipulated" allogeneic BMT, who do not have clinically evident GVHD, also have less leukemic relapse than the recipients of T cell depleted allogeneic BMT, indicating an important role for T cells in the "antileukemic" effect.

A number of biologic mechanisms could account for these observations. Leukemia specific T lymphocytes may be playing a role. Alternatively, T lymphocytes specific for alloantigens might be recognizing a variety of leukemic and nonleukemic cells, but having a quantitatively greater destructive effect on leukemia cells because of their potentially greater susceptibility. Separate mechanisms could involve immune release of cytokines such as interleukin-2 (IL-2), to activate a variety of nonspecific cell populations (such as NK cells, macrophages, etc.). Despite the clear evidence for a graft vs. leukemia effect in the clinical BMT setting, it has been difficult to characterize in individual patients the mechanism of the "GVL effect" or to quantitate whether a "GVL reaction" is underway.[2]

T CELL REACTIVITY TO HUMAN CANCERS

Attempts to dissect immune reactivity to human tumors have been pursued with *in vitro* analyses. Many attempts to identify "tumor specific" T cells have yielded lymphocytes that may destroy autologous or HLA identical tumor cells, but also destroy certain other tissues, reminiscent of the LAK (lymphocyte activated killer) phenomenon of activated NK cells that do not mediate the immunologically exquisite specificity of alpha/beta MHC restricted T cells.[3] While exceptions do exist for certain individual patients,[4] for most neoplasms, reproducible tumor specific T cells reactive with autologous tumor have been difficult to document. A clear exception to this rule is that of metastatic melanoma where several laboratories have shown peripheral blood lymphocytes or tumor infiltrating lymphocytes from certain patients appear to be tumor specific MHC restricted T cells.[5] Even so, analyses of T cell receptor genes within tumor infiltrating lymphocytes of melanomas indicates that the *de novo* immune response is not a potent expansion of a single tumor reactive T cell clone.[6]

To further evaluate the "allogeneic" component of the "GVL" reaction, we have stimulated lymphocytes with leukemia cells from unrelated allogeneic individuals. These cultures, of course, contain T cells potently reactive to foreign MHC antigens and thus destroy both leukemia and remission cells from the sensitizing leukemia patient.[7] However, cloning of limiting dilution populations from these alloactivated cultures has enabled the identification of cell lines[7] and clones[8] that are potently able to destroy the leukemia cells *in vitro*, while causing little or no destruction of the remission cells from the same patient. In seven of seven leukemia patients where these alloreactive cultures have been extensively evaluated, it has been possible to differentiate the "alloreactive" clones which mediate equal killing of the leukemic and remission cells, from the "leukemia specific" clones that preferentially destroy the leukemia cells. These clones are alpha/beta T cells that, usually, bear the CD4 molecule and appear to be class II MHC restricted. The nature of the specificity mediated by these clones, the target antigens recognized by them, and the stability of this specificity all require further analyses *in vitro*. If analogous clones could induce a "GVL" reaction *in vivo* in murine models, without causing severe GVH, such *in vitro* screened allogeneic human clones could potentially provide a form of allogeneic anti-tumor reactivity for clinical testing.[9].

NON-MHC RESTRICTED KILLING

Just as cloning of allogeneic T cells enabled differentiation of effector cells with varying degrees of tumor specificity, we have taken this approach for analyses of non-MHC restricted effector

cells,[10,11] predominantly NK cells found in peripheral blood lymphocytes (PBL). Further analyses of the specificity pattern of different clones that mediate "non-MHC restricted killing" showed a
reproducible pattern of destruction of lymphoma target cells by
gamma/delta T cells vs. NK cells. Specifically, the gamma/delta T
cells destroyed Daudi but not Raji lymphoma cells while the NK clones
destroyed both.[12] These Daudi reactive T cells were virtually all of
the V gamma 9/V delta 2 subtype.[13] Paul Fisch documented that these
Daudi reactive T cell clones also recognized an antigen present in
mycobacterial extract.[14] Furthermore, the same subpopulation of
gamma/delta cells in fresh PBL could respond to Daudi cells or the
mycobacterial extract.[14] Antibody blocking studies and immunoprecipitation indicate that these gamma/delta cells are recognizing a molecule on Daudi and in the mycobacterial extract that is immunologically cross reactive with the GroEL family of heat shock proteins.[14]
This observation now raises many intriguing possibilities for the
role of gamma/delta cells and heat shock proteins in a variety of
auto immune and tumor immune reactions.

IN VIVO ACTIVATION OF EFFECTOR LYMPHOCYTES

While in vitro analyses of T cells and NK cells provide insight
as to potential antitumor approaches, it is their antitumor activity
in vivo that is sought. Numerous clinical regimens have been testing
Interleukin-2 as an effector cell activator for in vivo cancer treatment, stimulated by the pioneering work of Rosenberg and colleagues
at the National Cancer Institute. Our clinical testing has focused
on approaches towards in vivo activation of effector lymphocyte
function.[15] Well tolerated doses of human recombinant IL-2, given as
single agent therapy, clearly induce in vivo the activation of NK
cells to mediate the LAK phenomenon[16] in an IL-2 dependent manner.[17]
Antitumor responses in patients with renal cell carcinoma and melanoma have been observed.[18,19] In our studies the addition of
exogenous in vitro activated "LAK cells" does not appear to substantially add to the antitumor effect, while significantly increasing
the toxicity of this otherwise well tolerated IL-2 regimen.[20]

Despite the documented antitumor responses observed using a
variety of IL-2 based regimens (with or without LAK cell infusions),
the majority of patients treated do not show measurable antitumor
effects, while virtually all patients show dose dependent IL-2
related immune mediated toxicity. Clearly, murine studies show more
effective immune mediated antitumor effects are usually obtained if
the immune therapy is used in the "micrometastatic" stage, prior to
detection of "bulky" neoplasms. Thus, "adjuvant" testing of these
approaches might show a protective effect that could exceed the
"tumor response rate" in Phase II trials for patients with bulky
refractory disease. Even so, murine and in vitro studies provide
numerous clues to mechanisms whereby the IL-2 induced immune activation could be further augmented by combination with a variety of
other approaches.

T CELLS

Murine studies document the greater potency of tumor specific T
cells than of "LAK cells" in vivo, when combined with IL-2.
Approaches underway elsewhere are utilizing tumor infiltrating
lymphocytes (TIL) from patients with melanoma in order to expand, for
some patients, in vitro activated populations of cells that appear to
show some degree of tumor specific T cell reactivity.[21] Clinical
responses have been observed in some patients treated with such cells
together with IL-2. However, many patients with melanoma, and the
majority of patients with other histologic tumor types, do not
generate in vitro distinct tumor specific T lymphocyte populations
from their TIL populations grown by these methods.[22] Even so, if it
would be possible to activate these same populations directly in
vivo, such an approach would have greater applicability and avoid the

complex and tedious *in vitro* TIL expansion.[6,22] Several teams are successfully pursuing *in vivo* immunization schemes to potentially expand these same tumor specific T lymphocytes. Intriguingly, single agent treatment with IL-2, despite anticipated T cell activation, appears to have a depressive effect on many T cell functions.[23] *In vitro* activation with anti CD3 antibody together with IL-2 can cause a profound T cell expansion.[24] Murine studies[25] have shown *in vivo* treatment with anti CD3 antibody at low dose can augment antitumor T cell function; *in vitro* studies with human lymphocytes from patients receiving IL-2 corroborate this result.[26] Thus, *in vivo* treatment with anti-CD3 may be one additional means to activate endogenous T cells, possibly in combination with IL-2 or other treatments. Clinical testing of this possibility is now underway.

COMBINATION WITH MONOCLONAL ANTIBODIES

The toxicity of IL-2 is dose related and directly due to the activated lymphocytes. Therefore, in order to obtain an improved antitumor effect without simultaneously causing greater toxicity to normal tissues, it will be essential to increase the specificity of the lymphocyte-tumor interaction. Using lymphocytes activated *in vivo* by IL-2, the degree of tumor destruction *in vitro* can be dramatically enhanced when antibodies having the correct conformation to enable antibody dependent cell cytotoxicity (ADCC) are added.[27] A variety of murine and chimeric monoclonal antibodies potent at ADCC are becoming available for clinical trials. Combining IL-2 with *in vivo* infusion of tumor specific antibodies may provide the combined lymphocyte activation and augmented specificity to allow better tumor destruction of tumors such as melanoma, and potentially enable lymphocyte mediated destruction of tumors previously felt unresponsive to *in vivo* IL-2 therapy, such as breast or lung cancer.[27]

COMBINATIONS INVOLVING MULTIPLE AGENTS

Effective cancer treatments are now available for a variety of malignancies. Particularly in the pediatric setting, combined multimodal approaches utilizing surgery, radiation therapy, and combinations of multiple chemotherapeutic agents, are proving effective.[28] Given the complex and constantly changing biologic behavior of growing neoplasms, it seems unlikely that a single biologic treatment modality will prove effective for patients with rapidly progressive malignancies refractory to all other approaches. In fact, it seems remarkable that any clinical antitumor responses have been observed using the approaches tested to date. Both clinical and laboratory models would suggest that integration of combined biologic approaches having an antitumor effect at the cellular level will be most effective when integrated into standard treatment regimens. Thus, one could imagine clinical treatment of an otherwise refractory malignancy to potentially involve the following sequential steps:

1) surgical removal of resectable tumor;

2) local radiation therapy to known non-resectable areas and to the "tumor field";

3) multi-agent chemotherapy to provide "cytoreduction" of chemotherapy responsive metastatic malignant cells;

4) hematopoietic supportive therapy (i.e. autologous stem cells or recombinant colony stimulating factors) to prevent severe myelosuppression and facilitate initiation of immunologic therapy;

5) combined "immunologic" therapy utilizing:

   a) effector cell activators (IL-2); b) modifiers (such as interferon or tumor necrosis factor) to modify susceptibility of tumor cell to immune destruction and increase expression of surface membrane antigens and adhesion molecules that might influence antibody or lymphocyte binding; c) infusion of a "cocktail" of biologically distinct monoclonal antibodies, each binding to different "tumor selective" antigens on the tumor cells, and able to either facilitate lymphocyte destruction of tumor, or deliver drug or toxin to tumor;

6)   initiate an "immunization" regimen with purified "tumor antigen" to activate protective endogenous immunity able to prevent subsequent recurrence.

Obviously, each of the steps in the above scenario involves multiple variables, any of which could have a major impact on the ultimate efficacy of the approach. However, because the antitumor efficacy of the individual components of this "combined approach" might not be dramatic or easily measured in clinical trials, it will be important to test these variables in protocols combining these distinct approaches.[29] Clearly the biologic reagents are becoming available, and "current standard therapy" is not effective for all too many patients with malignancies. Close interactions between clinical research teams, biotechnical companies providing reagents, and federal regulatory agencies enabling the combined clinical testing of reagents from a variety of sources, are absolutely essential in order to make these important large steps during the current decade.

ACKNOWLEDGEMENTS

This work has been supported by American Cancer Society Grant CH-237, and NIH Grants CA-32685, CM-47669, CA-53441, CM-87290, and RR-03186. Thanks are also due to the many laboratory and clinical colleagues and collaborators who have made the above reviewed research possible, particularly Dr. Jacquelyn A. Hank who has been instrumental in all of these studies, and to Judith Andreson and Mary Pankratz for preparation of this manuscript.

REFERENCES

1. M.M. Horowitz, R.P. Gale, P.M. Sondel, J.M. Goldman, J. Kersey, H-J. Kolb, A.A. Rimm, O. Ringden, C. Rozman, B. Speck, R.L. Truitt, F.E. Zwaan, and M.M. Bortin. Graft-vs-leukemia reactions following bone marrow transplantation. Blood 75:555 (1990).

2. P.M. Sondel, J.A. Hank, J. Molenda, J. Blank, W. Borcherding, W. Longo, M.E. Trigg, R. Hong, and M.J. Bozdech. Relapse of host leukemic lymphoblasts following engraftment by an HLA-mismatched marrow transplant: mechanisms of escape from the "graft versus leukemia" effect. Exper. Hematol. 13:782 (1985).

3. P.M. Sondel, J.A. Hank, P.C. Kohler, B.P. Chen, D.Z. Minkoff, and J. Molenda. Destruction of autologous human lymphocytes by interleukin-2-activated cytotoxic cells. J. Immunol. 137:502 (1986).

4. P. Fisch, G. Weil-Hillman, M. Uppenkamp, J.A. Hank, B.P. Chen, J.A. Sosman, A. Bridges, O.R. Colamonici, and P.M. Sondel. Antigen-specific recognition of autologous leukemia cells and allogeneic class-I MHC antigens by IL-2 activated cytotoxic T-cells from a patient with acute T-cell leukemia. Blood 74:343 (1989).

5. K. Itoh, C. Platsoucas, and C. Balch. Autologous tumor specific cytoxic T lymphocytes in the infiltrate of human metastatic melanoma. J. Exper. Med. 168:1419 (1988).

6. M.R. Albertini, J.A. Nicklas, B.F. Chastenay, T.C. Hunter, R.J. Albertini, J.A. Hank, and P.M. Sondel. Analysis of T-cell receptor gamma and beta genes from peripheral blood, regional lymph nodes and tumor infiltrating lymphocyte clones from melanoma patients. Cancer Immunol. Immunother. 32:325 (1991).

7. J.A. Sosman, K.R. Oettel, J.A. Hank, P. Fisch, and P.M. Sondel. Specific recognition of human leukemic cells by allogeneic T cell lines. Transplantation 48:486 (1989).

8. J.A. Sosman, K. Oettel, S.D. Smith, J.A. Hank, P. Fisch, and P.M. Sondel. Specific recognition of human leukemic cells by allogeneic T cells: II. Evidence for HLA-D restricted unique determinants on leukemic cells which are cross-reactive with determinants present on unrelated non-leukemic cells. Blood 75:2005 (1990).

9. J.A. Sosman and P.M. Sondel. The Graft Versus Leukemia Effect: Possible mechanisms and clinical significance to the Biologic Therapy of Leukemia. Bone Marrow Transplantation, In press, 1991.

10. B.P. Chen, M. Malkovsky, J.A. Hank, J.A. Molenda, and P.M. Sondel. Nonrestricted cytotoxicity mediated by interleukin-2 expanded leukocytes is inhibited by anti-LFA-1 monoclonal antibodies (MoAb) but potentiated by anti-CD3 MoAb. Cellular Immunol. 110:282 (1987).

11. B.P. Chen, J.A. Hank, E.E. Kraus, and P.M. Sondel. Selective lysis of target cells by interleukin-2 expanded peripheral blood mononuclear leukocyte clones. Cellular Immunol. 118:458 (1989).

12. P. Fisch, M. Malkovsky, E. Braakman, R.L.H. Bolhuis, A. Prieve, J.A. Sosman, V.A. Lam, and P.M. Sondel PM. Gamma/delta T-cell clones and natural killer-cell clones mediate distinct patterns of non-major histocompatibility complex-restricted cytolysis. J. Exp. Med. 171:1567 (1990).

13. E. Sturm, E. Braakman, P. Fisch, R.J. Vreugdenhil, P.M. Sondel, and R.L.H. Bolhuis. MCH unrestricted cytotoxic activity of cloned human TCR lymphocytes: Specific lysis of Daudi cells correlates with the usage of a gamma 9-delta 2 TCR gene-rearrangement. J. Immunol. 145:3202 (1990).

14. P. Fisch, M. Malkovsky, S. Kovats, E. Sturm, E. Braakman, B.S. Klein, S.D. Voss, L.W. Morrissey, R. DeMars, W.J. Welch, R.L.H. Bolhuis, and P.M. Sondel. Recognition by Human V-gamma 9/V-delta 2 T cells of a GroEL homolog on Daudi Burkitt's lymphoma cells. Science 250:1269 (1990).

15. P.M. Sondel, P.C. Kohler, J.A. Hank, K.H. Moore, N. Rosenthal, J. Sosman, R. Bechhofer, and B. Storer. Clinical and immunologic effects of recombinant interleukin-2 given by repetitive weekly cycles to patients with cancer. Cancer Res. 48:2561 (1988).

16. J.A. Hank, P.C. Kohler, G.W. Hillman, N. Rosenthal, K.H. Moore, B. Storer, D. Minkoff, J. Bradshaw, R. Bechhofer, and P.M. Sondel. In vivo induction of the lymphokine-activated killer phenomenon: Interleukin 2-dependent human non-major histocompatibility complex-restricted cytotoxicity generated in vivo during administration of human recombinant interleukin 2. Cancer Res. 48:1965 (1988).

17. J.A. Hank, G.W. Hillman, J.E. Surfus, J.A. Sosman, and P.M. Sondel. Addition of interleukin-2 in vitro augments detection of lymphokine-activated killer activity generated in vivo. Cancer Immunol. Immunother. 31:53 (1990).

18. J.A. Sosman, P.C. Kohler, J.A. Hank, K.H. Moore, R. Bechhofer, B. Storer, and P.M. Sondel. Repetitive weekly cycles of recombinant human interleukin-2: Responses of renal carcinoma with acceptable toxicity. J. Natl. Cancer Inst. 80:60 (1988).

19. J.A. Sosman, P.C. Kohler, J.A. Hank, K.H. Moore, R. Bechhofer, B. Storer, and P.M. Sondel. Repetitive weekly cycles of interleukin-2. II. Clinical and immunologic effects of dose, schedule and indomethacin. J. Natl. Cancer Inst. 80:1451 (1988).

20. M.R. Albertini, J.A. Sosman, J.A. Hank, K.H. Moore, A. Borchert, K. Schell, P.C. Kohler, R. Bechhofer, B. Storer, and P.M. Sondel. The influence of autologous lymphokine-activated killer-cell infusions on the toxicity and antitumor effect of repetitive cycles of interleukin-2. Cancer 66:2457 (1990).

21. S.A. Rosenberg, B. Packard, P. Aebersold, et al. Use of tumor infiltrating lymphocytes and interleukin-2 in the immunotherapy of patients with metastatic melanoma. New Engl. J. Med. 319:1676 (1988).

22. P.M. Sondel, J.A. Sosman, J.A. Hank, P.C. Kohler, and B. Storer. Tumor infiltrating lymphocytes and interleukin-2 in melanomas. New Engl. J. Med. (letter) 320:1418 (1989).

23. J.A. Hank, J.A. Sosman, P.C. Kohler, R. Bechhofer, B. Storer, and P.M. Sondel. Depressed *in vitro* T cell responses concomitant with augmented interleukin-2 responses by lymphocytes from cancer patients following *in vivo* treatment with IL-2. J. Biol. Resp. Mod. 9:5 (1990).

24. A.C. Ochoa, G. Gromo, B.J. Alter, P.M. Sondel, and F.H. Bach. Long-term growth of lymphokine activated killer (LAK) cells: Role of anti-CD3, Beta-IL 1, interferon-Gamma and -Beta. J. Immunol. 138:2728 (1987).

25. J.D.I. Ellenhorn, R. Hirsch, H. Schreiber, and J.A. Bluestone. *In vivo* administration of anti CD-3 prevents malignant progressor tumor growth. Science 242:569 (1988).

26. G. Weil-Hillman, K. Schell, D.M. Segal, J.A. Hank, J.A. Sosman, and P.M. Sondel. Activation of human T cells obtained pre and post IL-2 therapy by anti-CD3 monoclonal antibody plus IL-2: anti CD3 treatment prior to *in vivo* IL-2 therapy induces greater T cell activation. J. Immunother., in press, 1991.

27. J.A. Hank, R.R. Robinson, J. Surfus, B.M. Mueller, R.A. Reisfeld, N.K. Cheung, and P.M. Sondel. Augmentation of antibody dependent cell mediated cytotoxicity following *in vivo* therapy with recombinant interleukin-2. Cancer Res. 50:5234 (1990).

28. W.A. Bleyer. The impact of childhood cancer on the United States and the world. CA-A Cancer J. for Clinicians. 40:355 (1990).

29. P.M. Sondel, J.A. Hank, G. Weil-Hillman, P. Fisch, M. Albertini, S. Voss, and J.A. Sosman. The immunotherapy of cancer: Prospects for more specific antitumor efficacy. in: "The Cellular Immunology and Immunotherapy of Cancer," O. Finn and M. Lotze, eds., Alan R. Liss Inc., New York, p. 413 (1990).

ABNORMAL IMMUNOREGULATION IN HUMAN CANCER AT THE ACTUAL TUMOR SITE

Jules E. Harris and Donald P. Braun

Section of Medical Oncology
Rush Presbyterian St. Luke's Medical Center
Chicago, IL, 60612

INTRODUCTION

Studies evaluating the function of monocytes and macrophages in animal and human tumor systems have revealed that these cells can play diverse, and oftentimes, conflicting roles in tumor growth.   Thus, macrophages may contribute to tumor control by exerting antiproliferative or cytotoxic responses (1-3), but may also facilitate tumor cell embolization and metastasis (4,5). Macrophages also play a principal role in modulating the development and expression of antitumor immunity by other cell types including T cells, NK cells and LAK cells (6-9). Once again, however, this effect can be positive (i.e. promoting the development of antitumor immunity) or negative.

Recently, efforts have been made to control the function of macrophages from cancer patients in vivo through the use of biological response modifying agents. Preliminary results from these trials have demonstrated that macrophage function can be modulated in vivo, albeit with inconsistent and unpredictable results (10-13). But these studies are just beginning and a number of obstacles remain to be overcome. One of the key obstacles that has yet to be adequately addressed is the question of how biological response modifiers influence the function of macrophages that are actually located at the tumor site. The purpose of the present investigation was to evaluate the development of tumoricidal function in response to different macrophage activators in alveolar macrophages (AM) from lung cancer patients and in peritoneal macrophages (PM) from ovarian cancer patients.

Combination Therapies, Edited by A.L. Goldstein and
E. Garaci, Plenum Press, New York, 1992

METHODS

1. _Patient population._ The lung cancer patient population which provided alveolar macrophages and peripheral blood monocytes for these studies consisted of 25 patients with non-small cell lung cancer (15 adenocarcinomas, 8 squamous cell carcinomas and 2 large cell undifferentiated tumors) together with 30 patients with non-malignant lung diseases (primarily patients with chronic inflammatory lung diseases or chronic cough, no acute inflammatory diseases or sepsis) . In addition, 15 patients with epithelial ovarian carcinomas and 22 patients with endometriosis provided peritoneal macrophages and peripheral blood monocytes for these studies. All patients were tested at initial clinical presentation prior to initiation of definitive therapy.

2. _Macrophage activation and tumoricidal function._ The method used to evaluate the development of tumoricidal function in AM, PM and PBM from the study population is as we have previously described (14) Briefly: Alveolar fluids, peritoneal fluids, and peripheral blood were subjected to isopycnic gradient centrifugation on Lymphocyte Separation Medium to obtain mononuclear cells. The percentage of monocytes and macrophages was estimated in the sample by latex ingestion. Subsequently, macrophages were isolated by a 2 hour adherence to plastic microtiter wells, followed by extensive washing to remove non-adherent cells. Adherent cell cultures were then stimulated with different macrophage activators overnight, followed by washing to remove the activators. Next, ^{51}Cr-labelled Chang Hepatoma cells, an NK-insensitive target cell were added in the presence and absence of endotoxin and the cells were cultured for an additional 24 hours. Finally, supernatants were harvested and ^{51}Cr-release determined.

RESULTS

1. _The development of tumoricidal function in AM and PBM from patients with_
malignant and non-malignant lung diseases.

AM from lung cancer patients did not develop significant tumoricidal function in response to gamma IFN + LPS, GM-CSF or Phorbol Myristate Acetate under conditions which elicited significant tumoricidal function in the corresponding PBM from these patients (Table 1). The difference between AM and PBM for each activator was statistically significant at the $p<0.001$ level. The failure of AM from lung cancer patients to develop tumoricidal function was not due to a general impairment of responsiveness to these activators by alveolar macrophages. Thus, AM from control (non-cancer) patients can be activated by gamma IFN+LPS or GM-CSF to express substantial tumoricidal activity.

The difference in tumoricidal function in AM from cancer patients and AM from controls for each of these activation conditions was statistically significant at the p<0.01 level.

Table 1. Alveolar Macrophage (AM) and Peripheral Blood Monocyte (PBM) Cytotoxicity in Patients with Lung Diseases

NON-SMALL CELL LUNG CANCER

ACTIVATOR	NUMBER	AM[1]	PBM	
Medium	15	2.9±3	18.8±14	p<0.001
γ-IFN+LPS	15	6.4±4	43.6±20	p<0.001
GM-CSF	12	4.6±3	27.4±15	p<0.01
PMA	5	3.4±4	35.3±12	p<0.01

NON-MALIGNANT LUNG DISEASES

ACTIVATOR	NUMBER	AM	PBM	
MEDIUM	14	14.2±13	15.8±8	N.S.
γ-IFN+LPS	14	26.0±12	42.0±15	P<0.05
GM-CSF	6	21.6±15	25.6±11	N.S.

[1]mean % cytotoxicity ± standard deviation

2. <u>The development of tumoricidal function in PM and PBM from patients with malignant and non-malignant gynecological diseases.</u> The Tumoricidal function of PM from ovarian cancer patients was significantly reduced compared to the tumoricidal function of the PBM from the same patients. This was true for both gamma IFN + LPS and for GM-CSF under conditions which elicited enhanced tumoricidal function in the corresponding PBM from these patients (Table 2).

Table 2. Peritoneal Macrophage (PM) and Peripheral Blood Monocyte (PBM) Cytotoxicity in Patients with Gynecological Diseases

OVARIAN CANCER

ACTIVATOR	NUMBER	PM[1]	PBM	
MEDIUM	10	12.3±9	22.9±12	p<0.05
γ-IFN+LPS	10	14.4±10	37.7±11	p<0.02
GM-CSF	4	14.8±8	27.3±12	p<0.05

ENDOMETRIOSIS

ACTIVATOR	NUMBER	PM	PBM	
MEDIUM	16	17.8±12	25.2±9	N.S.
γ-IFN+LPS	16	28.2±17	44.4±21	N.S.

[1]mean % cytotoxicity ± standard deviation

The failure of PM from ovarian cancer patients to develop enhanced tumoricidal function was not due to a general impairment of responsiveness to these activators by PM. Thus, PM from endometriosis patients can be activated by gamma IFN+LPS to express significantly enhanced tumoricidal activity. The difference in tumoricidal function in PM from ovarian cancer and endometriosis patients for IFN + LPS was statistically significant at the p<0.02 level.

3. **The effect of Indomethacin, a prostaglandin antagonist, on the development of tumoricidal function in AM and PM from cancer patients.** These studies were based on our previous demonstration of the regulatory effects of prostaglandins on different aspects of macrophage function (9). The results of these studies demonstrated that the prostaglandin antagonist, indomethacin, could significantly enhance the development of tumoricidal function in the PM from ovarian cancer patients but not in the AM from lung cancer patients (Figure 1).

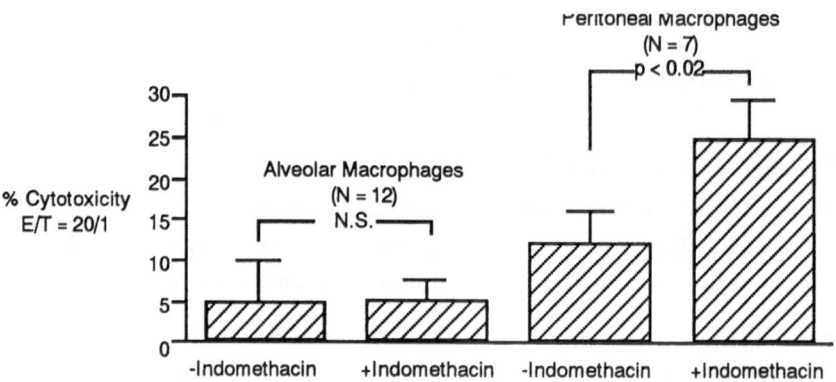

Figure 1. The Effect of Indomethacin on Tumoricidal Function in IFN-Treated Alveolar and Peritoneal Macrophages from Cancer Patients

4. **The development of tumoricidal function in AM and PM treated with anti-lymphocyte antibodies.** Although the adherent cells used in these studies were greater than 95% positive for latex ingestion and macrophage morphology, the possibility that a minor contaminating cell population was downregulating the response to the macrophage activators was considered. Accordingly, adherent macrophage cultures were treated with antibodies against T cells (anti-CD3+) or NK cells (anti-CD56 and anti-CD57) (Table 3). The initial results demonstrated that treatment with anti-CD3 antibodies + complement significantly augmented the development of cytotoxicity in non-cytotoxic alveolar macrophages from lung cancer patients and ovarian cancer patients whereas treatment with anti-CD56 or anti-CD57 antibodies failed to do so. We interpreted that to indicate that

a CD3+ cell was inhibiting the development of cytotoxicity in tumor-associated macrophages from cancer patients. However, control cultures revealed that complement was not needed for the augmentation of cytotoxicity by anti-CD3 monoclonal antibodies nor was stimlation with γ-IFN. Thus, it appeared that the elimination of a CD3+ cell might not have been responsible for the augmentation of tumoricidal function seen in anti-CD3-treated macrophages, and additional studies were needed.

Table 3. The Effect of Anti-Lymphocyte Antibodies on Tumoricidal Function of Alveolar Macrophages From Lung Cancer Patients

CULTURE CONDITIONS	NUMBER	% CYTOTOXICITY[1]	
γ-IFN	4	6.4$\pm$ 2	
γ-IFN + ANTI-CD3 + COMPLEMENT	4	28.8$\pm$ 4	p<0.01
γ-IFN + ANTI-CD56+ COMPLEMENT	2	6.7$\pm$ 2	
γ-IFN + ANTI-CD57+ COMPLEMENT	4	7.8$\pm$ 3	
γ-IFN + ANTI-CD3	3	26.6$\pm$ 2	p<0.01
MEDIA + ANTI-CD3	4	28.6$\pm$ 4	p<0.01
COMPLEMENT	3	7.2$\pm$ 6	

[1]mean % cytotoxicity $\pm$ standard deviation

Thus, further attempts were undertaken to characterize the ability of anti-CD3 monoclonal antibodies to augment macrophage tumoricidal function (Figure 2). In these studies, augmentation of tumoricidal function was observed in tumor-associated macrophages that had been treated with monoclonal anti-CD3 antibodies of the IgG2a isotype but not with anti-CD3 antibodies of the IgG1 isotype.

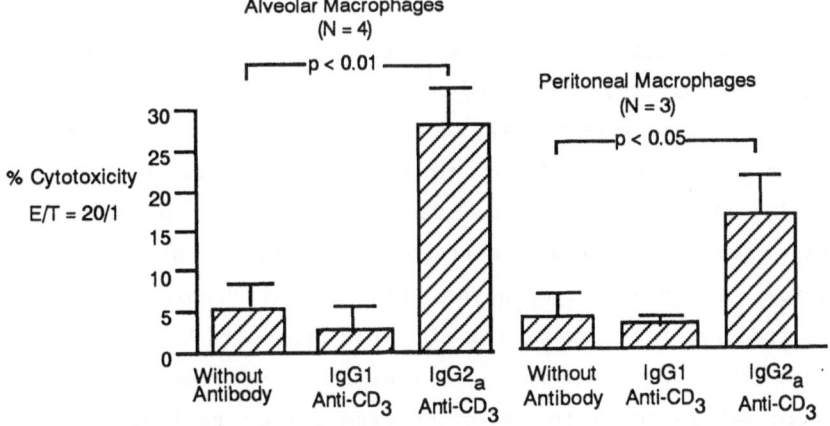

Figure 2. The Effect of Anti-CD3 Mouse Monoclonal Antibodies on Tumoricidal Function in Alveolar and Peritoneal Macrophages from Cancer Patients

This result was seen for both AM from lung cancer patients and PM from ovarian cancer patients. Based on these somewhat unexpected results, it appears that activation through the Fcγ-RI receptor on tumor-associated macrophages, which binds mouse IgG2a antibodies, is responsible for the augmentation of tumoricidal function observed and not the elimination of a CD3+ cell type. Furthermore, these results also suggest that IgG1 binding through the Fcγ-RII receptor on macrophages does not activate or augment tumoricidal function in alveolar or peritoneal macrophages.

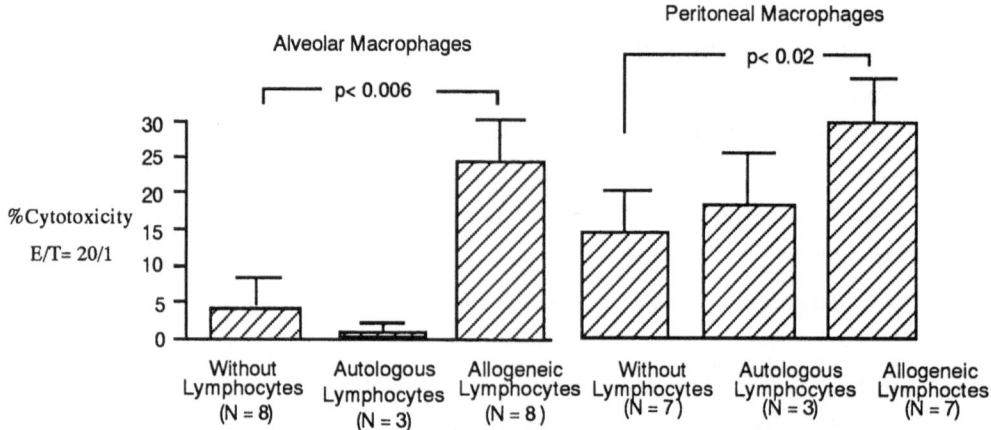

Figure 3. The Effect of Allogeneic or Autologous Lymphocytes on The Development of Tumoricidal Function in IFN-treated Alveolar Macrophages and Peritoneal Macrophages from Lung Cancer and Ovarian Cancer Patients

5. The development of tumoricidal function in AM and PM treated with allogeneic lymphocytes. The possibility that critical regulatory factors necessary for responsiveness to macrophage activators are deficient in macrophages obtained from tumor microenvironments was also considered. Accordingly, attempts to add such factors during the "priming" phase of macrophage activation were undertaken. Initially, and primarily for convenience, allogeneic lymphocytes from normal donors which could be purified and cryopreserved were used. This proved to be fortuitous since allogeneic lymphocytes were found to significantly increase the development of tumoricidal function in AM or PM from cancer patients. Somewhat surprisingly, autologous lymphocytes from lung cancer or ovarian cancer patients were unable to augment tumoricidal function in tumor-associated macrophages. The results of these studies are presented in Figure 3.

Subsequent studies (not presented) were undertaken which have demonstrated that:

1) Allogeneic lymphocytes cultured with activators in the absence of macrophages do not exhibit cytotoxicity against the NK-insensitive, Chang Hepatoma cell line;

2) Antibody + complement treatment to remove residual allogeneic lymphocytes following cocultivation with macrophages did not reduce the augmented cytotoxicity elicited in tumor-associated macrophages; and

3) Supernatants from cocultures of alveolar macrophages + allogeneic lymhocytes also can potentiate the development of tumoricidal function in alveolar macrophages from lung cancer patients.

These results provide further evidence that the cytotoxicity which has been elicited in cocultures of tumor-associated macrophages and allogeneic lymphocytes is due to the macrophages themselves, and not to residual lymphocytes.

6. <u>Attempts to augment the development of tumoricidal function against autoglous tumors.</u> In a limited number of cases, the strategies for augmenting the tumoricidal function of tumor-associated macrophages have been tested against autologous tumor cells from ovarian cancer patients. The results of an experiment which is representative of results with 3 ovarian cancer specimens is presented in Table 4. Treatment of peritoneal macrophages with either allogeneic lymphocytes or the cyclooxygenase inhibitor indomethacin significantly augmented tumor cell cytotoxicity against both the Chang hepatoma targets, and against the patient's own tumor cells. The possibility that these 2 different activation strategies may synergize to produce even greater levels of autologous tumoricidal function in peritoneal macrophages from ovarian cancer patients is currently being evaluated.

Table 4. The Effect of Indomethacin or Allogeneic Lymphocytes on the Development of Autologous Tumor Cell Cytotoxicity in Peritoneal Macrophages

	% CYTOTOXICITY	
CULTURE CONDITIONS	CHANG HEPATOMA	AUTOLOGOUS TUMOR
MEDIA	2.1	3.4
γ-IFN+LPS	3.5	5.8
γ-IFN+LPS+INDOMETHACIN	23.3	19.1
γ-IFN+ALLOGENEIC LYMPHOCYTES	15.9	14.7

DISCUSSION

The results of this investigation demonstrate that the tumoricidal function of AM from lung cancer patients or PM from ovarian cancer patients is reduced significantly compared to the tumoricidal function of the peripheral blood monocytes from the same patients. This was consistent for macrophages stimulated with multiple conventional macrophage activators and under diverse culture conditions. The impaired development of tumoricidal function in tumor-associated macrophages was not due to a general inability of these activators to stimulate tumoricidal function in AM or PM since the same activation conditions elicited significant tumoricidal function in AM or PM from patients with non-malignant diseases. However, significant tumoricidal function could be elicited in tumor-associated macrophages from cancer patients by several novel activation strategies including (i) suppression of cyclooxygenase activity with indomethacin (PM but not AM); (ii) allogeneic cell stimulation during priming (PM and AM); and (iii) treatment with murine IgG2a, anti-CD3 monoclonal antibodies (PM and AM). These strategies which were developed using an NK insensitive target cell line were also found to be effective in potentiating the development of autologous tumoricidal function in the PM from ovarian cancer patients.

The results suggest that the failure of conventional macrophage activators to stimulate tumoricidal function in tumor-associated macrophages is not due to an intrinsic deficiency in these cells. Rather, it appears that abnormal immunregulation in tumor microenvironments is responsible for this failure. The alternative activation strategies which were developed during the course of this investigation appear to overcome abnormal immunoregulation and permit the development of significant tumoricidal function. This result suggests that these alternative activation strategies may utilize different signal transduction pathways or elicit different cytokine responses in tumor-associated macrophages than are stimulated by conventional biological response modifiers currently in use for cancer therapy. It is possible that these alternative activation strategies may be exploited therapeutically for the treatment of human malignant disease.

REFERENCES

1.   Gerrard TL, Terz JJ, Kaplan AM (1980) Cytotoxicity to tumor cells of monocytes from normal individuals and cancer patients. Int J Cancer 26: 585.

2. Fidler IJ, Kleinerman ES (1984) Lymphokine-activated human blood monocytes destroy tumor cells but not normal cells under cocultivation conditions. J Clin Oncol 2:937.

3. Mantovani A, Polentarutti N, Peri G, Shavit ZB, Vecchi A, Bolis G, Mangioni C (1980) Cytotoxicity on tumor cells of peripheral blood monocytes and tumor-associated macrophages in patients with ascites ovarian tumor J Natl Cancer Inst 64:1307.

4. Polverini PJ, Leibovich SJ (1984) Induction of neovascularization in vivo and endothelial proliferation in vitro by tumor-associated macrophages. Lab Invest 51:635.

5. DeBaetselier P, Kapon A, Katzav S, Tzehoval E, Dekegel D, Segal S, Feldman M (1985) Selecting, accelerating and suppressing interactions between macrophages and tumor cells. Invasion Metastasis 5:106.

6. Bloom ET, Babbitt JT (1985) Monocyte-mediated augmentaton of human natural cell-mediated cytotoxicity. Cell Immunol 91:21.

7. DeBoer KP, Braun DP, Harris JE (1982) Natural cytotoxicity and antibody-dependent cytotoxicity in solid tumor cancer patients: regulation by adherent cells. Clin Immunol Immunopathol 23: 133.

8. Schulof RS, Michitsch RW, Livingston PO, Gupta S (1981) Monocyte-mediated suppression of lymphocyte cytotoxic activity for cultured autologous melanoma cells. Cell Immunol 57:529.

9. Roth MD, Golub SH (1988) Inhibition of lymphokine-activiated killer cell function by alveolar macrophages. Chest 94:44.

10. Huddlestone JR, Merigan TC Jr, Oldstone MBA (1979) Induction and kinetics of natural killer cells in humans following interferon therapy. Nature 282:417.

11. Krown SE, Real FX, Cunningham-Rundles S, Myskowski PL, Koziner B, Fein S, Mittelman A, Oettgen HF, Safai B (1983) Preliminary observations on the effect of recombinant leukocyte A interferon in homosexual men with Kaposi's sarcoma. N Engl J Med 308:107112.

12. McMannis JD, Fisher RI, Creekmore SP, Braun DP, Harris JE, Ellis TM (1988) In vivo effects of recombinant IL-2. I. Isolation of circulating Leu-19[+]lymphokine activated killer effector cells from cancer patients receiving recombinant IL-2. J Immunol 140: 1335.

13. Gabrilove JL, Starnes A, Begas A, Casper E et al. (1987) A phase I study of intravenously administered recombinant tumor necrosis factor alpha in patients with advanced cancer. Proc Am Soc Clin Oncol 6: 247.

14. Braun DP, Siziopikou KP, Casey LC, Harris JE (1990). The in vitro development of cytotoxicity in response to granulocyte/macrophage-colony-stimulating factor or interferon γ in the peripheral blood

monocytes of patients with solid tumors: Modulation by arachidonic
acid metabolic inhibitors.

THE IMMUNOBIOLOGY OF HUMAN MACROPHAGE Fc$_\gamma$ RECEPTORS

Alan D. Schreiber, Arnold I. Levinson, Milton D. Rossman

The University of Pennsylvania School of Medicine
Philadelphia, PA

At least three biochemically distinct Fc$_\gamma$ receptor classes have been described on human cells. These receptors have been designated Fc$_\gamma$RI, Fc$_\gamma$RII and Fc$_\gamma$RIII. They are membrane glycoproteins with extracellular domains that contain immunoglobulin-like regions. Therefore, they are members of the immunoglobulin gene superfamily. They appear to be located on human chromosome 1 and may have arisen from gene duplication. All three Fc$_\gamma$ receptors are present on the surface of human macrophages.

Fc$_\gamma$RI (CD64) was initially isolated from a human monocyte/macrophage cell line as a 72 kD glycoprotein (1). Equilibrium binding studies with monomeric IgG indicated that human Fc$_\gamma$RI binds monomeric IgG with high affinity (2-8) and subclasses IgG1 and IgG3 with higher affinity than IgG2 and IgG4 (9-13). Similar Fc$_\gamma$RI IgG isotype specificity appears to be present on inflammatory peritoneal macrophages and the monocyte cell line U-937 (6,12).

The Fc domain recognized by Fc$_\gamma$RI is localized to the IgG CH2 region. Fc$_\gamma$RI also binds relatively specifically to monomeric mouse IgG of the subclass IgG2a. Several monoclonal antibodies have been iolated which recognize distinct epitopes on Fc$_\gamma$RI (14-16).

The gene for human Fc$_\gamma$RI has recently been cloned (11). The extracellular region of Fc$_\gamma$RI consists of three immunoglobulin-like domains, two of which share homology with other Fc$_\gamma$ receptors. This unique third domain is likely responsible for the ability of Fc$_\gamma$RI to bind monomeric IgG and to exhibit high affinity. Transfection studies in COS cells reveal a single species of approximately 70 kD. Northern blot analysis with an Fc$_\gamma$RI DNA probe demonstrates a single 1.7 kb RNA transcript in monocytes and macrophages. In U-937 cells, both a 1.7 kb and 1.6 kb transcript have been noted, each of which increases following incubation with γ-interferon. Polymorphisms have been observed among Fc$_\gamma$RI cDNAs obtained from a single patient, suggesting that there may be more than one gene encoding Fc$_\gamma$RI. The predicted polypeptide sequence shows a hydrophobic signal sequence, a 21-residue hydrophobic transmembrane region and a charged cytoplasmic domain. Recent evidence indicates that there are two Fc$_\gamma$RI genes.

Our data indicate that both γ-interferon and glucocorticoids modulate the expression of Fc$_\gamma$RI (3,17,20). In addition, Northern blot analysis reveals that the steady state levels of mRNA are influenced by these two mediators (19-20). Our hypothesis is that the interaction of glucocorticoid hormone with its receptor (a DNA binding protein) may decrease Fc$_\gamma$RI mRNA levels by inducing a gene regulatory protein which differentially affects the transcription of Fc$_\gamma$RI. Alternatively, glucocorticoid

Combination Therapies, Edited by A.L. Goldstein and
E. Garaci, Plenum Press, New York, 1992

hormone interaction with its DNA binding protein receptor may lead to an association with Fc$_\gamma$RI DNA. This in turn could regulate the binding and/or activation of Fc$_\gamma$RI RNA polymerase. One possibility is that binding to or activation of RNA polymerase on Fc$_\gamma$RI DNA is inhibited by glucocorticoids. With γ-interferon, the effect of RNA polymerase on Fc$_\gamma$RI transcription may be enhanced.

Since monocytes and macrophages are exposed to high concentrations of circulating IgG, under most circumstances Fc$_\gamma$RI is likely saturated with IgG monomer. Thus, the *raison d'etre* for Fc$_\gamma$RI is at present uncertain. However, a compelling argument for the importance of Fc$_\gamma$RI can be made by the ease with which the number and the density of these surface receptors are modulated. Interferon-γ will increase both the number and the surface density of Fc$_\gamma$RI on monocytes (17,21-24). An increased number of Fc$_\gamma$RI appears within 8-12 hours and persists for at least 7 days. The increase in Fc$_\gamma$RI due to γ-interferon has been demonstrated both by immunofluorescent and monomeric IgG binding studies. Interferon-α and -β appear to have little or no effect on macrophage Fc$_\gamma$R1(23).

Fc$_\gamma$RII (CD32) was initially isolated by affinity chromatography using anti-Fc$_\gamma$ receptor antibody (1). Anti-Fc$_\gamma$RII monoclonal antibody (25) immunoprecipitated a 40 kD protein present on monocytes, neutrophils, platelets, B-cells, and several hematopoetic cell lines. Fc$_\gamma$RII does not bind monomeric IgG, but binds oligomeric IgG with low affinity (association constant for trimeric IgG = ~ 1×10^7 M-1) (26). Murine immunoglobulin isotypes IgG1 and IgG2b bind to Fc$_\gamma$RII with relative specificity (27). On U-937 cells, aggregates of mouse IgG2b exhibit enhanced binding to Fc$_\gamma$RII under conditions of low ionic strength and low temperature. We have observed that similar conditions facilitate human oligomeric IgG binding to platelets and HEL cells which express Fc$_\gamma$RII as their only Fc$_\gamma$ receptor (28,29,31).

Fc$_\gamma$RII plays a role in the human T cell proliferative response to mouse IgG1 anti-T cell antibodies (33). Monocytes from approximately 30% of normal individuals fail to stimulate T cell proliferation (non-responders) in the presence of IgG1 anti-T cell antibody (34). When purified monocyte Fc$_\gamma$RII from responder and non-responder individuals was compared, no differences in their electrophoretic mobility on SDS-polyacrylamide gels was observed (33). However, after isoelectric focusing different patterns were observed. The data led to the observation that this Fc$_\gamma$RII gene has two alleles which differ in their interaction with IgG1.

Fc$_\gamma$RII was the first human Fc$_\gamma$ receptor gene cloned (35-37). Subsequent to the original publications, Fc$_\gamma$RII clones have been reported by several laboratories (38). It appears that Fc$_\gamma$RII is encoded by at least three genes (Fc$_\gamma$RIIA, Fc$_\gamma$RIIB and Fc$_\gamma$RIIC). The extracellular domains of Fc$_\gamma$RII are closely homologous to the extracellular domains of Fc$_\gamma$RI and Fc$_\gamma$RIII and to the extracellular domains of the analogous murine Fc$_\gamma$ receptor. Similarly, the transmembrane domain of Fc$_\gamma$RII is homologous to that of murine Fc$_\gamma$RIIβ. Differences exist in the transmembrane region and considerable differences in the intracellular domain of the Fc$_\gamma$RII genes when compared to those of Fc$_\gamma$RI and Fc$_\gamma$RIII. The differences in the cytoplasmic domains suggest that intracellular signalling events may differ considerably among these three human Fc$_\gamma$ receptors. Northern blot analysis reveals two major transcripts of 2.4 and 1.6 kb in most of the cells thus far examined which express Fc$_\gamma$RII. Work on the genomic structure of Fc$_\gamma$RII has begun and the transcriptional starts sites and the 5'-flanking transcriptional regulatory region of Fc$_\gamma$RIIA have been defined (32). Of particular interest is the identification of elements which may mediate the response of glucocorticoids and γ-interferon that we have observed earlier.

Fc$_\gamma$RII is the only Fc$_\gamma$ receptor present on human platelets. Fc$_\gamma$RII has been cloned from a cDNA library prepared from the megakaryocyte/platelet like cell line HEL (38,39). One of these Fc$_\gamma$RII cDNA clones is of particular note. This clone, 2.1 kb in size, is identical to published sequences in the extracellular region, but has an important difference downstream. There is an in-frame deletion of 123 nucleotides eliminating the DNA for the entire transmembrane region, suggesting alternative splicing of the primary transcript which removes this specific sequence. The 2.1 kb clone does not share structural features with Fc$_\gamma$RI or Fc$_\gamma$RIII, based on nucleotide and amino acid sequence comparison. This clone may encode for a soluble form of Fc$_\gamma$RII, and using the polymerase chain reaction we have noted that it is identified in platelet, monocyte, HEL cell and U-937 cell Fc$_\gamma$RII mRNA (38,39).

The precise function of Fc$_\gamma$RII on monocytes and macrophages is being characterized. We have observed that Fc$_\gamma$RIIA in the absence of any other Fc$_\gamma$ receptors can mediate a phagocytic signal (55). Furthermore we have observed that stimulation of Fc$_\gamma$RIIA leads to phosphorylation of Fc$_\gamma$RIIA on tyrosine (56). Monocyte Fc$_\gamma$RII can induce IgG antibody induced cell-mediated cytotoxicity (40). A rise in intracellular calcium can be induced in U-937 cells and monocytes by both IgG1 and anti-Fc$_\gamma$RII (41). This may require a tripartite cross-linking of Fc and (Fab')$_2$, since calcium mobilization does not occur with F(ab')$_2$ fragments in the absence of the Fc domain (41). In addition, superoxide production after Fc$_\gamma$RII cross-linking has been noted, but only after γ-interferon priming of U-937 cells or monocytes. The hierarchy of human IgG subclass binding to Fc$_\gamma$RII appears to be IgG1 > IgG2 $\geq$ IgG4 > IgG3 (37).

Fc$_\gamma$RII expression can be regulated by GM-CSF on U-937 cells, an effect which requires protein synthesis (26). We have observed a stimulatory effect of GM-CSF on human monocyte Fc$_\gamma$RII protein and mRNA (42). G-CSF and γ-interferon also have been noted to increase Fc$_\gamma$RII protein expression on U-937 cells (26,20). Northern blot analysis reveals that U-937 cells treated with interferon-γ exhibit a 2.5-fold increase in Fc$_\gamma$RII mRNA levels that is maximal at 14 hours and declines to 1.4-fold over baseline by 48 hours of incubation (20). Treatment with glucocorticoids induces a small, but significant, decrease in Fc$_\gamma$RII protein, and dexamethasone is also able to inhibit by 20-60% the induction of Fc$_\gamma$RII by interferon-γ. Modulation by dexamethasone and interferon-γ of Fc$_\gamma$RII protein expression on U-937 cells is markedly different from that of Fc$_\gamma$RI in both magnitude and kinetics (20,43). Interferon-γ increases Fc$_\gamma$RI expression by 240% at 16 hours, while Fc$_\gamma$RI remains elevated through 48 hours. In contrast, expression of Fc$_\gamma$RII protein on U-937 cells is increased 56-72% after 16-24 hours of interferon-γ treatment and is minimal after 48 hours incubation. Thus, the modulation of Fc$_\gamma$RII on U-937 cells is at least in part due to changes in steady state levels of Fc$_\gamma$RII mRNA and we have recently shown that this is due to an effect on Fc$_\gamma$RII transcription (43). Furthermore, the difference between the magnitude of the changes in Fc$_\gamma$RII mRNA and protein suggests that some translational or post-translational control is involved in regulating the expression of Fc$_\gamma$RII. Since Fc$_\gamma$RI and Fc$_\gamma$RII bind related ligands, mediate similar functions, and appear to have similar changes in mRNA levels following interferon-γ treatment, it is possible the transcription of both genes is coordinately regulated. Isolation of the genomic sequences for Fc$_\gamma$RI and Fc$_\gamma$RII and analyses of 5'- and 3'-flanking sequencesis has revealed some common potential regulatory sequences (32).

A third Fc$_\gamma$ receptor class (Fc$_\gamma$RIII or CD 16) is present on tissue macrophages (Fc$_\gamma$RIIIA), neutrophils (Fc$_\gamma$RIIIB), and natural killer (NK) cells (Fc$_\gamma$RIIIA). This receptor has a low affinity for IgG and binds human IgG1 and IgG3 more effectively than IgG2 and IgG4. When isolated by immunoprecipitation, Fc$_\gamma$RIII has a broad electrophoretic mobility on SDS-polyacrylamide gel electrophoresis (51-73 kD). Fc$_\gamma$RIII appears on monocytes after *in vitro* culture for one to two weeks and has been identified on freshly isolated peritoneal and alveolar macrophages (44-46). Fc$_\gamma$RII is not detectable on U-937 cells or on uninduced HL-60 cells.

Several different monoclonal antibodies (3G8, 4F7, B73.1, Leu-11a,b, and VEP-13) have been defined which react with Fc$_\gamma$RIII. On neutrophils, it has been observed that the blood group antigens NA1 and NA2 represent alloantigens of Fc$_\gamma$RIII (47). Several different anti-Fc$_\gamma$RIII monoclonal antibodies have been identified based on their reactivity with NA1 and NA2 on neutrophils and NK cells (48).

Fc$_\gamma$RIII on neutrophils appears to be a phosphatidyl inositol (PI)-anchored protein and the expression of Fc$_\gamma$RIII is markedly diminished on neutrophils from patients with PNH, a disorder in which the expression of PI-anchored proteins is reduced (also see below)(47). In addition, treatment of normal neutrophils with glycosyl-phosphatidyl-inositol-specific phopholipase C, an enzyme which disrupts PI-linkages, reduces the expression of Fc$_\gamma$RIII. Evidence that Fc$_\gamma$RIII on neutrophils differs from Fc$_\gamma$RIII on macrophages comes from immunoprecipitation studies with anti-Fc$_\gamma$RIII monoclonal antibody (44,45). Neutrophil immunoprecipitated Fc$_\gamma$RIII had a broader electrophoretic mobility on SDS-PAGE than Fc$_\gamma$RIII isolated from *in vitro* cultured monocytes. In addition, after digestion with N-glycanase, neutrophil Fc$_\gamma$RIII is cleaved to a 33,000 M_r protein core, while the *in vitro* cultured monocyte protein is not altered by N-glycanase and is a 55,000 M_r molecule.

Fc$_\gamma$RIII (Fc$_\gamma$RIIIB) has been cloned by Seed and co-workers, the same laboratory which cloned the genes for Fc$_\gamma$RI and Fc$_\gamma$RII (50). These investigators employed a cDNA library from human placenta, presumably a source of monocytes and macrophages and their transcripts. The data indicate that the extracellular domain of Fc$_\gamma$RIII is closely homologous to that of Fc$_\gamma$RI and Fc$_\gamma$RII. However, in contrast to Fc$_\gamma$RII, which bears greatest homology to the murine Fc$_\gamma$RIIβ gene, Fc$_\gamma$RIII is most homologous with the α form of the murine Fc$_\gamma$RII gene. The extracellular domain of Fc$_\gamma$RIII ends in a short 200-220 residue hydrophobic domain followed by four hydrophobic residues, of which one is charged. A similar structure and a similar hyrophobicity profile of the predicted amino acid sequence is characteristic of membrane proteins bearing glycosyl phosphotidylinositol phospholipid (P-I) linked carboxyl termini. This indicates that Fc$_\gamma$RIII is a phospholipid anchored protein on at least some human cells in which it is expressed. In fact it has been established that Fc$_\gamma$RIII on human granulocytes is a P-I linked protein which is the product of the Fc$_\gamma$RIIIB gene.

It has been determined from our studies and those of others that Fc$_\gamma$RIII on tissue macrophages is not a P-I linked molecule (51). Patients with PNH have a deficiency in P-I linked proteins and their granulocytes are substantially deficient in Fc$_\gamma$RIII. Nevertheless, it has been our experience and the experience of others that patients with PNH do not have a substantial increase in their incidence of infection. This may be due to active Fc$_\gamma$RI and/or Fc$_\gamma$RII function in host defense in these patients. Alternatively, Fc$_\gamma$RIII may not be uniformly deficient in these patients, and their macrophages, as opposed to their neutrophiles, may express Fc$_\gamma$RIII. The data indicate that Fc$_\gamma$RIII is present on cells of the monocyte/macrophage lineage in PNH, as well as in normal individuals as a conventional transmembrane non-P-I linked form of Fc$_\gamma$RIII (51). This is the product of a distinct Fc$_\gamma$RIII gene, Fc$_\gamma$RIIIA.

Because Fc$_\gamma$RIII is not abundant on freshly isolated monocytes, there have only been limited studies to define the function of Fc$_\gamma$RIII on human macrophages. Clarkson et al (50) employed anti-Fc$_\gamma$RIII monoclonal antibody to inhibit the clearance IgG coated platelets in immune thrombocytopenic purpura (52,53). Since the clearance of platelets in immune thrombocytopenia is mediated by splenic macrophage Fc$_\gamma$ receptors, the rise in platelet count after infusion of anti-Fc$_\gamma$RIII is probably due to its inhibition of these macrophage receptors. Dr. Randi Isaacs in our laboratory has recently observed that Fc$_\gamma$RIII with its associated γ chain can mediate a phagocytic signal in the absence of any other Fc$_\gamma$ receptors (57).

Monocytes and alveolar macrophages grown in the presence of fibroblast supernatant express increased levels of Fc$_\gamma$RIII (46). On the other hand, glucocorticoids and γ-interferon do not appear to alter the expression of Fc$_\gamma$RIII *in vitro* (24). We have observed that M-CSF and serum factors play a role in regulating the expression of Fc$_\gamma$RIII on human monocytes/macrophages (54).

In summary, human macrophage Fc$_\gamma$ receptors are a hetergeneous group of glycoproteins, of which three distinct biochemical classes have been defined encoded for by at least seven genes. With the cloning of the human Fc$_\gamma$ receptor genes and their biochemical characterization, emphasis will now focus on their likely diverse functions in host defense, immune complex recognition and intracellular signaling. In addition, the further characterization of soluble Fc$_\gamma$ receptors and their potential immunoregulatory significance will become an increasing area of focus.

ACKNOWLEDGEMENT

The authors thank Ms. Ruth Rowan for her excellent assistance in preparing this manuscript for publication.

REFERENCES

1. Anderson, CL. Isolation of the receptor for IgG from a human monocyte cell line (U937) and from human peripheral blood monocytes. J Exp Med 1982;156:1794-1806.

2. Anderson CL, Spence JM, Edward TS and Nusbacher J. Characterization of a polyvalent antibody directed against the IgG Fc receptor of human mononuclear phagocytes. J Immunol 1985;134:465-470.

3. Rossman MD, Chien P, Cassizzi-Cprek A, Elias JA, Holian A, and Schreiber AD. The binding of monomeric IgG to human blood monocytes and alveolar macrophages. Am Rev Resp Dis 1986;133:292-297.

4. Kurlander RJ, Batker J. The binding of human Immunoglobulin G1 monomer and small, covalently cross-linked polymers of immunoglobulin G1 to human peripheral blood monocytes and polymorphonuclear leukocytes. J Clin Invest 1982;69:1-8.

5. Fries LF, Brickman CM, Frank MM. Monocyte receptors for the Fc portion of IgG increase in number in auto-immune hemolytic anemia and other hemolytic states are decreased by glucocorticoid therapy. J Immunol 1983;131:1240-1245.

6. Anderson CL, Abraham GN. Characterization of the Fc receptor for IgG on a human macrophage cell line, U937. J Immunol 1980;125:2735-41.

7. Chien P., Pixley A, Stumpo LG, Colman RW, and Schreiber AD. Modulation of the human monocyte binding site for monomeric immunoglobulin G by activated Hageman Factor. J Clin Invest 1988;82:1554-1559.

8. Schreiber, AD, Chien P, Tomaski A, and Cines DB. Effect of Danazol in immune thrombocytopenic purpura. N Eng J Med 1987;316:503-508.

9. Huber H, Fudenber HH. The interaction of monocytes and macropahges with immunoglobulines and complement. Ser Haematol 1970;3:160-175.

10. Huber H, Douglas SD, Nusbacher J, Kochwa S and Rosenfield RE. IgG subclass specificity of human monocyte receptor sites. Nature 1971;229:419-420.

11. Allen JM and Seed B. Isolation and expression of functional high-affinity Fc receptor complementary DNAs. Science 1989;243:378-381.

12. Kurlander RJ, Haney AF, and Gartrell J. Human peritoneal macrophages possess two populations of IgG Fc receptors. Cellular Immunol 1984;86:479-490.

13. Lubeck MD, Steplewski Z, Baglia F, Klein MH, Dorrington KJ, Koprowski H. The interaction of murine IgG subclass proteins with human monocyte Fc$_\gamma$ receptors. J Immunol 1985;135:1299-1304.

14. Anderson CL, Guyre PM, Shitin JC, Ryan DH, Looney RJ, and Fanger MW. Monoclonal antibodies to Fc receptors for IgG on human mononuclear phagocytes. Antibody characterization and induction of superoxide production in a monocyte cell line. J Biol Chem 1986;261:12856-12864.

15. Frey, J, Engelhardt W. Characterization and structural analysis of Fc$_\gamma$ receptors of human monocytes, a monoblast cell line (U937) and a myeloblast cell line (HL-60) by a monoclonal antibody. Eur J Immunol 1987;17:583-591.

16. Dougherty GJ, Selvendran Y, Murdoch S, Palmer DG, and Hogog N. The human mononuclear phagocyte high affinity Fc receptor, FcRI, defined by a monoclonal antibody, 10.1. Eur J Immunol 1987;17:1453-1459.

17. Rossman MD, Chen E, Chien P, and Schreiber AD. Modulation of Fc$_\gamma$ receptors on the human macrophage cell line U937. Cellular Immunol 1989;119:174-187.

18. Schreiber AD, Parsons J, McDermott P, Cooper RA. Effect of corticosteroids on the human monocyte receptors for IgG and complement. J Clin Invest 1975; 56:1189-1197.

19. Comber PG, Rossman MD, and Schreiber AD. Receptors for the Fc portion of IgG (Fc$_\gamma$R) on human monocytes and macrophages. In: Biochemistry of the Acute Allergic Reactins, Fifth International Symposium. Wintroub, Tauber, eds. Alan R. Liss, Inc., New York, 1988.

20. Comber PG, Rossman MD, Rappaport EF, Chien P, Hogarth PM, Schreiber AD. Modulation of human mononuclear phagocyte Fc$_\gamma$ receptors by glucocorticoids and interferon-γ. Cellular Immunol 1989;124:292-307.

21. Guyre PM, Morganelli PM and Miller R. Recombinant immune interferon increases immunoglobulin G Fc receptors on cultured human mononuclear phagocytes. J Clin Invest 1983;72:393-397.

22. Akiyama Y, Lubeck MD, Steplewsky A and Koprowski H. Induction of mouse IgG2a and IgG3 dependent cellular cytotoxicity in the human monocytttic cells (U937) by immune interferon. Cancer Res 1984;44:5127-5131.

23. Perussia B, Dayton ET, Lazarus R, Fanning V, and Trinchieri G. Immune interferon induces the receptor for monomeric IgG1 on human monocyte and myeloid cells. J. Exp Med 1983;158:1092-1113.

24. Girard MT, Hjaltadottir S, Fejes-Toth AN and Guyre PM. Glucocorticoids enhance the gamma-interferon augmentation of human monocyte immunoglobulin G Fc receptor expression. J Immunol 1987;138:3235-3241.

25. Rosenfeld SI, Looney RJ, Leddy JP, Phipps DC, Abraham GN and Anderson CL. Human platelet Fc receptor for immunoglobulin G. Identification of 40,000-molecular weight membrane protein shared by monocytes. J Clin Invest 1985;76:2317-2322.

26. Liesveld JC, Abboud CN, Looney JR, Ryan DH and Brennan JK. Expression of IgG Fc receptors in myeloid leukemic cell lines. J Immunol 1988;140:1527-1533.

27. Jones DHK, Looney RJ, Anderson CL. Two distinct classes of IgG Fc receptors on a human monocyte line (U937) defined by differences in binding of murine IgG subclasses at low ionic strength. J Immunol 1985;135:3348-3353.

28. King M , P. McDermott and Schreiber AD. Characterization of the Fc$_\gamma$ receptor on human platelets. Cellular Immunol 1990;128:262-479.

29. King, M., Comber, P., Chien, P., Ruiz, P. and Schreiber, A.D. Characterization of Fc$_\gamma$ receptors on a human erytholeukemia (HEL) cell line. Exp. Hematology, in press.

30. Rossman MD, Chen E, Chien P, Rottem M, Cprek A, and Schreiber AD. Fc$_\gamma$ receptor recognition of IgG ligand by human monocytes and macrophages. Am J Respiratory Cell and Molecular Biology. 1989;1:211-220.

31. Gomez, FP, Chien P, King, M, McDermott P, Rossman, MD and Schreiber, AD. Monocyte Fc$_\gamma$ receptor recognition of cell bound and aggregated IgG. Blood 1989;74:1058-1065.

32. McKenzie, SE, Keller, MA, Cassel, DL, Schreiber, AD, Schwartz, E, Surrey, S. and Rappaport EF. Submitted for publication.

33. Anderson CL, Ryan DH, Looney RJ, Leary PC. Structural polymorphism of the human monocyte 40 kilodalton Fc receptor for IgG. J Immunol 1987;138:2254-56.

34. Tax WJ, Hermes FF, Willems RW, Capel PJ, Koene RA. Fc receptors for mouse IgG1 on human monocytes: polymorphism and role in antibody-induced T cell proliferaton. J Immunol 1984;133:1185-89.

35. Stewart SG, Trounstine ML, Vaux DJT, Koch T, Martens CL, Mellman I and Moore KW. Isolation and expression of cDNA clones encoding a human receptor for IgG (Fc$_\gamma$RII). J Exp Med 1987;166:1668-1684.

36. Hibbs ML, Bonadonna L, Scott BM, McKenzie IF and Hogarth PM. Molecular cloning of a human immunoglobulin G Fc receptor. Proc Nat Acad Sci 1988;85:2240-2244.

37. Stengelin S, Stamenkovic I, and Seed B. Isolation of two distinct human Fc receptors by ligand affinity cloning. The Embo J 1988;7:1053-1059.

38. Rappaport, EF., Cassel, EF, McKenzie, SE, Surrey, S, Schwartz, E and Schreiber, AD. Expression of Fc$_\gamma$RII in hematopoietic cells: Analysis of transcripts encoding the soluble and membrane-associated molecular forms. Clin Res 1991;39:151a.

39. Rapparport, E, Cassel, D, Meister, R, Walterhouse, D, Schreiber, AD and Schwartz, E. Isolation and characterization of a cDNA clone coding for a potential soluble form of the Fc$_\gamma$ receptor, Fc$_\gamma$RII. Submitted for publication.

40. Fanger MW, Shen L, Granziana RF and Guyre PM. Cytotoxicity mediated by human Fc receptors for IgG. Immunol Today 1989;10:92-99.

41. Macintyre EA, Roberts PJ, Abdul-Gaffar R, O'Flynn K, Pilkington GR, Farace F, Morgan J, Linch DC. Mechanism of human monocyte activation via the 40-kDa Fc receptor for IgG. J Immunol 1988;141:4333-4343.

42 Rossman, MD, Ruiz, P, Gomez F, Chien, P, Rottem, M and Schreiber AD. Modualtion of macrophage Fc$_\gamma$ receptors by rGM-CSF. Submitted for publication.

43. Comber, PG, Lentz, V, and Schreiber, AD. Modulation of the transcriptional rate of Fc$_\gamma$ receptor mRNA in human mononuclear phagocytes by interferon-γ and dexamethasone. Submitted for publication.

44. Fleit HB, Wright SD, Unkeless JC. Human neutrophile Fc$_\gamma$ receptor distribution and structure. Proc Natl Acad Sci USA 1982;79:3275-3279.

45. Clarkson SB, Ory PA CD 16: Developmental regulated IgG Fc receptors on cultured monocytes. J Exp Med 1988;167:408-417.

46. Baumgartner I, Scheiner O, Holzinger C, Boltz-Nitulescu G, Klech H, Lassmann H, Rumpold H, Forster O, and Kraft D. Expression of VEP13 antigen (CD16) on native human alveolar macrophages and cultured blood monocytes. Immunobiology 1988;177:317-326.

47. Werner G, von dem Borne AEG Kr, Fos MJE, Tromp JF, van der Plas-van Dalen CM, Visser FJ, Engelfriet CP, Tetteroo PAT. Localization of the human NA1 alloantigen on neutrophil Fc-γ receptors. In Leukocyte Typing II, Vol. 3. Human Myeloid and

Hematopoietic Cells ed E.L. Reinherz Haynes BF, Nadler LM, Bernstein ID. 1986;109-121.

48. Tetteroo PAT, van det Schoot CE, Bos MJE, von dem Borne AEG Kr. Three different types of Fc receptors on human leukocytes defined by workshop antibodies: $Fc_\gamma RI_{10}$ of K/Nk lymphocytes and $Fc_\gamma RII$. In Leulocyte Typing III, vol 3. Human Myeloid and Hematopoietic Cells, eds. McMichael A, Oxford Univ Press. 1987.

49. Huizinga TWJ, van der Schoot CE, Jost C, Klaasen R, Kleijer M, van dem Brone AEG Kr, Roos D, and Teteroo PAT. The PI-linked receptor FcRIII is released on stimulation of neutrophils. Nature 1988;333:667-9.

50. Simmons D and Seed B. The Fc_γ receptor of natural killer cells is a phospholipid-linked membrane protein. Nature 1988;133:568-570.

51. Darby, C, Chien P, Rossman, M and Schreiber, AD. Monocyte/macrophage $Fc_\gamma RIII$, unlike $Fc_\gamma RIII$ on neutrophils, is not PI-linked protein. Blood 1990;75:2396-2400.

52. Clarkson SB, Bussel JB, Kimberly RP, Valinsky JE, Nachman RL, and Unkeless JC. Treatment of refractory immune thrombocytopenic purpura with an anti-Fc gamma-receptor antibody. N Engl J Med 1986;314:1236-1239.

53. Clarkson SB, Kimberly KP, Bussel JB, Witner MD, Valinsky JE, Nachman RL, Unkeless JC. Treatment of refractory immune thrombocytopenic purpura with an anti-Fc_γ-receptor antibody N Eng J Med 1986;314:1236-39.

54. Darby, C, Chien, P, Kootstra, GJ and Schreiber, AD. Regulation of $Fc_\gamma RIII$ generation on cultured human monocytes. Submitted for publication.

55. Indik, Z, Kelly, C, Chien, P, Levinson, AI and Schreiber, AD. Human $Fc_\gamma RII$ in the absence of other Fc_γ receptors, mediates a phagocytic signal. J Clin Invest 119;1766-1771.

56. Huang, MM, Indik, Z, Brass, LF, Schreiber, AD and Brugge, JS. Stimulation of the platelets Fc_γ receptor ($Fc_\gamma RII$) activates tyrosine phosphorylation. J Biol Chem, in press.

57. Isaacs, R, Chien, P and Schreiber, AD. $Fc_\gamma RIIIA$ mediates phagocytosis of IgG-sensitized RBCs and transduces a calcium signal in COS-1 cells. Blood 1991;78:386a.

SYNERGY BETWEEN G-CSF AND WR-2721: EFFECTS ON ENHANCING HEMOPOIETIC RECONSTITUTION AND INCREASING SURVIVAL FOLLOWING EXPOSURE TO IONIZING RADIATION

M.L. Patchen, T.J. MacVittie, and L.M. Souza

*Armed Forces Radiobiology Research Institute, Bethesda, MD and #AMGen, Thousand Oaks, CA

INTRODUCTION

WR-2721 is one of the most effective exogenous radioprotectants discovered (1, 2). Mechanisms through which WR-2721 protects cells from radiation-induced lethality include free radical scavenging, hydrogen atom donation, and induction of hypoxia. As a survival-enhancer in experimental animals, WR-2721 is extremely effective when administered ~30 min before radiation exposure. However, because the survival-enhancing effects of WR-2721 are dose dependent, WR-2721 doses that produce the greatest radioprotection are also the most toxic (3, 4). We previously demonstrated that an alternate approach to the use of high (potentially toxic) doses of single radioprotectants is the use of low doses of multiple agents that act by different survival-enhancing mechanisms (5, 6). For example, we demonstrated that the survival-enhancing effects of low-dose WR-2721 could be increased when glucan, an immunomodulator and hemopoietic stimulant, was administered following irradiation. The enhanced survival observed with WR-2721 + glucan was attributed to sequential effects of cell protection mediated by WR-2721 and increased hemopoietic proliferation mediated by glucan. Because glucan is a potent inducer of hemopoietic cytokines (7, 8), we hypothesized that hemopoietic cytokines may be used in place of glucan to stimulate hemopoiesis and to increase the survival-enhancing effects of WR-2721. In these particular studies, the ability of granulocyte colony-stimulating factor (G-CSF) to increase the survival-enhancing effects of a low dose of WR-2721 are described.

METHODS AND MATERIALS

Mice

C3H/HeN female mice (~20 g) were purchased from Charles River Laboratories (Raleigh, NC). Mice were maintained at the Armed Forces Radiobiology Research Institute (AFRRI) in a facility accredited by the American Association for the Accreditation of Laboratory Animal Care (AAALAC). Mice were housed 10 per cage in Micro-Isolator cages on hardwood-chip, contact bedding and were provided commercial rodent chow and acidified water (pH 2.5) ad libitum. Animal rooms were equipped with full-spectrum light from 6 a.m. to 6 p.m. and were maintained at 70°F +/- 2°F with 50% +/- 10% relative humidity using at least 10 air changes per hour of 100% conditioned fresh air. Upon arrival, all mice were tested for Pseudomonas and quarantined until test results were obtained. Only healthy mice were released for experimentation. All animal experiments were approved by the Institute Animal Care and Use Committee prior to performance.

WR-2721 And G-CSF

Stock WR-2721 was obtained from Walter Reed Army Institute of Research (Washington, DC) and kept frozen at -20°C until use. Immediately before each use, WR-2721 was dissolved in sterile pyrogen-free saline. Exposure of the material to light was minimized. Thirty minutes before irradiation, mice were injected intraperitoneally (i.p.) with 4 mg of WR-2721 in a 0.5-ml volume. WR-2721 control mice received 0.5 ml of saline. Recombinant human G-CSF was provided by AMGen (Thousand Oaks, CA). The G-CSF was E. coli-derived and had a specific activity of 10^8 units/mg as assayed by a granulocyte-macrophage colony-forming unit assay using normal human bone marrow cells. Endotoxin contamination was less than 0.5 ng/mg protein as determined by the Limulus amebocyte lysate assay. G-CSF was administered subcutaneously (s.c.) once per day at a dose of 2.5 ug in a 0.1-ml volume on days 1-16 postirradiation. G-CSF controls were administered 0.1 ml of saline s.c.

Irradiation

Mice were placed in ventilated Plexiglas containers and exposed to bilateral total-body gamma rays at a dose rate of 0.4 Gy/min. The AFRRI ^{60}Co source was used for irradiations. Dosimetry was determined by ionization chambers as previously described (9) with calibration factors traceable to the National Institute of Standards and Technology. Before initiating animal experiments, the dose rate at the midline of an acrylic mouse phantom was measured using a 0.5-cm^3 tissue equivalent ionization chamber manufactured by Exradin (Lisle, IL). Before each experimental irradiation, the dose rate at the same location with the phantom removed was measured using a 50-cm^3 ionization chamber fabricated at AFRRI. The ratio of these two dose rates, the tissue-air ratio (TAR), was then used to ensure delivery of the midline dose desired for each animal exposure. The TAR used in these experiments was 1.001.

Survival Assays

Ten mice receiving each drug treatment were exposed to radiation doses ranging from 7 Gy to 14 Gy. Irradiated mice were returned to the animal facility and cared for routinely. Survival was monitored for 30 days; on day 31 surviving mice were euthanized by cervical dislocation. Experiments were repeated three times. The percentage of mice surviving each radiation dose at 30 days postexposure was used to construct a survival curve for each drug treatment. The radiation dose lethal for 50% of mice within 30 days postexposure (LD50/30) was extrapolated from each survival curve and used to calculate dose reduction factors (DRF's; LD50/30 of treated mice divided by LD50/30 of radiation control mice) for each drug treatment.

Spleen Colony-Forming Unit Assays

Endogenous and exogenous spleen colony-forming units were used to evaluate regeneration of pluripotent hemopoietic progenitor cells. Endogenous spleen colony-forming units (E-CFU) were evaluated using the method of Till and McCulloch (10). Mice from various treatment groups were exposed to 10.75 Gy total-body irradiation. Twelve days after irradiation, mice were euthanized by cervical dislocation and their spleens were removed. Spleens were fixed in Bouin's solution, and the number of grossly visible spleen colonies was counted. Exogenous spleen colony-forming units (CFU-s) were also evaluated by a method of Till and McCulloch (11). Recipient mice were exposed to 9.25 Gy of total-body irradiation to eradicate most endogenous hemopoietic stem cells. Three to five hours later, 1-5 x 10^4 bone marrow or 1-5 x 10^5 spleen cells from normal or treated mice were intravenously injected into the lateral tail veins of irradiated recipient mice. Twelve days after transplantation, the recipients were euthanized by cervical dislocation, the spleens were removed, and spleen colonies were counted as described for the E-CFU assay. The cell suspensions used for each CFU-s assay represented tissues from three normal, irradiated, G-CSF-treated, WR-2721-treated, or combination-treated mice at each time point. Cells were flushed from femurs with 3 ml of McCoy's 5A medium (Flow Labs, McLean, VA) containing 10% heat-inactivated fetal bovine serum (Hyclone Labs, Logan, UT). Spleens were pressed through stainless-steel mesh screen, and the cells were washed from the screen with 6 ml medium. The total number of nucleated cells in the suspensions was determined by Coulter counter. Experiments were repeated three times.

Granulocyte-Macrophage Colony-Forming Cell Assay

Hemopoietic progenitor cells committed to granulocyte and/or macrophage development were assayed using a previously described (5) agar granulocyte-macrophage colony-forming cell (GM-CFC) assay. Mouse endotoxin serum (5% v/v) was added to feeder layers as a source of colony-stimulating activity. Colonies (> 50 cells) were counted after 10 days of incubation in a 37°C humidified environment containing 5% CO_2. Triplicate plates were cultured for each cell suspension, and experiments were repeated three times. The cell suspensions used for each assay were prepared as described for the CFU-s assay.

Peripheral Blood Cell Counts

Blood was obtained from halothane-anesthetized mice by cardiac puncture using a heparinized syringe attached to a 20-gauge needle. White blood cell (WBC), red blood cell (RBC), and platelet (PLT) counts were performed using a Coulter counter.

Statistics

Results of replicate experiments were pooled and represent the mean +/- standard error of pooled data. Student's t-test was used to determine statistical differences in all but survival data. Survival data were analyzed using the method of Finney (12). Differences were considered significant when the p-value was less than 0.05.

RESULTS

Survival-Enhancing Effects of G-CSF, WR-2721, And WR-2721 + G-CSF

The ability of G-CSF, WR-2721, and WR-2721 + G-CSF to enhance survival in irradiated mice is illustrated in Figure 1. The LD50/30 for saline-treated mice was 7.85 Gy +/- 0.06 Gy. Preirradiation administration of 4 mg of WR-2721 significantly increased survival, resulting in an LD50/30 of 11.30 Gy +/- 0.15 Gy and a DRF of 1.44. Postirradiation treatment with G-CSF alone also slightly enhanced survival, yielding an LD50/30 of 8.30 Gy +/- 0.08 Gy and a DRF of 1.06. Administration of WR-2721 preirradiation and G-CSF postirradiation raised the LD50/30 to 12.85 Gy +/- 0.24 Gy, and resulted in a DRF of 1.64. This DRF was more than additive between the DRF's obtained with WR-2721 (1.44) and G-CSF (1.06) alone.

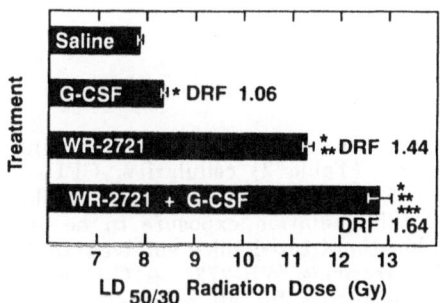

Figure 1. Effect of saline, G-CSF, WR-2721, and WR-2721 + G-CSF treatments on survival of irradiated mice. C3H/HeN mice were administered WR-2721 (4 mg/mouse, i.p.) 30 min before ^{60}Co irradiation and G-CSF (2.5 ug/mouse/day, s.c.) on days 1-16 after irradiation. * p < 0.05, with respect to saline values; ** p < 0.05, with respect to G-CSF values; *** p < 0.05, with respect to WR-2721 values.

The E-CFU assay was used in preliminary studies to identify hemopoietic differences among saline-, G-CSF-, WR-2721-, and combination-treated mice. In these studies a 10.75-Gy radiation dose was chosen because it was the highest radiation dose that would permit saline-treated mice to survive the 12 days postirradiation needed for performing the E-CFU assay. Figure 2 illustrates the E-CFU results obtained in mice exposed to 10.75 Gy. No E-CFU were detected in saline- or G-CSF-treated mice. WR-2721-treated mice exhibited only 1.8 +/- 0.1 E-CFU, while combination-treated mice exhibited 12.4 +/- 1.5 E-CFU. These data illustrate the ability of G-CSF to amplify the number of multipotent hemopoietic stem cells protected by preirradiation WR-2721 administration. The onset and duration of the hemopoietic responses induced by G-CSF, WR-2721, and WR-2721 +

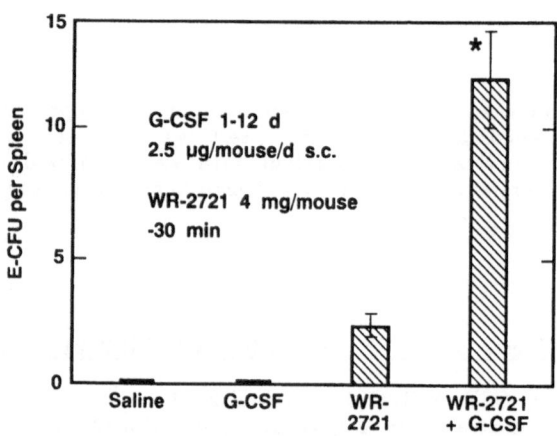

Figure 2. Effect of saline, G-CSF, WR-2721, and WR-2721 + G-CSF treatments on endogenous spleen colony formation (E-CFU) in mice exposed to 10.75 Gy. C3H/HeN mice were administered WR-2721 (4 mg/mouse, i.p.) 30 min before ^{60}Co irradiation and G-CSF (2.5 ug/mouse/day, s.c.) on days 1-12 (assay terminated on day 12) after irradiation. Data represented as the mean +/- standard error of values obtained from 15 mice in each treatment group. * $p < 0.05$, with respect to WR-2721 values.

G-CSF were further characterized by sequentially following the recovery of bone marrow (Table 1) and splenic (Table 2) cellularity, CFU-s, and GM-CFC on days 10, 17 and 24 after a 10.75-Gy radiation exposure. Although mice from all four treatment groups survived this radiation exposure to be evaluated at day 10, only WR-2721-treated and combination-treated mice survived to be evaluated on days 17 and 24 postexposure. Mice receiving WR-2721 + G-CSF consistently exhibited the most rapid and dramatic recoveries for all parameters evaluated. In addition to enhanced hemopoietic stem and progenitor cell recoveries, a more rapid recovery of mature peripheral blood WBC's, RBC's, and PLT's was also observed in mice receiving the combination WR-2721 + G-CSF treatment (Table 3).

Table 1

**Effect of G-CSF, WR-2721, and WR-2721 + G-CSF on
Bone Marrow Cellularity, CFU-s, and GM-CFC Following a
10.75 Gy Radiation Exposure[1]**

	Saline	G-CSF	WR-2721	WR-2721 + G-CSF
			Treatment	
Cells per Femur (x 10^6)				
Day 10	0.37 ± 0.02	0.52 ± 0.09	1.46 ± 0.15	2.32 ± 0.25^3
17	$-^2$	$-^2$	2.14 ± 0.38	2.91 ± 0.16
24	$-^2$	$-^2$	2.23 ± 0.27	5.23 ± 0.25^3
CFU-s per Femur				
Day 10	0 ± 0	0 ± 0	0 ± 0	0 ± 0
17	$-^2$	$-^2$	18.00 ± 4.00	84.00 ± 12.00^3
24	$-^2$	$-^2$	53.00 ± 11.00	381.00 ± 68.00^3
GM-CFC per Femur				
Day 10	0 ± 0	0 ± 0	0 ± 0	16.00 ± 5.00^3
17	$-^2$	$-^2$	38.00 ± 11.00	353.00 ± 46.00^3
24	$-^2$	$-^2$	234.00 ± 53.00	510.00 ± 57.00^3

[1] Mean ± standard error of values obtained for three experiments.

[2] No mice survived to be assayed at this time point.

[3] $p < 0.05$, with respect to WR-2721 values.

(In nonirradiated C_3H/HeN mice, Cellularity = 6.59 ± 0.32, CFU-s = 2787 ± 423, GM-CFC = 3366 ± 263).

Table 2

**Effect of G-CSF, WR-2721, and WR-2721 + G-CSF on Splenic Cellularity, CFU-s,
and GM-CFC Following a 10.75 Gy Radiation Exposure[1]**

	Saline	G-CSF	WR-2721	WR-2721 + G-CSF
			Treatment	
Cells per Spleen (x 10^6)				
Day 10	12.0 ± 0.2	13.0 ± 0.5	14.1 ± 0.6	15.2 ± 0.8
17	$-^2$	$-^2$	69.9 ± 1.9	223.3 ± 23.2^3
24	$-^2$	$-^2$	194.6 ± 16.3	153.4 ± 26.1
CFU-s per Spleen				
Day 10	0.8 ± 0.4	1.3 ± 0.2	4.7 ± 1.2	54.8 ± 6.8^3
17	$-^2$	$-^2$	488.0 ± 25.6	1382.0 ± 34.1^3
24	$-^2$	$-^2$	2473.0 ± 490.0	4193.0 ± 526.7^3
GM-CFC per Spleen				
Day 10	0 ± 0	0 ± 0	0 ± 0	0 ± 0
17	$-^2$	$-^2$	249.0 ± 35.5	13044.0 ± 1040.0^3
24	$-^2$	$-^2$	13132.0 ± 1015.0	17776.0 ± 1208.0^3

[1] Mean ± standard error of values obtained from three experiments.

[2] No mice survived to be assayed at this time point.

[3] $p < 0.05$, with respect to WR-2721 values.

(In nonirradiated C_3H/HeH mice, Cellularity = 147 ± 10, CFU-s = 6907 ± 779, GM-CFC = 1650 ± 118).

Table 3
Effect of WR-2721 and WR-2721 + G-CSF on
Peripheral Blood Cell Counts Following a
10.75 Gy Radiation Exposure[1]

	Treatment	
	WR-2721	WR-2721 + G-CSF
WBC per mm^3 (x 10^3)		
Day 10	1.4 ± 0.3	1.4 ± 0.2
17	2.3 ± 0.1	18.3 ± 3.1[2]
24	5.5 ± 0.3	28.4 ± 3.5[2]
RBC per mm^3 (x 10^6)		
Day 10	5.0 ± 0.5	4.3 ± 0.5
17	3.4 ± 0.3	4.0 ± 0.4
24	2.3 ± 0.6	6.0 ± 0.2[2]
PLT per mm^3 (x 10^3)		
Day 10	45.0 ± 9.0	170.0 ± 22.0[2]
17	100.0 ± 18.0	177.0 ± 13.0[2]
24	151.0 ± 15.0	435.0 ± 98.0[2]

[1] Mean ± standard error of values obtained from 3 experiments.

[2] $p < 0.05$, with respect to WR-2721 values.

(In nonirradiated C$_3$H/HeN mice, WBC = 6.2 ± 0.7; RBC = 6.3 ± 0.5 and PLT = 950 ± 38)

DISCUSSION

Hemopoietic injury and associated risks of infection and hemorrhage are common problems associated with radiation and radiomemetic drug therapies used in the treatment of cancer. Recent studies have demonstrated that the aminothiol WR-2721 can be administered prior to irradiation or chemotherapy to selectively protect normal cells, especially hemopoietic cells, and as a result reduce radiation- or drug-induced hemopoietic injury (14, 15, 16, 17, 18, 19, 20). Administration of the hemopoietic growth factor granulocyte colony-stimulating factor (G-CSF) after radiation or radiomimetic drug therapies also has been demonstrated to reduce the side effects of hemopoietic injury by accelerating hemopoietic regeneration (21, 22, 23, 24, 25, 26, 27, 28). In the studies reported here, we evaluated the survival and hemopoietic effects of WR-2721 and G-CSF used in combination in a murine radiation model.

In addition to reconfirming the ability of both WR-2721 and G-CSF to individually enhance survival in irradiated mice (2, 5, 6, 24), our data clearly illustrate the benefit of using these two agents in combination. The enhanced survival observed in combination-treated mice (Figure 1) appeared to result from the ability of G-CSF to accelerate regeneration of mature hemopoietic elements (Table 3) by amplification of multipotent and committed progenitor cells protected by the WR-2721 treatment (Tables 2 and 3).

In conclusion, we have demonstrated that the use of WR-2721 + G-CSF in combination can synergize to further mitigate hemopoietic injury and lethality associated with radiation exposure. Postirradiation use of hemopoietic growth factors in combination with classical radioprotectants may prove to be a valuable adjunctive therapy in the treatment of cancer.

ACKNOWLEDGMENTS

We are grateful to Mr. Brian Solberg and Ms. Barbara Calabro for excellent technical assistance and to Ms. Carolyn Wooden and Ms. Catharine Sund for editorial assistance. This work was supported by the Armed Forces Radiobiology Research Institute, Defense Nuclear Agency, under Research Work Unit 00132. Views presented in this paper are those of the authors; no endorsement by the Defense Nuclear Agency has been given or should be inferred. Research was conducted according to the principles enunciated in the Guide for the Care and Use of Laboratory Animals prepared by the Institute of Laboratory Animal Resources, National Research Council.

REFERENCES

1. D.Q. Brown, W.J. Graham, L.J. MacKenzie, J.W. Pittock, and L.M. Shaw, Can WR-2721 be improved upon? Pharmacol. Ther. 39:157 (1988).

2. D.E. Davidson, M.M. Grenan, and T.R. Sweeney, Biological characteristics of some improved radioprotectors, in: "Radiation Sensitizers: Their Use in the Clinical Management of Cancer", L.W. Brady, ed., Masson Publishing, New York (1980).

3. M.R. Landauer, H.D. Davis, J.A. Dominitz, and J.F. Weiss, Dose and time relationships of the radioprotector WR-2721 on locomotor activity in mice. Pharmacol. Biochem. Behav. 27:573 (1987).

4. J.M. Yuhas, Biological factors affecting the radioprotective efficiency of s-2[3-aminopropylamino]ethyl phosphorothioic acid (WR-2721): LD50/30 doses. Radiat. Res. 44:621 (1970).

5. M.L. Patchen, T.J. MacVittie, and W.E. Jackson, Postirradiation glucan administration enhances the radioprotective effects of WR-2721. Radiat. Res. 117:59 (1989).

6. M.L. Patchen, T.J. MacVittie, and J.F. Weiss, Combined modality radioprotection: The use of glucan and selenium with WR-2721. Int. J. Radiat. Oncol. Biol. Phys. 18:1069 (1990).

7. M.L. Patchen and T.J. MacVittie, Hemopoietic effects of intravenous soluble glucan administration. J. Immunopharmacol. 8:407 (1986).

8. E.R. Sherwood, D.L. Williams, R. McNamee, E. Jones, W. Browder, and N.R. DiLuzio, Enhancement of interleukin-1 and interleukin-2 production by soluble glucan. Int. J. Immunopharmacol. 9:261 (1987).

9. J. Schulz, P.R. Almond, J.R. Cunningham, J.G. Holt, R. Loevinger, N. Suntharalingam, K.A. Wright, R. Nath, and D. Lempert, A protocol for the determination of absorbed dose for high energy photon and electron beams. Med. Phys. 10:741 (1983).

10. J.E. Till and E.A. McCulloch, Early repair processes in marrow cells irradiated and proliferating in vivo. Radiat. Res. 18:96 (1963).

11. J.E. Till and E.A. McCulloch, A direct measurement of the radiation sensitivity of normal mouse bone marrow cells. Radiat. Res. 14:213 (1961).

12. D.J. Finney, "Statistical Methods in Biological Assays", MacMillan Press, New York (1978).

13. G.S. Peters, C.L. van der Wilt, F. Gyergyay, J. van Laar, and H.M. Pinedo, Protection by WR-2721 of the toxicity induced by the combination of cisplatin and 5-fluorouracil. Proceedings of the 7th International Conference on Chemical Modifiers (In Press).

14. J.H. Wasserman, T.L. Phillips, G. Ross, and L.J. Kane, Differential protection against cytotoxic chemotherapeutic effects on bone marrow CFU's by WR-2721. Cancer Clin. Trials. 4:3 (1981).

15. J.M. Yuhas, J.M. Spellman and F. Culo, The role of WR-2721 in radiotherapy and/or chemotherapy. in: "Radiation Sensitizers: Their Use in the Clinical Management of Cancer", L.W. Brady, ed., Masson Publishing, New York (1980).

16. D.J. Grdina and C.P. Sigdestad, Radiation protectors: the unexpected benefits. Drug Metabol. Rev. 20:1342 (1989).

17. L. Milas, N. Hunter, C. Stephens, and L.J. Peters, Inhibition of radiation carcinogenesis in mice by s-2-(3-aminopropylamino)-ethyl phosphorothioic acid. Cancer Res. 44:5567 (1984).

18. B. Nagy, P.J. Dale, and D.J. Grdina, Protection against cis diaminodichloroplatinum cytotoxicity and mutagenicity in V79 cells by 2-[(aminopropyl)-amino]ethanethiol. Cancer Res. 46:1132 (1986).

19. D. Glover, S. Grabelsky, K. Fox, C. Weiler, L. Cannon, and J. Glick, Clinical trials of WR-2721 and cis-platinum. Int. J. Radiat. Oncol. Biol.Phys. 16:1201 (1989).

20. A.T. Turrisi, M.M. Kligerman, D.J. Glover, J.H. Glick, L. Norfleet, and M. Gramkowski, Experience with Phase I trials of WR-2721 preceeding radiation therapy. in: "Radioprotectors and Anticarcinogens", O.F. Nygaard and M.G. Simic, eds., Academic Press, New York (1983).

21. C.A. Sieff, Hematopoietic growth factors. J. Clin. Invest. 79:1549 (1987).

22. Y. Kobayashi, T. Okabe, A. Urabe, N. Suzuki, and F. Takaku, Human granulocyte colony-stimulating factor produced by Escherichia coli shortens the period of granulocytopenia induced by irradiation in mice. Jpn. J. Cancer Res. 78:763 (1987).

23. T.J. MacVittie, R.L. Monroy, M.L. Patchen, and L.M. Souza, Therapeutic use of recombinant human G-CSF (rhG-CSF) in a canine model of sublethal and lethal whole-body irradiation. Int. J. Radiat. Biol. 57:723 (1990).

24. M.L. Patchen, T.J. MacVittie, B.D. Solberg, and L.M. Souza, Therapeutic administration of recombinant human granulocyte colony-stimulating factor accelerates hemopoietic regeneration and enhances survival in a murine model of radiation-induced myelosuppression. Int. J. Cell Cloning 8:107 (1990).

25. J.E. Talmadge, H. Tribble, R. Pennington, O. Bowersox, M.A. Schneider, P. Castelli, P.L. Black, and F. Abe, Protective, restorative, and therapeutic properties of recombinant colony-stimulating factors. Blood 73:2093 (1989).

26. M.A. Bonilla, A.P. Gillio, M. Ruggerio, N.A. Kernan, J.A. Brochstein, M. Abboud, L. Fumagalli, M. Vincent, J.L. Gabrilove, K. Welte, L.M. Souza, and R.J. O'Reilly, Effects of recombinant human granulocyte colony-stimulating factor on neutropenia in patients with congenital agranulocytosis. N. Engl. J. Med. 320:1574 (1989).

27. M.H. Bronchurd, J.H. Scarffe, N. Thatcher, D. Crowther, L.M. Souza, N.K. Alton, N.G. Testa, and T.M. Dexter, Phase I/II study of recombinant human granulocyte colony-stimulating factor in patients receiving intensive chemotherapy for small cell lung cancer. Br. J. Cancer. 56:809 (1987).

28. J.A. Glaspy and D.W. Golde, Clinical trials of myeloid growth factors. Exp. Hematol. 18:1137 (1990).

ST 789, A CANDIDATE FOR COMBINATION THERAPIES OF INFECTIONS AND CANCER

C. De Simone, E. Arrigoni Martelli*,
G. Famularo#, P. Foresta*, V. Ruggiero*,
R. Giacomelli#, G. Tonietti#, and
E. Jirillo##

Infectious Dieseases, Dept. Exp. Medicine
University of L'Aquila, L'Aquila
*Sigma-Tau, Pomezia
#Internal Medicine, L'Aquila
##Immunology, Bari, Italy

INTRODUCTION

ST 789 is a synthetic compound which belongs to a new family of hypoxanthine derivatives exhibiting an aminoacidic function at the N-9 position of the purine ring (Cornaglia-Ferraris et al., 1984). Available literature indicates that hypoxanthine derivatives exhibit well established immunomodulant properties (Cornaglia-Ferraris et al., 1984). Furthermore, the addition of arginine to these molecules proved able to strongly enhance their immunomodulant activity. We review here the immunomodulant properties of both arginine and arginine-containing compounds, and mostly of ST 789. Furthermore, we report the results of preliminary experiments performed in our laboratory to better understand the mechanisms accounting for the immunomodulant activity of ST 789.

EFFECTS OF ARGININE ON IMMUNE RESPONSE

As far as the effects of arginine on immune response are concerned a large body of experimental evidence has been accumulated since the early report of the arginine role in the recovery of wound healing capacity in experimentally injured rats (Seifter et al., 1978). Diet arginine supplementation recently proved in animal models to enhance peripheral blood T lymphocyte responsiveness to both mitogens and antigens (Barbul et al., 1980) as well as to increase thymic weight and cellularity in otherwise normal rats (Daly et al., 1990). Arginine supplementation has also been shown to increase the T-cell antitumor activity (Reynolds et al., 1990; Lowell et al., 1990) and natural killer (NK)- and macrophage-dependent cytotoxicity (Lowell et al., 1990; Reynolds et al., 1988; Daly et al., 1988). Furthermore, the arginine supplementation in surgical patients has been reported to increase both the surface expression of CD4 antigen and lymphocyte responsiveness to mitogens (Daly et al., 1988).

The ability of arginine to enhance immune functions has been shown also in *in vitro* studies. In fact, the pretreatment of peripheral blood lymphocytes with arginine either alone or in combination with lysine in concentrations as similar as those obtained by *in vivo* administration resulted in a strong enhancement of both T- and spleen-cell activation following mitogens (Reynolds et al., 1988; Fabris et al., 1991). Conflicting data have been recently reported about the role of arginine in modulating NK activity. In fact, arginine supplementation seems to be able to recover the low endogenous NK activity (Fabris et al., 1991). Furthermore, preliminary data suggest that arginine supplementation is also unable to restore cytotoxicity in the normal range in animals with reduced NK responsiveness to IL-2 boosting, whereas a strong enhancement has been found following interferon (IFN) stimulation (Fabris et al., 1991).

Moreover, arginine concentrations lower than plasma levels commonly obtained throughout *in vivo* administration enhance macrophage functions, such as phagocytosis, bacterial *killing* and monokine production, whereas higher arginine concentrations exhibit strong inhibitory properties (Albi et al., 1989; Fabris et al., 1991). Furthermore, arginine is strictly required by monocyte-macrophages for producing reactive nitrogen intermediates, at least in certain macrophage-target cell combinations (Keller et al., 1990).

Several mechanisms could be indirectly involved in mediating the immuno-modulating effects of arginine. Arginine has a secretagogue action on growth hormone (GH) (Isidori et al., 1981; Fabris et al., 1988) and GH modulates various immune functions (Barbul et al., 1983). Furthermore, in rat models the enhancement of allograft rejection by arginine administration (Reynolds et al., 1990) strictly requires an intact pituitary-thymus axis (Fabris et al., 1988; Goldstein et al., 1977) as well as the recovery of thymus weight following injury is abrogated by previous hypophysectomy and restored by GH treatment (Fabris et al., 1988; Goldstein et al. 1977). This hypothesis is further supported by the recently reported arginine ability to enhance thymic endocrine activity, as demonstrated by the recovery of reduced plasma thymulin levels in both experimental animals (Fabris et al., 1991) and human cancer patients (Fabris et al., 1991; Giovarelli et al., 1987) following *in vivo* arginine administration.

EFFECTS OF ST 789 ON IMMUNE RESPONSE

ST 789, formerly PCF 39, an L-Arg synthetic derivative (N-alpha-5 (5, 6-dihydro-6-oxo-0-purinyl) pentyloxy/carbonyl-L-Arginine) has been reported to influence T lymphoproliferative responses and to induce the expression of Thy 1.2 antigen, which is an important differentiation marker of precursor T cells, on lymphocytes from *nu/nu* mice (Giovarelli et al., 1987; Baldinelli et al., 1991). These data, together with the requirement of substances potentially interesting as immunoregulatory drugs since their ability to enhance the production of mature immunocompetent cells by acting on thymocyte differentiation, prompted Baldinelli et al. to investigate the effects of ST 789 on thymocytes obtained from normal adult mice (Baldinelli et al., 1991). These authors evaluated the coordinate expression of CD4 and CD8 antigens as well as of p55 chain of IL-2 receptor (Tac antigen) in thymocyte short-term cultures upon incubation with ST 789 alone or in conjunction with PHA. The ability of ST 789 to rise intracellular free calcium ions, which is strictly correlated with lymphocyte activation, was also investigated. ST 789 was ineffective in modifying the frequency of thymocyte subsets, as determined by using dual color flow cytometry, and did not induce the appearance of p55 chain on cortical thymocytes. On the contrary, PHA resulted in a dramatic dose-dependent decrease of CD4+CD8+ thymocyte subset, which has not affected by ST 789. Finally, PHA promptly increased thymocyte free intracellular calcium ion levels, whereas ST 789 did not. Therefore, ST 789 is likely to not affect the thymocyte activation/differentiation pathway, at least in normal adult mice. However, further studies will need to evaluate the effects of ST 789 on human thymocytes.

The reported ability of ST 789 to affect both *in vitro* and *in vivo* T, NK, and phagocytic cell activity, which is strictly dependent under normal conditions on cytokine release, prompted several authors to evaluate the effects of ST 789 on the *in vitro* production of IL-1, IL-2, IL-4, IL-6, and IFN-gamma by peripheral blood mononuclear cells (PBMCs) from healthy subjects (Munno et al., 1991; Famularo et al., 1991). These experiments clearly demonstrated that ST 789 was not able per se to induce cytokine release . Furthermore, PBMC costimulation with ST 789 plus LPS, PHA and ConA did not modify IL-1, IL-2, IL-4, and IFN-gamma release in terms of either enhancement or inhibition as compared to PBMCs activated by lectins alone. However, an unexpected finding was that the addition of ST 789 to PHA-driven PBMCs resulted in strongly increased IL-6 levels in supernatants harvested following 48 hrs of culture (Famularo et al., 1991). Therefore, ST 789 seems to be a strong inducer of IL-6 production. However, currently available data did not yet address the question of which mononuclear cell subset, T or B or NK cells or monocytes, which are all capable of producing IL-6 (Hirano et al., 1990; Kishimoto, 1989), is mostly involved in ST 789-dependent enhancement of *in vitro* IL-6 release. The discrepancy between the strongly increased IL-6 levels by culturing PBMCs in the presence of both ST 789 and PHA in spite of the non affected IL-1 levels has not been fully explained since IL-6 production as a rule is strictly related to IL-1 in both *in vitro* and *in vivo* models (Hirano et al., 1990; Kishimoto, 1989). Therefore, further studies are currently in progress in our laboratory to answer this question.

A direct effect of ST 789 possibly accounting, at least in part, for the ability of enhancing lymphocyte proliferative responsiveness to both mitogens and antigens has been raised by the finding of increased intracellular levels of cyclic GMP in PBMC *in vitro* treated with substituted purines (Cornaglia-Ferraris et al., 1984). Furthermore, hypoxanthine derivatives have been recently suggested to mimic inosine ribose moiety thus acting on putative inosine receptors on both T and NK cells and modulating cellular functions (Stradi et al., 1990). However, more detailed studies will be required to better understand this issue.

The putative immunoenhancing properties of ST 789 have been strongly pointed out by demonstrating that *in vivo* administered ST 789 is able to restore immune response in immunocompromised hosts and to protect against pathogens. The treatment with cyclophosphamide (Cy), which strongly suppresses host's immune responses, has been reported to be a valuable model of immunosuppression in both animals and humans (Matsumoto et al., 1987). We recently investigated whether the pretreatment of Cy-immunosuppressed CD1 and Balb/c mice with ST 789 improved survival following the experimental infection with both bacterial

(*Klebsiella oxytoca*, *K. pneumoniae* 7823, *Escherichia coli* ESM, *Serratia marcescens* A/1, *Salmonella typhimurium*, *Proteus mirabilis*, *Pseudomonas aeruginosa*) and fungal pathogens (*Candida albicans*, *Aspergillus* (A.) *fumigatus*) (Foresta et al., l991) (Table 1).

Our data clearly demonstrate that ST 789 proved highly effective in prolonging survival of infected mice. However, the administration routes strictly affected our results. In fact, it turned out that i.p. treatment was protective, whereas both s.c. and p.o. ST 789 did not in spite of administering strongly increased doses.

Table 1 - *Protective effects of ST 789 in mice immunosuppressed with Cyclophosphamide and infected with Escherichia coli ISM.*

Treatment	Administration route	D/T $\approx LD_{10}$◆
CTR	-	7/85 (8.2%)
CTR immunosup.	-	65/85 (76.4%)
ST 789 100 mg/Kg	p.os	6/9 (66.7%)
ST 789 0.2 mg/Kg	s.c.	38/55 (69.0%)
ST 789 2 mg/Kg	s.c.	14/20 (70.0%)
ST 789 50 mg/Kg	s.c.	22/30 (73.3%)
ST 789 0.2 mg/Kg	i.p.	31/65 (47.6%)*
ST 789 2 mg/Kg	i.p.	7/30 (23.3%)*
ST 789 25 mg/Kg	i.p.	9/85 (10.5%)*

ST 789 was administered by daily injection for 5 consecutive days to mice experimentally with cyclophosphamide (100 mg/Kg,i.p.) 2 hours before starting ST 789 treatment. Treated and untreated mice were both infected 24h after the last ST 789 administration.
◆: inoculum corresponding approx. to 1.35 x 10^3 microbial cells
χ^2: * = p ≤ 0.001

Furthermore, preliminary experiments performed in our laboratory indicate that the combined administration of ST 789 and ceftazidime at doses per se completely ineffective (0.05 mg/Kg/day and 0.02 mg/Kg, for ST 789 and ceftazidime, respectively) proved to strongly protect Cy-immunosuppressed mice in the *K. oxytoca* model of experimental infection. ST 789 and amphotericin B exhibited a similar synergism in the treatment of both *C. albicans* and *A. fumigatus* experimental infections as well as ST 789 and gentamicin were synergistic in treating Cy-immunosuppressed mice following the challenge with *P. aeruginosa*. Therefore, ST 789 either alone or in combination with antibiotics such as ceftazidime, amphotericin B, and gentamicin enhances host's defenses against several pathogens, at least in animal models of immunosuppression.

The mechanisms accounting for these effects of ST 789 are yet poorly understood. The reported ST 789 ability in restoring the proliferative responsiveness to mitogens of lymphocytes from Cy-treated mice (Ruggiero et al., 1991) is likely to play a major role. However, other cellular targets could mediate the immunomodulant activity of ST 789. In fact, ST 789 treatment proved to expand the bone marrow NK progenitor cells *in vivo*, thus strongly enhancing the regeneration of murine NK cell activity (Riccardi et al., 1991).

Furthermore, since Cy-treatment severely reduces circulating granulocytes (Matsumoto et al., 1987), the capacity of ST 789 to protect Cy-treated mice against pathogens might depend on recruitment of granulocytes, and possibly, monocytes. A role of granulocyte-colony-stimulating factor in mediating this effect of ST 789 has not been yet demonstrated; thus, further studies are currently in progress in our laboratory to better understand this issue.

ANTITUMOR ACTIVITY OF ST 789

A clear-cut antitumor activity of ST 789 has been demonstrated. In fact, mice parenterally administered with ST 789 exhibited a significant resistance to the growth of two syngeneic tumors regardless of the presence of spleen cells mixed with tumor cells (Giovarelli et al., 1987). It is worth to emphasize that tumor inhibition mediated by IL-2 and IFN-gamma has been shown to be strictly dependent on the presence of splenocyte (Forni et al., 1985; Giovarelli et al., 1986). Furthermore, these data indirectly support the results of previous experiments assaying the ability of ST 789 to induce U-937 and HL-60 human leukemic cell lines to differentiate. In fact, ST 789 did not result into differentiation, whereas IFN-gamma and 12-O-tetradecanoyl-13-phorbol-acetate (TPA) led to U-937 and HL-60 cell line activation, as shown by morphologic and phenotypic changes (Ponzoni et al., 1987). Therefore, we suggest that the antitumor activity of ST 789 is mediated by a different pathway as compared to IL-2 and IFN-gamma. Finally, available literature indicates that the arginine residue of ST789 molecule is likely to play a pivotal role in mediating the antitumor activity of ST 789 by increasing T-lymphocyte cytotoxicity (Reynolds et al., 1990; Lowellet al., 1990) as well as NK and macrophage cytotoxicity (Lowell et al., 1990; Reynolds et al., 1988; Daly et al., 1988). Furthermore, a significant absolute increase of CD4+ cells was found in cancer patients following the treatment with arginine-lysine combination (Fabris et al., 1991).

REFERENCES

Albina, J. E., Caldwell, M. D., Henry, W. L. Jr, Mills, C.D.,1989, Regulation of macrophage functions by L-Arginine, J Exp Med 169: 1021-1029.

Baldinelli, L., Biselli, R., Fattorossi, A., 1991 (in press),Influence of ST 789 on murine thymocytes: a flow cytometry study of thymocyte subset distribution and of intracellular free Ca++ increase upon activation, Thymus.

Barbui, A., Wasserkrug, H. L., Seifter, E., Rettura, G., Levenson, S. M., Efron, G., 1980, Immunostimulatory effects of arginine in normal and injured rats, J Surg Res 29: 228-235.

Barbul, A., Rettura, G., Levenson, S. M., Seifter, E., Wound healing and thymotrophic effects of arginine: a pituitary mechanism of action, 1983, Am J Clin Nutr 37: 786-794.

Cornaglia-Ferraris, P., Coffey, R. G., Hadden, J.W., Substituted purines as immunomodulators: speculative considerations, 1984, J Immunol Immunopharmacol 2: 134-141.

Cornaglia-Ferraris,P., 1985, Immunomodulatory properties of a N-9 arginyl hypo-xantine derivative (PCF-39), Int J Immunopharmacol 7: 338-346.

Daly, J. M., Reynolds, J. V., Thon, A. K., Kinsley, L., Dietrich-Gallagher, M., Shou, J., Ruggieri, B., 1988, Immune and metabolic effects of arginine in the surgical patient, Am Surgery 208: 512-533.

Daly, J. M., Reynolds, J., Sigal, R. K., Shou, J., Liberman, M. D., 1990, Effect of dietary protein and amino-acids on immune function, Crit Care Med 18: 86-93. y

Fabris, N., Moccheggiani, E., Muzzioli, M., Provinciali, M.,19881, Neuroedocrine-thymus interactions: perspectives for intervention in aging, Ann NY Acad Sci 521: 72-87.

Fabris, N., Moccheggiani, E., 1991 (in press), Arginine-containing compounds and thymic endocrine activity, Thymus.

Famularo, G., Giacomelli, R., Valdarnini, D., De Simone, C., Tonietti, G., 1991 (in press), Modulation by ST 789 of *in vitro* lymphocyte activation and cytokine production, Thymus.

Foresta, P., Riccardi, C., 1991 (in press), Immunorestorative properties of ST 789 on experimentally immunosuppressed and infected mice, 1991 (in press), Thymus.

Forni, G., Giovarelli, M., Santoni, A., 1985, Lymphokine-activated tumor inhibition in vivo. The local administration of interleukin 2 triggers nonreactive lymphocytes from tumor bearing mice to inhibit tumor growth, J Immunol, 134: 1305-1311.

Giovarelli, M., Cofano, F., Vecchi, A., Forni, M., Landolfo, S., Forni, G., 1986, Interferon-activated tumor inhibition in vivo: small amounts of interferon-gamma inhibit tumor growth by eliciting host systemic immunoreactivity, Int J Cancer 37: 141-148.

Giovarelli, M., Arione, R., Jemma, C., Musso, T., Benetton, G., Forni, G., Cornaglia-Ferraris, P., 1987, In vitro and in vivo immunomodulatory activity of an N-9 arginyl hypoxantine derivative (PCF-39) Int J Immunopharmacol 9: 659-667.

Goldstein, A. L., Low, T.L.K., Mc Adoo, M., 1977, Thymosin alpha 1. Isolation and seuence analysis of an immunological active thymic polypeptide, Proc Natl Acad Sci USA 74: 711-715.

Hirano, T., Akira, S., Taga, T., Kishimoto, T., 1990, Biological and clinical aspects of interleukin 6, Immunol Today 11: 443-449.

Isidori, A., Lo Monaco, A., Cappa, M., 1981, A study of growth hormone release in man after oral administration of amino acids, Curr Med Opin 7: 475-481.

Keller, R., Geiges, M., Keist, R., 1990, L-arginine-dependent reactive intermediates as mediator of tumor cell killing by activated macrophages, Cancer Res 50: 1421-1425.

Kishimoto, T., 1989, The biology of interleukin-6, Blood 74: 1-10.

Lowell, J. A., Parnes, H. L., Blackborn, G. L., 1990, Dietary immunomodulation: beneficial effects on oncogenesis and tumor growth, Crit Care Med 18: 145-148.

Matsumoto, M., Matsubara, S., Matsuno, T., 1987, Protective effect of human granulocyte colony-stimulating factor on microbial infections in neutropenic mice, Infect Immunol 55: 2715-2722.

Munno, I., Pellegrino, N. M., Marcuccio, C., De Simone, C., Jirillo, E., 1991 (in press) Influence of ST 789 on interleukin-1, interleukin-2 and interferon-gamma production from normal human peripheral blood mononuclear cells, Thymus.

Ponzoni, M., Cirillo, C., Perezzani, L. S., Cornaglia-Ferraris, P., 1987, Immunomodulatory properties of a new hypoxantine derivative, PCF-39. II. Comparison with other agents promoting the differentiation of human myeloid or monocyte-like cell lines, EOS J Immunol Immunopharmacol 7: 166-171.

Reynolds, J. V., Daly, J. M., Zhang, S. M., Ziegler, M. M., Nasi, A., 1988, Arginine, protein malnutrition and cancer, J Surgery Res 45: 513-522.

Reynolds, J. V., Daly, J. M., Shou, J., Sigal, R., Ziegler, M. M., Naji,A., 1990, Immunological effects of arginine supplementation in tumor bearing and non tumor-bearing hosts. Ann Surg 211: 202-210.

Riccardi, C., Migliorati, G., 1991 (in press), Enhancement of murine NK cell activity generation by ST 789, Thymus.

Ruggiero, V., Albertoni, C., Manganello, S., Foresta, P., Arrigoni-Martelli E., 1991 (in press), Modulation of splenic lymphocyte activities by a new hypoxantine derivative (ST 789) in immunosuppressed mice, Agents Act.

Seifter, E., Rettura, G., Barbui, A., Levenson, S. M., 1978, Arginine: an essential aminoacid for injured rats, Surgery 84: 224-230.

Stradi, R., Rossi, E., Perezzani, L., Migliorati, G., Riccardi, C., Cornaglia-Ferraris, P., 1990, Synthetic biological response modifiers.Part I. Synthesis and immunomodulatory properties of some N2-(w-(hypoxanthin-9-YL)alkoxycarbonyl)-L-arginines, Il Farmaco 45: 39-47.

QS-21 AUGMENTS THE ANTIBODY RESPONSE TO A SYNTHETIC PEPTIDE

VACCINE COMPARED TO ALUM

J.E. Kirkley, Paul H. Naylor, Dante J. Marciani*,
Charlotte R. Kensil*, Mark Newman*, and
A.L. Goldstein

Dept. of Biochemistry and Molecular Biology,
The George Washington University Medical Center,
Washington, D.C.
*Cambridge Biotech Corp., Worcester, MA

INTRODUCTION

The immunomodulating ability of adjuvants has been
shown to enhance immune responses directed both specifically
and non-specifically against tumor development and growth
and to increase immune response to weak antigens. This
study compared two adjuvants, alum and QS-21, given
separately and together in a candidate p17-based subunit
AIDS vaccine, HGP-30-KLH. Alum, the only adjuvant approved
for human use, confers a particulate appearance to the
immunogen by adsorbing it and retains the immunogen in the
body.[1] QS-21 is a pure triterpene glycoside saponin
adjuvant,[2] and is purified from the total saponin fraction
of Quillaja saponaria Molina. Crude mixtures of Quillaja
saponaria saponins serve as the matrix component of the
immunostimulating complex (ISCOM).[3] The study's hypothesis
was that these two adjuvants function by different means to
increase antibody titer to a synthetic peptide immunogen.
QS-21, with its biochemical as well as physical properties,
was expected to generate a greater antibody response than
alum, and the two combined may be additive or synergistic.
HGP-30 is a synthetic peptide representing a 30-amino
acid stretch (aa85-114) near the C-terminal of HIV-1 p17 gag
protein. This peptide was selected as the basis of a
candidate AIDS vaccine for a number of reasons. It contains
predicted and demonstrated human T- and B-cell epitopes and
has been shown to contain a neutralizing epitope.[4-10] Its
immunogenicity and non-toxicity, when conjugated to KLH and
administered in alum, has been demonstrated in a variety of
animals. The prototype HGP-30-KLH/alum construct, which has
begun phase 1 trials in California, has already been tested
in phase 1 trials in England, in which it was shown to be
safe and immunogenic.[11] With respect to adjuvant activity,
it represents a clinically useful example of a peptide-
carrier model to allow comparison of effects on both peptide
and carrier.

METHODS AND MATERIALS

Immunization and serum collection

Groups of Balb/c mice (n=9-10) were injected subcutaneously in the scruff of the neck with 25ug of HGP-30-KLH conjugate mixed with alum (3:1 adjuvant:conjugate ratio by mass), QS-21 (4:5), or alum and QS-21 (3:1 and 4:5). HGP-30, manufactured by Alpha 1 Biomedicals Inc. and supplied by Viral Technologies Inc., was conjugated via glutaraldehyde-induced lysine linkage to Calbiochem KLH (keyhole limpet hemocyanin) as previously described.[12] QS-21 was supplied by Cambridge Biotech Corp. Aluminum hydroxide gel (alum) was obtained from Superfos S/A. Mice were housed in an AALRC-approved facility, and all procedures were approved by the Institutional Animal Care Committee. Serum samples were obtained by bleeding the mice through the tail vein, allowing the blood to clot at room temperature, centrifuging the clotted samples, and drawing off the supernatant sera which were stored frozen at a 1/10 dilution in phosphate buffered salt solution (PBS) until the time of assay.

Measurement of serum antibodies

Serum samples were diluted in PBS and measured for the presence of IgG antibodies to the peptide, HGP-30, and the carrier, KLH, by enzyme linked immunosorbent assay (ELISA). Nunc Maxisorp 96-well plates were coated overnight at room temperature with 50ul/well of 10ug/ml HGP-30 or KLH diluted in PBS, obtained from the sources named above. Between each step, the plates were washed 5 times in a Skatron A/S Microwash II with a PBS solution containing Sigma Chemical Co. Tween 20 and thimerosal as a preservative ('E buffer'). The plates were blocked for 2 hours at 37°C with 200ul/well 5% powdered milk dissolved in E buffer. The serum samples were plated 50ul/well and incubated 1 hour at 37°C. Goat anti-mouse IgG peroxidase-conjugated second antibody (Kirkegaard and Perry Laboratories Inc.) was diluted 1/2000 in E containing 1% w/v bovine serum albumin (Sigma Chemical Co.) and plated at 50ul/well, and incubated 1 hour at 37°. Color was developed by adding 50ul/well TMB Microwell Peroxidase Substrate System substrate (Kirkegaard and Perry) and stopped with 50ul/well H_3PO_4 diluted to 1M (Fisher Scientific). Plates were read on a Dynatech Laboratories Inc. MR650 plate reader at an absorbance wavelength of 405nm. Data were captured with Dynatech Immunosoft Version 3.0 and analyzed with Lotus 1-2-3. Serum samples for each collection point were assayed at a 1/400 dilution to yield a time course of antibody production. The 8-week serum samples were serially diluted from 1/400 to 1/25600 and analyzed by ELISA for HGP-30- and KLH-specific titers. Results are reported as the group average optical density of the 9-10 individual serum samples from each treatment. Statistical analysis was performed using an NIH open software program (Blossom).

RESULTS

At all time points after the initial immunization, the

CHOICE OF ADJUVANT AFFECTS ANTIBODY RESPONSE

A: QS21 with or without Alum raises more antibody
   to HGP-30 than does Alum alone.

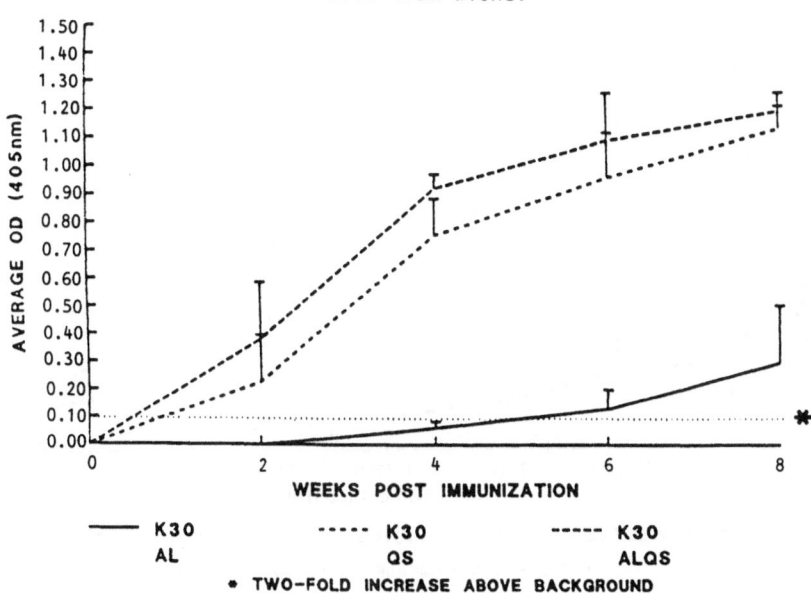

B: Anti-KLH antibody response is enhanced by QS21
   or QS21 plus Alum compared to Alum.

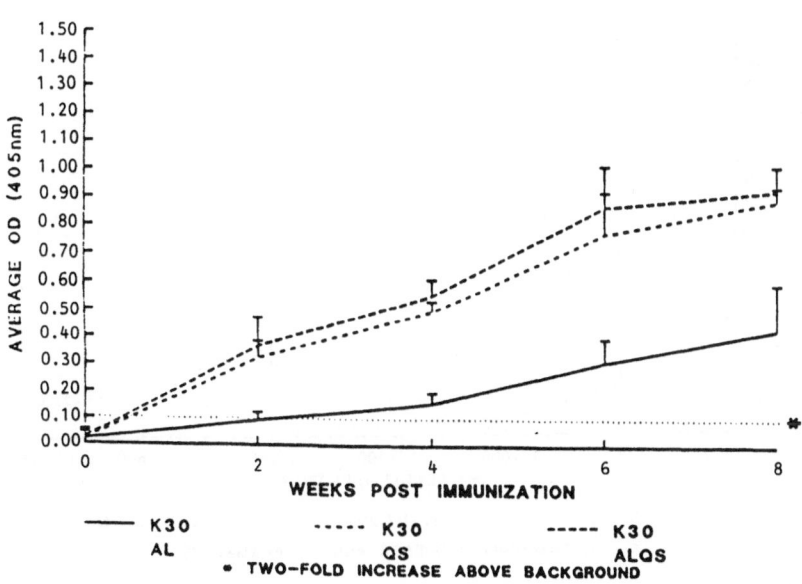

Figure 1. Balb/c mice were immunized SQ with 25ug/mouse KLH-
HGP-30 administered in the alum (K30/AL), QS-21 (K30/QS), or
alum plus QS-21 (K30/ALQS). Serum samples taken at two-week
intervals were measured at a 1/400 dilution for anti-HGP-30
(Fig. 1a) or anti-KLH (Fig. 1b) IgG by ELISA. Results are
expressed as average optical density, measured at 405nm, of
9-10 animals per group. Statistical significance of differences in group averages was analyzed by ANOVA.

A: Anti-HGP-30 titer raised by QS-21 is higher
than the titer generated by Alum.

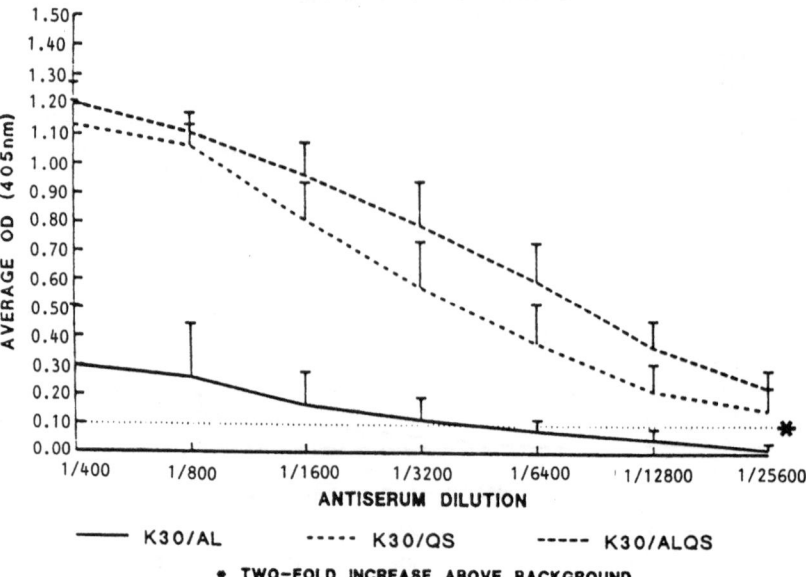

B: QS-21 with or without Alum induces a higher titer
anti-carrier response than does Alum alone.

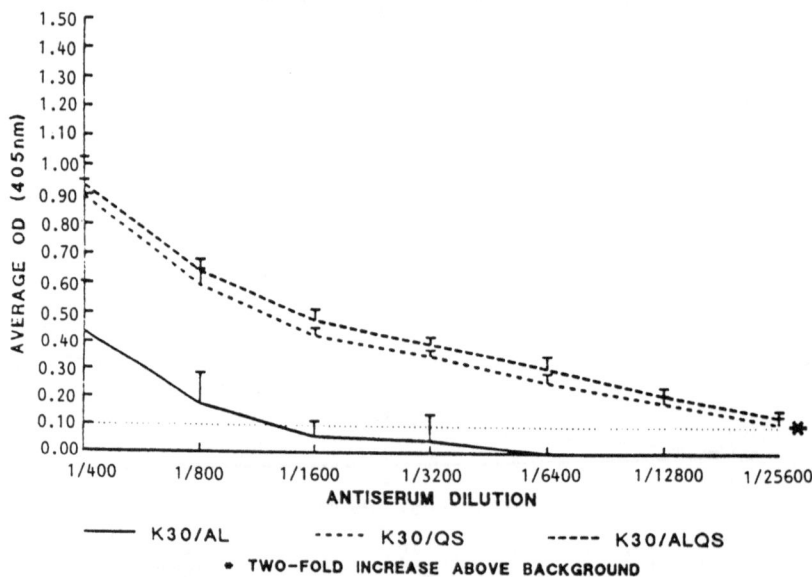

Figure 2. Balb/c mice were immunized SQ with 25ug/mouse KLH-
HGP-30 administered in alum (K30/Al), QS-21 (K30/QS), or alum
plus QS-21 (K30/ALQS). Serum samples taken at the maximum
antibody response, which occurred 8 weeks post immunization,
were diluted in two-fold increments from 1/400 to 1/25600.
Antibodies to HGP-30 (Fig. 2a) and to KLH (Fig. 2b) were
measured by ELISA. The data are expressed as the average
optical density, measured at 405nm, of 9-10 animals per group.
Statistical significance of differences in group averages was
analyzed by ANOVA.

mice who received conjugate in alum produced significantly weaker anti-peptide and anti-carrier responses than did the mice who received conjugate in either QS-21 or QS-21 plus alum (Fig. 1). Early in the time course, QS-21 plus alum produced a stronger antibody response in serum diluted to 1/400 at the two- and four-week points than QS-21 did, but this advantage disappeared at the two later time points as the QS-21-induced response increased.

A serial dilution of the 8-week sera confirmed that the antibody response generated by QS-21 with or without alum was greater than that generated by alum alone (Fig. 2). The anti-HGP-30 titer, defined as the serum dilution giving an optical density two-fold above background, of the QS-21 treatment was 1/25600, compared to 1/3200 for the alum treatment, while the titer produced by the QS-21+alum treatment was estimated at 1/51200. Results were similar when the antibody response against the carrier was analyzed.

CONCLUSION

QS-21 was a more potent adjuvant than alum when the antibody response to either the peptide hapten, HGP-30, or the carrier, KLH, was examined. As part of the immunizing complex, the QS-21 was well tolerated by the animals, and there were no significant differences in reactions at the injection site between QS-21, QS-21 plus alum, and alum alone. While the addition of alum to QS-21 modestly augmented the anti-peptide titer, it did not have a sizeable effect on the response generated by QS-21, nor did it negatively affect the adjuvant activity of the stronger QS-21. Thus QS-21 would appear to be a useful adjuvant for inclusion in settings where an increase in immunogenicity is desired.

ACKNOWLEDGMENTS

This study was supported in part by a grant from Viral Technologies, Inc., and by gifts from the Institute for Advanced Studies in Immunology and Aging. JEK is the recipient of the Missy Tracy Fellowship from the IASIA.

REFERENCES

1. Warren, H.S., Vogel, F.R., and Chedid, L.A., 'Current status of immunological adjuvants,' Ann. Rev. Immun. 4:369-388, 1986.

2. Kensil, C.R., Patel, U., Lennick, M., and Marciani, D., "Separation and characterization of saponins with adjuvant activity from Quillaja saponaria Molina cortex," J. Immunology 146:431-437, 1991.

3. Morein, B., Sundquist, B., Hoglund, S., Dalsgaard, K., and Osterhaus, A., 'Iscom, a novel structure for antigenic presentation of membrane proteins from enveloped viruses,' Nature 308:457, 1984.

4. Coates, A.R.M., Cookson, J., Barton, G.J., Zvelebil,

M.H., and Sternberg, M.J., 'AIDS vaccine predictions,' Nature 326:549-550, 1987.

5. Jaing, J.D., Chu, F.N., Naylor, P., Kirkley, J., Mandelli, J., Wallace, J.I., Sarin, P., Goldstein, A., and Bekesi, J.G., 'Antibody responses to synthetic epitopes of HIV-1 gag p17 in different stages of HIV-1 infection in homosexuals and IV drug abusers,' Proc. Natl. Acad. Sci. (submitted).

6. Wahren, B., Rosen, J., Sandstrom, E., Mathiesen, T., Modrow, S., and Wigzell, H., 'HIV-1 peptides induce a proliferative response in lymphocytes from infected persons,' J. AIDS 4:448-456, 1989.

7. Achour, A., Picard, O., Zagury, D., Sarin, P.S., Gallo, R.C., Naylor, P.H., and Goldstein, A.L., 'HGP-30, a synthetic analogue of human immunodeficiency virus (HIV) p17, is a target for cytotoxic lymphocytes in HIV-infected individuals,' PNAS 87:7045-7049, 1990.

8. Goldstein, A.L., Naylor, P.H., Sarin, P.S., Kirkley, J.E., Stambuk, D., and Rios, A., 'Progress in the development of a p17 based HIV vaccine: immunogenicity of HGP-30 in humans,' Abstract S.A.76, VI International Conference on AIDS, San Francisco, Calif., U.S.A., 1990.

9. Boucher, A.B., Krone, W.J.A., Goudsmit, J., Meloen, R.H., Naylor, P.H., Goldstein, A.L., Sun, D.K., and Sarin, P.S., 'Immune response and epitope mapping of a candidate HIV p17 vaccine HGP-30,' J. Clin. Lab. An. 4:43-47, 1990.

10. Papsidero, L.D., Sheu, M., and Ruscetti, F.W., 'Human immunodeficiency virus type 1 neutralizing monoclonal antibodies which react with p17 core protein. Characterization and epitope mapping,' J. Virol. 63:267-272, 1989.

11. Goldstein, A.L., Naylor, P.H., Kirkley, J.E., Naylor, C.W., Gibbs, C.J., and Sarin, P.S., 'Evaluation of a synthetic HIV-1 p17-based candidate AIDS vaccine, HGP-30,' Abstract M.C.P.13, V International Conference on AIDS, Montreal, Quebec, Canada, 1989.

12. Naylor, P.H., Naylor, C.W., Badamchian, M., Wada, S., Goldstein, A.L., Wang, S.-S., Sun, D., Thorton, A.H., and Sarin, P., 'Human immunodeficiency virus containing an epitope immunoreactive with thymosin alpha 1 and the thirty amino acid synthetic p17 group specific antigen peptide HGP-30,' PNAS 84:2951-2955, 1986.

236

SYNERGISTIC REGULATION OF LAK LYMPHOCYTE CYTOTOXICITY BY

COMBINATION CYTOKINE AND CISPLATIN TREATMENT

Charles H. Evans, Paulette M. Furbert-Harris, Anath A. Flugelman,
Craig D. Woodworth and Joseph A. DiPaolo

Laboratory of Biology
National Cancer Institute
Bethesda, Maryland 20892

The purpose of this investigation is to define if combination lymphokine and chemotherapeutic drug treatment can enhance the sensitivity of human papillomavirus (HPV) DNA immortalized dysplastic and HPV DNA containing cervical carcinoma cells to destruction by natural killer (NK) and lymphokine activated killer (LAK) lymphocytes. Human papilloma viruses infect squamous epithelium and are associated with the development of benign and malignant epithelial tumors.[1-3] HPV type 16 is a suspected etiologic agent in the pathogenesis of cervical intraepithelial dysplasia and malignancy.[4] In most premalignant and benign cervical lesions, HPV DNA exists in an episomal form, while in cervical cancers it is found integrated into the cellular genome.[5] The cell-mediated effector arm of the immune response may have a key role in host defense against HPV infection and the possible development of neoplastia. Support for this is the presence of T lymphocytes, and the absence of a significant number of B lymphocytes, in cervical metaplasia and in normal cervical epithelium.[6] However, in HPV infections and cervical intraepithelial neoplasia there is a general depletion of intraepithelial T lymphocytes with T4$^+$ helper lymphocytes being more depleted than T8$^+$ suppressor lymphocytes.[6]

Because specific T lymphocyte reactivity is partially or completely absent in patients with HPV infections and cervical intraepithelial neoplasia, and because substantial evidence exists for the role of NK lymphocytes in both viral infections and in neoplasia,[7-9] investigation of the presence and function of this component of natural lymphocytotoxicity in these virus associated diseases is relevant. Toward this end, Tay et al.,[10] have evaluated the presence of NK lymphocytes in tissue specimens from patients with HPV infection and cervical intraepithelial neoplasia. NK lymphocytes, positive for both the leu 7 (HNK-1) and leu 11 (NK-15) surface antigens, were present in most HPV infections and in half of the cervical intraepithelial neoplasia specimens tested.

Several lymphokines are known to modulate the sensitivity of NK susceptible target cells. Interferons down-regulate[11] and leukoregulin up-regulates[12] tumor cell sensitivity to NK lymphocytotoxicity. Interferons have recently been introduced in the treatment of HPV infections and cervical intraepithelial neoplasia because the response rate to conventional chemotherapeutic treatment is highly variable and in most cases is less than 50%.[13,14] Interferons are well known for their anti-viral activity and their immunomodulatory functions. Most interferon therapy of HPV infections and cervical intraepithelial neoplasia has been performed with IFNα and IFNβ.[15] More recently, clinical trials have begun with IFNγ.[16,17] It is important, therefore, in the design of both preventive and therapeutic strategies for

Combination Therapies, Edited by A.L. Goldstein and
E. Garaci, Plenum Press, New York, 1992

cell by cytokines such as the interferons and leukoregulin affects or is a result of viral DNA expression and function.

HPV16-immortalized human cervical epithelial (HCX) cell lines have been developed in the Laboratory of Biology as a model for studying the role of HPV in the development of cervical cancer.[18] Important characteristics of this model are that HPV16 DNA is integrated and transcriptionally active, and although the cells are not tumorigenic in nude mice, they acquire additional transformed properties with cultivation. In this respect, these cells resemble dysplastic cervical epithelial cells.[18] Leukoregulin is a lymphokine produced by activated lymphocytes, which increases tumor cell membrane permeability[19,20] and drug uptake[21], inhibits tumor cell replication[20] and up-regulates the sensitivity of tumor cells to killing by NK and LAK lymphocytes.[12,22] Leukoregulin has been shown to differentially up-regulate the sensitivity of HPV16 DNA immortalized cervical cells to lymphocytotoxicity with up-regulation to LAK lymphocytotoxicity being greater than to NK lymphocytotoxicity.[23] The objectives of the present study are to evaluate whether the addition of a chemotherapeutic drug will further up-regulate the sensitivity of the cells to lymphocytotoxicity.

Several HPV immortalized cervical lines are being studied. In the establishment of the cell lines, secondary cultures of normal human exocervical epithelial cells were transfected with a recombinant human papilloma virus DNA[18] which contained the neomycin gene[24] and were selected for resistance to the antibiotic G418 (Gibco, Grand Is., N.Y.). Cell lines were derived by pooling cells from several resistant colonies and subculturing at 1:10 in chemically defined medium (MCDB153-LB).[24] Subsequently, sublines resistant to terminal differentiation were selected by culturing cells in MCDB153-LB + 5% fetal bovine serum (FBS) (Gibco, Grand Island, N.Y.). Serum-selected cells were chosen to compare with the HPV16-positive cervical carcinoma line, QGU[25], because QGU cells are normally grown in medium containing FBS. A tumor producing derivative of HPV16 DNA immortalized HCX16-2 cells obtained after transfection of the HCX16-2 cells with v-Ha-*ras* is also being evaluated. All cells are maintained in monolayer cultures in 100mm plastic tissue culture dishes.

Leukoregulin is isolated from phytohemagglutinin (PHA)-stimulated normal human peripheral blood lymphocytes.[20] Briefly, Ficoll-Hypaque (LSM, Organon Teknika Corp., Durham, N.C.)-isolated normal mononuclear leukocytes are cultured at $1x10^6$ cells/ml in serum free RPMI 1640 with PHA (Sigma Chemical Co., St. Louis, MO) at 10 μg/ml in 2 liter plastic cell culture roller bottles (Corning Glass Works, Corning, N.Y.) at 37^0C in a 5% CO_2, 95% air atmosphere for 48 hr. The lymphokine containing culture medium is separated from the cells by filtration through a Millipore GVLP 0.4μm membrane and concentrated 50-fold by ultrafiltration over a YM10 Amicon membrane (Amicon, Inc., Danvers, MA). The lymphokine concentrates are diafiltered against pH 7.4, 0.01M sodium phosphate buffered saline-0.1% PEG, sterilized by filtration through a 0.22 μm Millex-GV filter unit (Millipore Corp., Bedford, MA) and stored at -30°C. Leukoregulin is purified by sequential DEAE ion-exchange, isoelectric focusing, and HPLC molecular sizing chromatography and its activity quantitated by growth inhibition of human K562 erythroleukemia cells[20]. By definition, one leukoregulin cytostatic unit produces 50% growth inhibition of $2x10^4$ K562 cells after 3 day culture of the cells with leukoregulin.[20]

Nylon wool (Fenwal Laboratories, Morton's Grove, IL) nonadherent mononuclear lymphocytes are isolated from Ficoll-Hypaque-fractionated fresh human apheresis mononuclear leukocyte collections from normal individuals at the National Institutes of Health Blood Bank and serve as NK effector lymphocytes.[20] Ficoll-Hypaque-fractionated mononuclear cells are cultured at $1x10^6$ cells/ml in RPMI 1640 medium containing human recombinant interleukin 2 (rIL-2) (Collaborative Research, Boston, MA), (100 u/ml) and 5% human AB serum for 7 days at 37^0C in a 5% CO_2, 95% air in water saturated atmosphere and are used as LAK effector lymphocytes.[26]

Confluent monolayer cultures of normal cervical epithelial cells, HPV16-immortalized cervical epithelial cells and HPV16 positive cervical epithelial tumor cells are incubated with 100 µCi ^{51}sodium chromate (New England Nuclear, Wilmington, DE) for 16-18 hr. The cells are washed with 10 ml RPMI 1640 medium-10% FBS and incubated with 5 ml RPMI 1640 medium containing 1% FBS or the same medium containing leukoregulin (2.5 u/ml) for 1 hr. The cells are trypsinized (0.1% trypsin + 25 ml PBS, pH 7.4 + 25 ml EDTA Versene, 1:5000 - Gibco, Grand Island, N.Y.) for 5 min and single cell suspensions washed in 50 ml RPMI 1640 medium-10% FBS and adjusted to 1x10^5 target cells/ml.

A 4 hr ^{51}Cr release cytotoxicity assay is used in these studies.[22] Briefly, 100 µl of effector lymphocytes at 5x10^6, 2.5x10^6, 1x10^6, 2.5x10^5 and 1x10^5/ml are mixed with 100 µl of epithelial target cells to yield effector to target (E:T) cell ratios of 50:1, 25:1, 10:1, 2.5:1 and 1:1. Experiments are performed in triplicate in 12x75 mm Falcon polystyrene culture tubes, (Becton Dickinson and Co., Lincoln Park, N.J.). The tubes are centrifuged at 50 X G for 3 min, and incubated at 37^{0}C in a 5% CO_2, 95% air in water saturated atmosphere for 4 hr. Chromium release in the culture supernatants is quantitated in a LKB gamma counter (LKB Products Inc., Bromma, Sweden). Spontaneous release (target cells + medium) ranges between 5 and 15%. Percent specific release is calculated as follows:

$$\% \text{ Specific Release} = \frac{(\text{Test cpm - spontaneous cpm})}{(\text{Total cpm - spontaneous cpm})} \times 100$$

LAK cell cytotoxicity is evaluated using the same procedures. Each experiment is performed in triplicate and the standard error of the mean (SE) of all experiments is 5% or less. The results presented are representative of 4 or more experiments.

Early passage HPV16 DNA immortalized human cervical epithelial cells have been evaluated after culturing for 11 to 18 weeks, while the later passage cells have been examined after 30 weeks in culture. Both early and late passage HPV16-immortalized cervical epithelial cells are resistant to NK lymphocytotoxicity (Figure 1).

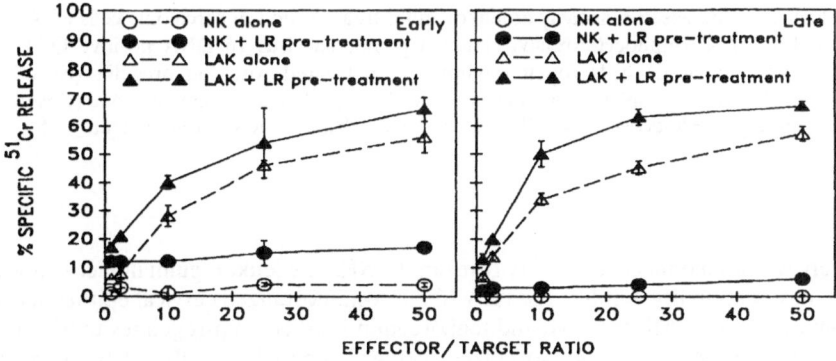

Figure 1. Sensitivity of early and late passage leukoregulin-treated HPV16 DNA-transfected cervical epithelial cells to NK and to LAK lymphocytotoxicity. A HPV16 DNA positive cervical epithelial cell line (HCX16-2) at passages 15 (early) and 35 (late) was treated with leukoregulin at 2.5 U/ml (open symbols) for 1 hr and incubated with NK (solid circles) or LAK (solid triangles) lymphocytes in a 4 hr ^{51}Cr release assay. This leukoregulin concentration increases K562 leukemia cell sensitivity to NK cytotoxicity 2-5 fold and to LAK cytotoxicity 1-3 fold. Values shown are the mean +2 SE and are typical responses.[23]

Leukoregulin causes a slight increase (P = <0.05) in susceptibility to NK lymphocytotoxicity in the early passage HCX16-2 cervical cells. Late passage cells are more resistant to NK lymphocytotoxicity and their NK sensitivity is not up-regulated by leukoregulin. On the other hand, both early and late passage immortalized cervical epithelial cells are sensitive to LAK lymphocyte cytotoxicity. Leukoregulin markedly up-regulates the sensitivity to LAK lymphocytotoxicity, more so with the late passage cervical epithelial cells at lymphocyte/target cell ratios of 10:1 and 25:1.

Although leukoregulin's slight augmentation of sensitivity to NK lymphocytotoxicity is seen only with the early passage cells, leukoregulin increases the sensitivity of both the early and late passage HPV-immortalized cervical epithelial cells to LAK lymphocytotoxicity with the increased susceptibility to LAK lymphocytotoxicity being 1.5 to 4-fold higher for the late passage compared to the early passage HPV-immortalized cervical epithelial cells.[23] The response of the early passage HPV16-immortalized cervical cells to leukoregulin is very similar to that of cervical epithelial cells not transfected with HPV16 DNA, while the response of the late passage HPV16-transfected cervical cells is similar to that of HPV16 positive QGU cervical carcinoma cells (Figure 2).

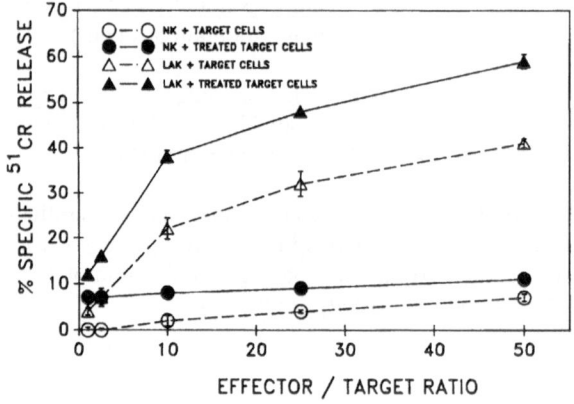

Figure 2. Increased sensitivity of leukoregulin-treated cervical carcinoma cells to NK and to LAK lymphocytotoxicity. Human papilloma virus 16 DNA positive QGU cervical carcinoma cells (open symbols) were treated with leukoregulin (closed symbols) at 2.5 U/ml for 1hr, incubated with NK (closed circles) or LAK (closed triangles) lymphocytes in a 4hr ^{51}Cr release assay. Values shown are the mean ± 2 SE.

QGU cervical carcinoma cells are very resistant to NK, and leukoregulin induces only a slight increase in susceptibility, but like the HPV16 DNA-immortalized cervical epithelial cells, the carcinoma cells are LAK sensitive and leukoregulin markedly up-regulates their sensitivity. Thus, late passage HPV16-immortalized cervical epithelial cells, exhibits a greater leukoregulin up-regulation in sensitivity to LAK than to NK lymphocyte cytotoxicity, mimicking the pattern of leukoregulin-induced up-regulation observed with the HPV16 positive cervical carcinoma cells.

Because leukoregulin increases the sensitivity of tumor cells to NK and LAK lymphocyte cytotoxicity while concomitantly increasing the uptake of doxorubicin and other tumor inhibitory antibiotics[21] we are evaluating whether leukoregulin in combination with chemotherapeutic agents synergistically enhances the cytotoxicity of NK and LAK lymphocytes for HPV DNA containing cervical epithelial and carcinoma cells. Recent experiments with combination leukoregulin and cisplatin (CisPt) treatment of HPV16 DNA-immortalized cervical epithelial cells demonstrate enhancement of target cell sensitivity to NK and to LAK lymphocyte cytotoxicity above that exhibited by the cervical cells treated with either agent alone. Although HPV-immortalized cervical epithelial cells and HPV16 DNA positive cervical carcinoma cells are relatively resistant to NK lymphocytotoxicity (Figures 1 and 2), sensitivity to NK lymphocytotoxicity increases after combination treatment with leukoregulin and CisPt for one hour (Figure 3).

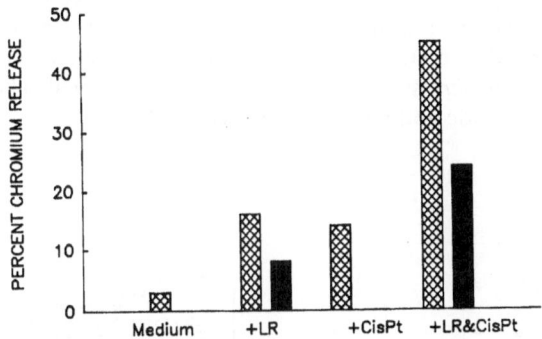

Figure 3. Enhancement of natural killer cytotoxicity for QGU cervical carcinoma (hatched bars) and HPV16 DNA immortalized HCX16-2 cervical epithelial cells (solid bars) following combination treatment of the target cells with 2.5 u/ml leukoregulin and 0.1 nM CisPt for one hour. Results are shown for a NK to target cell ratio of 10:1. When the cytotoxicity over a range of NK lymphocyte to QGU target cells is expressed in lytic units (LU), one lytic unit being the number of NK lymphocytes necessary to produce 30% target cell lysis, the LU/10^6 LAK lymphocytes is <10 for medium and for CisPt treated target cells, >20 for leukoregulin treated cells, and >200 for the combination CisPt and leukoregulin treatment is >200 LU.

Even greater increases in cytotoxicity are observed with LAK lymphocytes where in a typical experiment the LU/10^6 LAK lymphocytes for medium and CisPt treated QGU carcinoma cells are >200 compared to >1000 for the leukoregulin treatment and >3000 for the combination of CisPt and leukoregulin treatment. Similar enhancement of the sensitivity to LAK lymphocytotoxicity for HPV-immortalized and H-*ras* neoplastically transformed HPV-immortalized cervical epithelial cells is produced by combination CisPt and leukoregulin treatment as illustrated in Figure 4.

Most surprising is the observation that treatment of the HPV DNA immortalized cervical cells, the PH1 tumor producing v-Ha-*ras* transfected HPV16 DNA HCX-2 cells and the QGU cervical carcinoma cells when treated for just one hour with CisPt and γ-interferon lose their sensitivity to destruction by LAK lymphocytes (Figure 4). These are very important observations as current combination chemotherapy using conventional drugs is not encouraging in terms of response rate, toxicity and other side effects. Cisplatin remains one of the drugs of choice in cervical cancer, alone or in combination with other chemotherapeutic agents. Bonomi et al.,[44] however, find only a 22% response rate with combined cisplatin and 5FU treatment in a phase II study in cervical cancer patients although this combination of drugs produced an 88% response in squamous cell carcinoma of the head and neck. It is, therefore, important to determine the extent to which cytokines like leukoregulin and interferon up- or down-regulate the degree of NK and LAK lymphocyte cytotoxicity in the presence of anti-tumor chemotherapeutic agents. This is potentially a new therapeutic approach for the treatment of cervical dysplasia and neoplasia.

Our investigations demonstrate that HPV16-immortalized cervical epithelial cells lose their sensitivity to natural lymphocytotoxicity and undergo a differential cytokine-controllable increase in their sensitivity to natural lymphocytotoxicity during the weeks following transfection and immortalization with HPV16 DNA.[23] Leukoregulin increases the sensitivity of the immortalized cells to NK and to LAK lymphocytotoxicity 18-20 weeks after transfection with HPV16 DNA, with a greater degree of up-regulation by leukoregulin occurring for LAK compared to NK sensitivity. Tay et al.,[10] have shown that few NK cells are present in cervical epithelia with HPV infections and in cervical intraepithelial neoplasia. The resistance of HPV16-immortalized cervical epithelial cells, like HPV16 positive cervical carcinoma cells, to NK lymphocyte killing *in vitro* suggests that NK cells alone may also be ineffective *in vivo* in the destruction of dysplastic and neoplastic cervical cells.

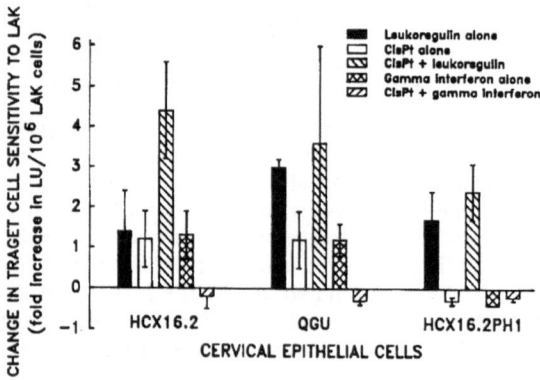

Figure 4. Modulation of cervical epithelial cell sensitivity to normal human LAK cytotoxicity by CisPt, leukoregulin, and γ-interferon combination treatment. The target cells were treated for one hour as in Figure 3 with 0.1 nM CisPt, 2.5 u leukoregulin, 100 u γ-interferon/ml or a combination of CisPt and cytokine and the net cytotoxicity at effector to target ratios of 1 to 10:1 converted to lytic units (LU) per one million LAK lymphocytes. Results shown are the mean ±S.E. of the change from the sensitivity observed without cytokine or CisPt treatment, e.g. the ratio of the LU for the cytokine, CisPt or combined cytokine+CisPt treatment, to the LU observed with no treatment.

NK lymphocytes, however, can function in an immunomodulatory capacity, not only modulating other effector cells, but by regulating their own activity. They do so by producing and releasing an assortment of cytokines, such as IFNγ,[27] IL-2,[28] and leukoregulin[20] which act to amplify and regulate the immune response. IFN[29] and IL-2[30,31] can act directly on the NK cells to enhance their killer activity. Leukoregulin in contrast to IFN and IL-2 modulates natural lymphocytotoxicity activity by up-regulating the sensitivity of tumor target cells to NK[22] and LAK[12] lymphocyte killing. Interferon, particularly IFNα, has been used in the clinical treatment of human genital papillomavirus infections.[15-17] The response rate of these patients to IFN treatment is dependent on the HPV type with HPV16/18 infections showing a lower response rate.[17] IFN can be applied topically but is usually administered systemically.

In the later situation, it is difficult to know whether IFN, which can both up-regulate effector lymphocytes[32] and down-regulate target cell sensitivity,[22,33,34] is acting directly on the abnormal target cell, or on the immune effector cell, or both.

Our studies show that leukoregulin treatment of late passage HPV-immortalized cells has very little effect on the sensitivity of the cells to NK lymphocytotoxicity. On the other hand, both the HPV-immortalized cells and the cervical carcinoma cells are very sensitive to IL2-activated LAK cells and this sensitivity is increased by leukoregulin. Since it has been shown that LAK precursor cells do exist *in vivo* and that their activity can be enhanced by exogenous IL-2,[35] it is possible that LAK cells may play a significant role *in vivo* in the immune response against cervical neoplasia. NK cells may function as immunomodulators, releasing substances that activate and amplify LAK cells, as evidenced by the *in vitro* reactivity of LAK cells to the cervical target cells and their corresponding modulation by leukoregulin which up-regulates target cell sensitivity to LAK lymphocytes.

Women with generalized immunodepression are reported to be at risk of developing cervical neoplasia.[36,37] However, cervical neoplasia is usually found in women who do not present clinically with systemic immunosuppression. Hence, if immunosuppression is an important factor in cervical carcinogenesis the suppression is probably localized. A contributory factor to local immunosuppression may be seminal fluid which contains a number of immunosuppressant agents[38] which exert a suppressive affect on both humoral and cellular immune responses,[39,40] including NK lymphocyte cytotoxicity.[41] The risk of cervical neoplasia increases with sexual promiscuity and with early onset of sexual activity. This results in a greater exposure to seminal fluid and an increased potential exposure to genitally-transmitted HPV16 virus which may itself be immunosuppressive.[42] The dramatic loss of antigen presenting Langerhans' cells in the cervix of women with HPV infection and cervical intraepithelial neoplasia[43] further supports the possibility of a localized immunodeficient state which would facilitate continued growth of the virus and its interaction with other factors in the progression of cervical cells to the neoplastic state.

In addition to leukoregulin-induced up-regulation of target cell sensitivity to NK and LAK lymphocytotoxicity, leukoregulin increases target cell plasma membrane permeability[19] and tumor cell uptake of anti-cancer drugs.[21] These observations suggest that leukoregulin alone or in combination with anti-viral or anti-cancer drugs has the potential to play a significant role in mediating the successful treatment of HPV16 infections and prevention of cervical dysplasia and neoplasia. The development of HPV-immortalized human cervical epithelial cells to study cervical carcinogenesis provides a valuable model system to define the physiological and biotherapeutic role of leukoregulin and other cytokines in combination with other anti-cancer therapeutics in the prevention and control of cervical dysplasia and neoplasia.

REFERENCES

1. Durst M, Gissman L, Ikenberg H, Zur Hausen H (1983). *Proc Natl Acad Sci* 80: 3812-3815.
2. Gissman L (1984). *Cancer Surv* 3: 161-181.
3. McCance DJ, Campion MJ, Clarkson PK, Chesters PM, Jenkins D, Singer A (1985). *Brit J Obstet Gynaecol* 92: 1101-1105.
4. Schneider HK, Schuhmann R, Gissman L (1985). *Int J Cancer* 35: 443-448.
5. Kadish QS, Burk RD, Kress Y, Calderin S, Romney SL (1986). *Human Pathol* 17: 384-392.
6. Tay SK, Jenkins D, Maddox P, Singer A (1987). *Brit J Obstet Gynaecol* 94: 16-21.
7. Herberman RB, Ortaldo JR (1981). *Science* 214: 24-30.
8. Lopez C, Kirkpatrick D, Fitzgerald P (1982). In: R.B. Herberman (ed.), *NK cells and Other Natural Effector Cells*, pp 1445-1450. New York: Academic Press, Inc.

9. West WH, Cannon GB, Kay HD, Bonnard GD, Herberman RB (1977). *J Immunol* 118: 355-361.

10. Tay SK, Jenkins D, Singer A (1987). *Brit J Obstet Gynaecol* 94: 901-906.

11. Trinchieri G, Santoli D (1978). *J Exp Med* 147: 1314.

12. Furbert-Harris P, Evans CH (1989). Leukoregulin up-regulation of tumor cell sensitivity to natural killer and lymphokine-activated killer cell cytotoxicity. *Cancer Immunol Immunother.* 30:86-91.

13. VonKrogh G (1981). *Acta derm venereol* (Stockh.) Suppl. 98:1-48.

14. Kirby P (1988). *JAMA* 258: 570-572.

15. Choo YC, Seto WH, HSU C, Merigan TC, Tan YH, MA HK, NG MH, (1986). *Brit J Obstet Gynaecol* 93: 372-379.

16. Kirby P, Wells D, Kiviat N, Corey L (1986). *J Invest Dermat* 86: 485.

17. Schneider A, Papendick U, Gissman L, DeVilliers E (1987). *Int J Cancer* 40: 610-614.

18. Woodworth CD, Waggoner S, Barnes W, Stoler MH, DiPaolo JA (1988). *Cancer Res* 50: 3709-3715.

19. Barnett SC, Evans CH (1986). *Cancer Res* 46: 2686-2692.

20. Ransom JH, Evans CH, McCabe RP, Pomato N, Heinbaugh JA, Chin M, Hanna Jr. MG (1985). *Cancer Res* 45: 851-862.

21. Evans CH, Baker PD (1988). *J Natl Cancer* Inst 80: 861-863.

22. Evans CH, Heinbaugh JA, Ransom JH (1987). *Lymphokine Res* 6: 277-297.

23. Furbert-Harris PM, Evans CH, Woodworth CD, DiPaolo JA (1989) Loss of leukoregulin up-regulation to NK but not LAK lymphocytotoxicity in human papilloma virus 16 DNA-immortalized cervical epithelial cells. *J. Natl. Cancer Inst.* 81: 1080-1085.

24. Pirisi L, Shigeru Y, Feller M, Doniger J, DiPaolo JA (1987). *J Virol* 61: 1061-1066.

25. Shirasawa H, Tomita Y, Sekiya S, Takamizawa H, Simizu B (1987). *J Gen Virol* 68: 583-591.

26. Grimm EA, Ramsey KM, Mazumder A, Wilson DJ, Djeu JY, Rosenberg SA (1983). *J Exp Med* 157: 884-897.

27. Djeu JY, Stocks N, Zoon K, Stanton GJ, Timonen T, Herberman RB (1982). *J Exp Med* 156: 1222-1234.

28. Kasahara T, Djeu JY, Dougherty SF, Oppenheim JJ (1983). *J Immunol* 131: 2379-2385.

29. Trinchieri G, Perussia B (1984). *Lab Invest* 50: 489-513.

30. Henney C, JuriBayashi K, Kern D, Gillis S (1981). *Nature* 291: 335.

31. Weck PK, Whisnant JK (1987). *Cancer Cells* 5: 393-402.

32. Herberman RB, Ortaldo JR, Bonnard GD (1979). *Nature* 277: 221-223.

33. Trinchieri G, Granata D, Perussia B (1978). *J Immunol* 126: 335-340.

34. Uchida A, Vanky F, Klein E (1985). *J Natl Cancer Inst* 75: 849-857.

35. Anderson TM, Ibayashi Y, Tokuda Y, Colquhoun SD, Holmes EC, Golub SH (1988). *Cancer Res* 48: 1180-1183.

36. Porrecco R, Penn I, Droegemueller W, Greer B, Makowski E (1975). *J Obstet Gynaecol* 45: 359-364.

37. Obalek S, Glinski W, Hafleck M, Orth G, Jablonska S (1980). *Dermatologica* 161: 73-83.

38. James K, Hargreave TB (1984). *Immunol Today* 5: 357-363.

39. Lord EM, Sensabaugh GF, Stites DP (1977). *J Immunol* 118: 1704-1711.

40. Majumddar S Bapna BC, Mapa MK, Gupta AN, Devi PK, Subrahmanyam D (1982). *Int J Fertil* 27: 224-228.

41. Rees RC, Valley P, Clegg A, Potter CW (1986). *Clin Exp Immunol* 63: 687-695.

42. Jablonska S, Orth G, Lutzner MA (1982). *Seminars Immunopath* 5: 33-62.

43. Tay SK, Jenkins D, Maddox P, Campion M, Singer A (1987). *Brit J Obstet Gynaecol* 94: 10-15.

44. Bonomi P, Blessing J, Ball H, Hanjani P, DiSaia PJ (1989). *Gynec Oncol* 34:357-359.

THE BIOLOGICAL RESPONSE MODIFIERS INTERLEUKIN-2 AND TUMOR NECROSIS FACTOR-α MODULATE THE CYTOTOXIC ACTIVITY OF TUMOR INFILTRATING LYMPHOCYTES AGAINST HUMAN COLON CANCER CELLS

Vito M. Stolfi, Jeffrey W. Milsom,
James H. Finke, Victor W. Fazio
Luca Ferraris and Claudio Fiocchi

Departments of Colorectal Surgery, Gastroenterology and Research Institute, The Cleveland Clinic Foundation, Cleveland Ohio, 44195

INTRODUCTION

Colorectal cancer is one of the most common malignancies in both men and women in the United States , and its incidence is still rising every year (1). At the time of initial diagnosis, less than 60% of the patients have localized disease which is amenable to surgical treatment, and the prognosis is even worse in the advanced stages of the disease. In addition to surgery, or when surgery is not indicated because of metastatic disease, alternate forms of therapy include chemotherapy and occasionally radiotherapy. Presently, 5-fluorouracil (5-FU) is the most effective chemotherapeutic agent, but response rate usually is not better than 20-30% (2). Other substances have been used in combination with 5-FU , such as leucovorin (folinic acid) and cis-platinum. These combinations only induce a modest increase in the response rates, but often result in severe drug-related toxicities, including 3-4% of drug related fatalities (3-5). Levamisole, an antihelmintic drug with immuno-enhancing properties, has been recently used in combination with 5-FU, and a moderate increase of survival rates has been reported (6).

Advances in the understanding of the biology and function of the soluble products of activated immune cells have lead to the novel concept of biological response modifiers (BRM). Because of their potent activity as immunomodulators, many of them are currently used as experimental drugs in the treatment of oncological diseases. The potentiation of the cytotoxic activity of immune cells has lead to the infusion of these cells with antitumor activity into a tumor-bearing host, an approach known as adoptive immunotherapy, which has proven to be efficacious in some experimental animal models (7-9). After obtaining encouraging results, this experimental system was transferred to humans, resulting in clinical trials where patients with metastatic cancer unresponsive to conventional therapy received infusions of large numbers of *in vitro* expanded autologous lymphokine-activated killer (LAK) cells and recombinant interleukin 2 (IL2) (10, 11). Variable results were observed ranging from a complete absence of response to a substantial diminution of the tumor mass. With this regimen, however, advanced colorectal cancer showed very limited or no response. More recently, another antineoplastic effector cell and an alternate form of adoptive immunotherapy has been developed: tumor infiltrating lymphocytes (TIL) are expanded *in vitro* and then infused into cancer patients (12). As occurred with LAK cells and IL2 treatment, clinical trials using TIL have been already implemented, and preliminary results have already been reported, showing a significant response rate in selected tumors such as malignant melanoma (13, 14).

Very little investigation has been done so far in regard to the use of BRM and activated immune cells in colorectal cancer, and TIL in particular. According to a recent study, freshly isolated human colorectal cancer TIL were weakly cytotoxic against autologous tumor cells, but proliferated better than peripheral blood lymphocytes (PBL), and displayed greater total cytotoxic activity per culture than PBL (15). In order to expand these preliminary observation, the present study was designed aiming at the isolation of TIL from human colorectal carcinomas, examination of their long-term growth in response to IL2 and IL2 plus tumor necrosis factor α (TNFα), as well as their cytotoxic activity under these culture conditions. Moreover, the proliferative and cytotoxic activities of TIL were assessed in parallel with those of autologous intestinal lamina propria mononuclear cells (LPMC), which represent the cell type most likely to mount a local immune response to large bowel tumors.

MATERIALS AND METHODS

Fifteen patients, 9 men and 6 women, aged 53-81 years, admitted to the Cleveland Clinic Hospital for resection of primary colorectal carcinomas, constituted the source of fresh tumor tissue and autologous bowel mucosa. The project was approved by the Institutional Review Board of The Cleveland Clinic Foundation. Immediately after procurement, the malignant tissue was rinsed to eliminate necrotic material, minced in 3 mm fragments, and transferred to an enzymatic solution containing calcium and magnesium-free Hank's balanced salt solution (HBSS), 2 mg/ml collagenase type III (Worthington, Freehold, NJ), O.3 mg/ml deoxyribonuclease type I (Sigma, St.Louis, MO), 5 µg/ml hyaluronidase (Sigma), and a combination of penicillin, streptomycin, and fungizone. After slow stirring for 30 minutes at room temperature, the cell-containing supernatant was aspirated, and the cells were harvested for assessment of number and viability. A new aliquot of fresh enzymatic solution was then added and the procedure was repeated 2-3 times, with harvesting of cells every 60-120 minutes. To isolate LPMC, a method previously described was employed (16).

The tumor cell suspension containing a mixture of TIL and cancer cells was cultured for five to eight weeks in culture medium containing RPMI 1640, 10% fetal calf serum, 2.5% penicillin-streptomycin-fungizone, 1.5% HEPES, 0.1% gentamycin, 1% L-glutamine (Gibco, Grand Island, NY), and 1,000 U/ml of human recombinant IL2, with and without 1,000 U/ml of human recombinant TNFα (Cetus, Emeryville, CA). Control cultures were also performed using TNFα alone. Autologous LPMC were cultured in parallel under identical conditions. All cultures were initiated at a cell density of 0.5×10^6/ml, checked for growth biweekly, and fed accordingly.

In order to assess TIL and LPMC cytotoxic activity (% specific lysis) of TIL and LPMC, these cells were tested against Daudi (a natural killer-resistant human lymphoid cell line) target cells, and the human colorectal cancer cell line HT-29, using a four hour ^{51}Cr-release assay.

Statistical analyses were performed using the signed rank test, the Student's t test, and the Wilcoxon method, and all values were expressed as mean±SEM.

RESULTS

Fifteen tumor specimens were obtained, with a wet weight of 1 to 9 g. Total cell recovery was $6\pm5\times10^6$/g of tumor, of which $1.8\pm0.3 \times 10^6$ were TIL (4 to 45%), and $4.2\pm0.1 \times10^6$ (55 to 96%) were tumor cells. Viability was assessed by 0.1% trypan blue staining. Recovery of autologous LPMC from normal colonic mucosa ranged from 3 to 10 x 10^6/g, and viability averaged 90% as previously reported (16).

When stimulated with IL2 or IL2 plus TNFα, all but two of the TIL cultures grew well, as so did all LPMC isolates. On the contrary, TNFα alone was insufficient to induce or sustain growth, and cell viability declined rapidly, preventing their use in functional assays. When cultured in the presence of IL2 alone, TIL grew significantly more than autologous LPMC (69 ± 55 vs 6 ± 1 fold expansion; $p<0.05$, at peak growth). The cell expansion of TIL was significantly enhanced when TNFα was added to IL2 as compared to the growth rate of the same cells exposed only to IL2 (fold expansion:198 ± 93 vs 51 ± 34; $p<0.01$). Under the influence of the IL2 plus TNFα combination, TIL continued to grow exponentially for 35 days when the cultures were terminated. In contrast, the growth of TIL cultured with IL2 alone peaked at 21 days. Contrary to TIL, the combination of IL2 and TNFα inhibited the growth of autologous LPMC when compared to the growth of the same cells cultured in the presence of IL2 alone (4 ± 1 vs 9 ± 1 fold expansion; $p=0.026$).

When tested for cytotoxic function, TIL and LPMC cultured in the presence of IL2 alone displayed comparable levels of lytic activity either against Daudi or HT-29 target cells at an effector-to-target ratio of 50 to 1 (Table). As observed for cell growth, a differential effect was noticed with regard to their cytotoxic activity when the same cells were cultured with the combination IL2 plus TNFα. When compared to the cytotoxicity of the same cells exposed only to IL2, this combination of BRM induced an increase in the level of cytotoxicity of TIL, while causing a decrease of LPMC cytotoxicity. At the same effector-to-target ratio of 50 to 1, the addition of TNFα to the cultures significantly (*$p<0.05$) enhanced the specific killing of TIL against Daudi, while that of LPMC decreased. In addition, at the same effector-to-target ratio, TIL became significantly (**$p=0.035$) more cytotoxic against Daudi target cells than the autologous LPMC. Similar results were obtained when TIL and LPMC were tested against HT-29 target cells (Table). When compared to IL2 alone, the combination of IL2 plus TNFα significantly (***$p<0.02$) enhanced the cytotoxicity of TIL against this colon cancer cell line, while depressing the cytotoxicity of LPMC against the same target .

Target cell	BRM	TIL	LPMC
Daudi	IL2	47±12%*	45±11%
HT-29	IL2	50±5%***	46±10%
Daudi	IL2+TNFα	64±8%*,**	37±10%**
HT-29	IL2+TNFα	64±6%***	31±8%

DISCUSSION

This study was aimed at the investigation of the potential antineoplastic activity of human colorectal cancer TIL by examining the effect of the two BRM IL2 and TNFα in promoting these cells' cytotoxic activity *in vitro*. In comparison with IL2 alone , this combination significantly increased both growth and cytotoxic activity of colorectal cancer TIL, whereas depressed the same activities of autologous intestinal LPMC.

Recombinant human IL2 is a cytokine routinely used for long-term expansion (17) and induction of cytotoxicity of TIL (18-21). Continuous advances in culturing human TIL with IL2 have allowed functional studies and clonal analysis of TIL populations, as well as provided additional information about the characteristics of these cells in a variety of solid tumors (18-23).

Tumor necrosis factor α has a variety of biological actions, including *in vitro* direct cytotoxic or cytostatic activity against selected cell lines, and can cause necrosis of some murine tumors *in vivo* (24). Among various other effects of this cytokine are included the enhancement of IL2 receptor expression , γ interferon production, and class II MHC antigen expression by activated lymphocytes (25, 26). Of particular relevance to this report are several observations of the cytotoxic potentiating activity of this cytokine. The addition of TNFα at the beginning of IL2-driven PBL cultures can cause a 10-fold increase in these cells' antitumor cytotoxic activity (27). In combination with low concentrations of IL2, TNFα induces non-MHC-restricted killer cells in cultures of PBL (28, 29) and synergizes with IL2 in promoting the generation of cytotoxic T lymphocytes in human mixed lymphocytes cultures (29, 30). Recently, the combination of IL2 and TNFα has also been shown to modulate the *in vitro* cytotoxicity of TIL, as reported for ovarian carcinoma TIL which become significantly more cytotoxic against autologous tumor cells in comparison to the same cells cultured with IL2 alone (31).

The results of our study clearly show that the combination of IL2 and TNFa selectively enhance growth and cytotoxic activity of human colorectal cancer TIL not only against Daudi but, also against the human colorectal cancer cell line HT-29. Enhancement of TIL cytotoxicity by this combination of BRM has been previously described in ovarian tumors (31), but this is the first time that the combination of IL2 plus TNFα has been demonstrated to enhance both growth and cytotoxic activity of human TIL. The use of LPMC for control and comparison is well justified. Intestinal LPMC represent a mix cell population which include a large number of T cells exposed to the unique micro-environment of the large bowel mucosa (32). These T cells are the most likely to infiltrate local neoplastic growths. However, the effect of the IL2 plus TNFα combination induced an opposite effect of intestinal LPMC as compared to TIL, suggesting that colorectal cancer TIL and LPMC-derived T cells are either two functionally different cell populations, or cells from the same population that have differentiated along different pathways.

Obviously, additional studies are needed to better characterize human colorectal cancer TIL grown in long-term culture under the influence of BRM combinations. These investigations should include a detailed phenotypic characterization, an expansion of the spectrum of cytotoxic activity and the induction of autologous tumor cell killing, and perhaps the use of other BRM alone or in combination with the ones used in this study. Nevertheless, the preliminary results strongly suggest that combinations of BRM rather than single agents appear to be more promising for the development of future adoptive immunotherapy with human colorectal cancer TIL.

REFERENCES

1. Boring CC, Squires TS, Tong T. Cancer Biostatistics 1991. Cancer **41**:19, 1991.

2. Hansen RM. Systemic therapy in metastatic colorectal cancer. Arch Int Med **150**:2265, 1990.

3. Abbruzzese JL and Levine B Treatment of advanced colorectal cancer. Hematol Oncol North Am **3**:135:1989.

4. Budd GT, Fleming TR, Bukowski RM, Mc Cracken JD, Rivkin SE, O'Brian RM, Balarzak SP and Mcdonald JS. 5-fluorouracil in the treatment of metastatic colorectal cancer: a randomized comparison. A Southwest Oncology Group Study. J Clin Oncol **5**:272,1987.

5. Abruck SG Overview of clinical trials using 5-fluorouracil and leucovorin for the treatment of colorectal cancer. Cancer **63** (6 suppl.): 1026, 1989.

6. Moertel CG, Fleming TR, McDonald JS, et al. Levamisole and fluorouracil for adjuvant therapy of resected colon carcinoma. N Engl J Med **332**: 352, 1990.

7. Mazumder A and Rosenberg SA. Successful immunotherapy of natural-killer resistant established pulmonary melanoma metastases by the intravenous adoptive transfer of syngeneic lymphocytes activated in vitro by interleukin 2. J Exp Med **159**:495, 1984.

8. Lafreniere R, Rosenberg SA. Adoptive immunotherapy of murine hepatic metastases with lymphokine-activated killer (LAK) cells and recombinant interleukin-2 (rIL2) can mediate the regression of both immunogenic and nonimmunogenic sarcomas and adeno-carcinomas. J Immunol **135**: 4273, 1985.

9. Mule JJ, Ettinghausen SE, Spiess PJ, Shu S, and Rosenberg SA. Antitumor efficacy of lymphokine-activated killer cells and recombinant interleukin-2 in vivo: survival benefit and mechanism of tumor escape in mice undergoing immunotherapy. Cancer Res **46**:676, 1986.

10. Rosenberg SA, Lotze MT, Muul LM, Chang AE, Avis FP, Leitman S Marston Linehan W, Robertson CN, Lee RE, Rubin JT, Seipp RN, Simpson CG and White DE. A progress report on the treatment of 157 patients with advanced cancer using lymphokine-activated killer cells and interleukin-2 or high dose interleukin-2 alone. N Eng J Med **316**:889, 1987.

11. West WH, Tauer KW, Yannelli JR, Marshall GD, Orr DW, Thurman GB and Oldham RK. Constant infusion recombinant interleukin-2 in adoptive immunotherapy of advanced cancer. N Eng J Med **316**:898, 1987.

12.   Rosenberg SA The development of new immunotherapies for the treatment of cancer using interleukin 2. Ann Surg **208**:121, 1988.

13.   Rosenberg SA, Packard BS, Aebersold PM, Solomon D, Topalian SL, Toy ST, Simon P, Lotze MT, Yang JC, Seipp CA, Simpson C, Carter C, Bock S, Schwartzentruber D, Wei JP, White DE. Use of tumor-infiltrating lymphocytes and interleukin 2 in the immunotherapy of patients with metastatic melanoma. N Engl J Med **316**:889, 1987.

14.   Kradin RL, Kurnick JT, Lazarus DS, Preffer FI, Dubinnet SM, Pinto GE, Gifford J, Davidson E, Grove B, Callahan RJ, Strauss HW Tumor-infiltrating lymphocytes and interleukin 2 in treatment of advanced cancer. Lancet **1**:577, 1989.

15.   Yoo YK, Heo DS, Hata K, Van Thiel DH and Whiteside TL Tumor-infiltrating lymphocytes from human colon carcinomas. Functional and phenotypic characteristic after long-term culture in recombinant interleukin 2. Gastroenterology **98** :259, 1990.

16.   Fiocchi C, Battisto JR and Farmer RG. Gut mucosal lymphocytes in inflammatory bowel disease. Isolation and preliminary functional characterization. Dig Dis Sci, **24**:705, 1979.

17.   Heo DS, Whiteside TL, Johnson JT, Chen K, Barnes EL and Herberman RB. Long-term interleukin 2-dependent growth and cytotoxic activity of tumor-infiltrating lymphocytes from human squamous carcinomas of the head and neck. Cancer Res **47**:6353, 1987.

18.   Kurnick JT, Kradin RL, Blumberg R, Schneeberger EE and Boyle LA. Functional characterization of T lymphocytes propagated from human lung carcinomas.   Clin Immunol Immunopathol **38**:367, 1986.

19.   Finke JH, Tubbs R, Connelly B, Pontes E and Montie J. Tumor-infiltrating lymphocytes in patients with renal cell carcinomas. Ann NY Acad Sci **532**:387, 1988.

20.   Muul LM, Spiess PJ, Director EP and Rosenberg SA. Identification of cytolytic immune responses against autologous tumor in humans bearing malignant melanoma. J Immunol **138**:989, 1987.

21.   Itoh K, Platsoukas CD and Balch CM. Autologous tumor-specific cytotoxic T lymphocytes in the infiltrate of human metastatic melanoma. Activation by interleukin 2 and autologous tumor cells, and involvement of the T cell receptor. J Exp Med **168**:1419, 1988.

22.   Vose BM, Quantitation of proliferation in cytotoxic precursor cells directed against human tumors: Limiting dilution analysis in peripheral blood and the tumor site. Int J Cancer **30**:135, 1982.

23.   Cozzolino F, Torcia M, Corossino AM, Giordani R, Selli C, Talini G, Readi E, Novelli A, Pistoia V and Ferrarini M. Characterization of cells from invaded lymph nodes in patients with solid tumors. J Exp Med **166**:303, 1987.

24. Carswell EA, Old LJ, Kassel RL, Green F, Fiore N and Williamson B. Endotoxin-induced serum factor that causes necrosis in tumors. Proc Natl Acad Sci USA **72**:3066, 1975.

25. Old LJ, Tumor Necrosis Factor and related cytotoxins. CIBA Foundation Symposium 131, New York: John Wiley & Sons, Inc. 1987.

26. Ramija P, Epstein LB. Tumor necrosis factor as immunoregulatory and mediator of monocyte cytotoxicity induced by itself, γ-interferon, and interleukin-1. Nature (Lond.) **323**:86, 1986.

27. Scheurich P, Thoma B, Ucer U and Pfizenmaier K. Immunoregulatory activity of recombinant human tumor necrosis factor (TNF-α): induction of TNF receptors on human T cells and TNF-α mediated enhancement of T cell responses. J Immunol **138**:1786, 1987.

28. Chouaib S, Bertoglio J, Blay JY, Marichiol-Founigault C and Fradelizi D. Generation of lymphokine-activated killer cells: synergy between tumor necrosis factor alpha and interleukin-2. Proc Natl Acad Sci USA, **85**:6875, 1988.

29. Owen-Shaub LE, Gutterman JU and Grimm EA. Synergy of tumor necrosis factor and interleukin-2 in the activation of human lymphokine-activated killer cells cytotoxicity. Cancer Res **48**:788, 1988.

30. Rangers GE, Figari IS, Espevick T and Palladino MA Jr. Inhibition of cytotoxic T cell development by transforming growth factor B and reversal by recombinant tumor necrosis factor alpha. J Exp Med **166**:991, 1987.

31. Yi Li W, Lusheng S, Kanbour A, Herberman RB and Whiteside TL. Lymphocytes infiltrating human ovarian tumors: synergy between tumor necrosis factor alpha and interleukin 2 in the generation of CD8+ effectors from tumor-infiltrating lymphocytes. Cancer Res **49**,5979, 1989.

32. Brandtzaeg P, Valnes K, Scott H, Rognum TO, Bjerke K and Baklien K. The human gastrointestinal secretory immune system in health and disease. Scand J Gastroenterol **97**:1562, 1989.

ISOLATION AND CHEMICAL CHARACTERIZATION OF A NOVEL THYMIC HORMONE THAT
SYNERGIZES WITH GRF AND TRH IN ENHANCING RELEASE OF GROWTH HORMONE AND
PROLACTIN

Mahnaz Badamchian, *Bryan L. Spangelo, and
Allan L. Goldstein

Dept. of Biochemistry & Molecular Biology, The George
Washington University, Washington, DC 20037; *Dept. of
Internal Medicine, University of Virginia, Charlottesville,
Virginia

INTRODUCTION

During the course of recent studies, we have discovered a major
thymus—brain connection. Our current research indicates that the
thymosins and the endocrine thymus may play a broader role in the
physiology of the body. The question of whether the thymus plays a more
general role by controlling the aging of other organ and endocrine
systems has been debated for some time. Now it appears that the thymus
may accomplish control over immunity and perhaps other systems by
influencing the functioning of T-cells and by feedback loops to the
brain. We have found that a number of novel thymosin peptides in TF5
can alone and/or in combination with pituitary releasing factors
stimulate the release of neuropeptides such as ACTH (Healy et al.,
1983), LRF (Rebar et al., 1981), GH (Spangelo et al.,1987; Badamchian et
al., 1990, 1991); PRL (Spangelo et al., 1987); β-END (Farah et al.,
1987), and TSH (Goya et al., 1988), thus establishing a direct link
between the endocrine thymus and neuroendocrine system. This new thymus
brain link opens up a number of interesting questions with regard to the
physiology of aging. It is possible that the decreased production of
hormones of the thymus, which occurs before the onset of puberty, may
provide a first signal to other endocrine and neuroendocrine systems to
begin the process of slowing down. Our current studies suggest that
these bioactive peptides, for which we have suggested the name
immunotransmitters (Hall et al., 1985), may hold a vital key to our
understanding of the physiological process of aging and diseases
associated with this process.

In the present study we report the isolation and characterization
of MB-35, a new peptide with hormone-releasing activity that has been
purified from TF5. This peptide is a highly charged basic molecule of
35 amino acid residues and a molecular weight of 3756. A computer-
assisted search of published protein sequences has revealed that this
peptide has a 100% homology with a region of the histone H2A.
Biological studies using rat pituitary cells have revealed that MB-35 is
active alone or in combination with growth hormone releasing factor
(GRF) or thyrotropin releasing hormone (TRH) and can increase the
production of GH and/or PRL beyond that achievable with GRF and TRH
alone. The observation that histone H2A, the parent molecule, is

Combination Therapies, Edited by A.L. Goldstein and
E. Garaci, Plenum Press, New York, 1992

without activity is of keen interest, since it suggests that nucleoproteins may have heretofore unknown physiological activities perhaps related to cell cycle and/or other events associated with DNA activation events.

MATERIALS AND METHODS

Purification of Natural Peptide MB-35

TF5 (1.5g) was applied to a Delata-prep HPLC system equipped with a Model 481 variable-wavelength detector with a semi-preparative flow-cell, set at 280 nm, and a 300 x 50-mm Delta-pak, 300 Å, 15-μm C_{18} column (Waters). Eluent A was 0.02 M ammonium acetate (pH 6.8), and eluent B was acetonitrile. A 60-min linear gradient from 0-80% B was run at a flow-rate of 80 ml/min (Figure 1 Panel A). TF5 was dissolved in the initial buffer and applied to the column through a port in the solvent delivery system. One min fractions were collected and assayed for hormone-releasing activity.

Our results indicated that the peak of hormone-releasing activity eluted in Fraction 46, which, therefore, was used for further purification (Figure 1 Panel A). Fraction 46 was fractionated further on a 150 X 3.9 mm-I.D. Delta-pak 300 Å, 5-μm C_{18} column using model 510 HPLC system (Waters), equipped with model 441 detector set at 214 nm. Eluent A was 0.1% TFA in water; eluent B was acetonitrile with 0.1% TFA. Separation of peptide MB-35 was achieved by a 10 min linear gradient from 0 to 29% B followed by a 25 min hold at 29% B. At 35.1 min the gradient was increased to 30% B, followed by a 20 min hold at 30% B. At 55.1 min the column was washed with 50% B for 10 min. One-half min fractions were collected and assayed for hormone-releasing activity using normal anterior pituitary cells. Results indicated that a peak of activity eluted in Fraction 49 (Figure 1, Panel B), which was concentrated to 300 μl to remove acetonitrile and chromatographed under the same conditions. The single homogeneous peptide peak was collected and identified as peptide MB-35 (Figure 1, Panel C) and subjected to SDS-PAGE, IEF, amino acid composition and sequence analysis. The yield of peptide MB-35 from TF5 is about 0.1%.

Purification of Synthetic Peptide MB-35

Peptide MB-35 has been synthesized using a solid phase procedure (Badamchian et al., 1990). The crude synthetic material was purified on a 150 x 3.9 mm Delta-Pak 300 Å 5 μm C_{18} column using model 510 HPLC system (Waters), equipped with model 441 detector set at 214 nm. Eluent A was 20 mM potassium phosphate buffer (pH 6.0) and eluent B was acetonitrile with 50% eluent A. Separation of synthetic peptide MB-35 was achieved with a 40 min linear gradient from 0 to 100% B with 10 min hold at 100% B (Figure. 2A). There were several minor components in addition to a major peak. The major peak was collected and concentrated to remove acetonitrile and subsequently chromatographed under the same conditions to give single peak of 0.17 g of homogeneous synthetic MB-35 (Figure 2B). The yield of the final purified product was 14%. HPLC purified synthetic MB-35 subjected to IEF, SDS-PAGE, amino acid sequence and composition analysis.

Electrophoresis

Analytical IEF in thin layer polyacrylamide gels was performed on Parmacia/LKB Pagplate. Pagplate provides a pH range of 3.5-9.5 and has

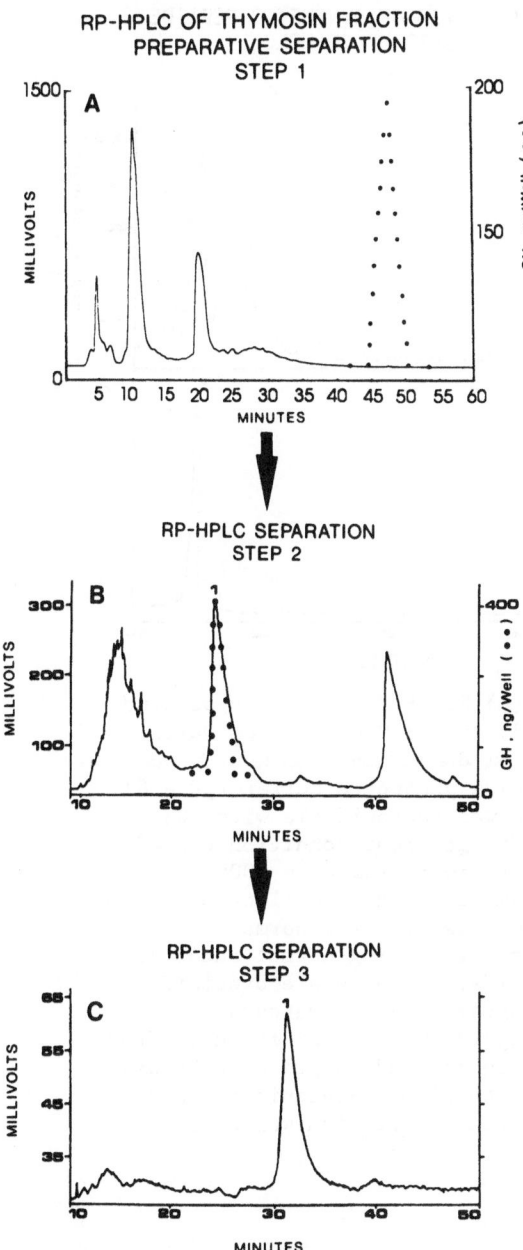

Figure 1. Flow diagram of the
fractionation of peptide MB–35 from
bovine thymosin fraction 5. Panel
A: RP–HPLC separation of 1.5 g of
TF5 (detection was at 280 nm).
Panel B: Rechromatography of the
active fraction from Panel A, used
for purifying peptide MB–35
(detection was at 214 nm). Panel C:
Rechromatography of the active
fraction (Peak 1) from panel B
(detection was at 214 nm). The
chromatographic condition is
described in Materials and Methods.

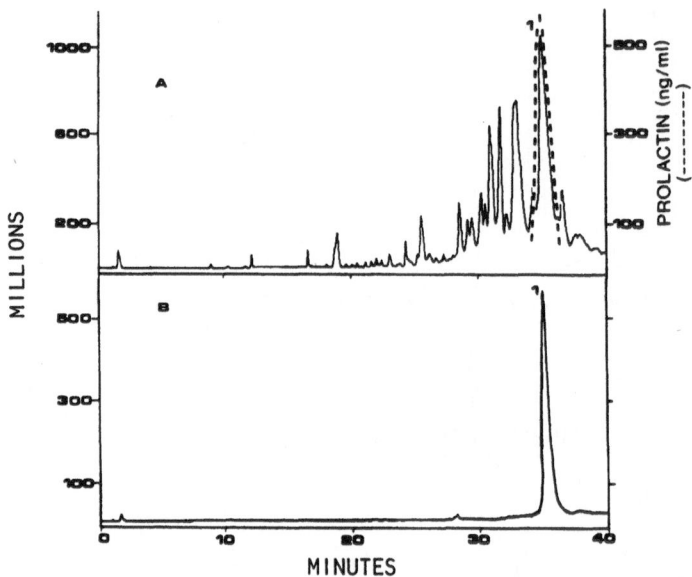

PURIFICATION OF SYNTHETIC PEPTIDE
MB-35 BY RP-HPLC

Figure 2. (A) RP-HPLC separation of crude peptide MB-35 on a 3.9 mm x 15 cm Delta-pak 300 Å 5 μm C_{18} column. Eluent A was 20 mM potassium phosphate buffer (pH 6.0) and eluent B was acetonitrile with 50% eluent A. The gradient condition was 40 min linear gradient from 0 to 100% B. Detection was at 214 nm. Collected fractions were assayed for hormone-releasing activity using normal anterior pituitary cells. Results are overlaid on the chromatogram. (B) Chromatography of synthetic peptide MB-35. Fraction 36 from the separation of crude peptide MB-35 was concentrated to remove acetonitrile and chromatographed. Detection was at 214 nm.

a gel concentration of 5% and degree of cross-linkage of 3%. The ampholine concentration is 2.4% (weight/volume). Peptide MB-35 samples (about 20-50 μg) were applied 2 cm from cathode strip. The electrolyte solutions used were 1 M NaOH for the cathode and 1 M H_3PO_4 for the anode. Isoelectric focusing was carried out for 90 min on a Pharmacia/LKB multiphor unit with cooling to 4°C. Constant power of 25 watts was supplied by a Pharmacia/LKB Model 2103 power supply set to a maximum current of 90 mA and a maximum potential of 1400 V. At the end of the run, gels were fixed in 20% trichloroacetic acid and 3.5% sulphosalicyclic acid for 1 h.

SDS-PAGE was performed using 12% polyacrylamide slab gels (16 cm x 18 cm x 1.5 mm), according to the method of Laemmli (1970). Peptide MB-35 samples (10-20 μg) were incubated at 90°C for 5 min before gel electrophoresis. Proteins were visualized in the gels using Coomassie Blue R-250. Molecular weight was estimated using low molecular weight standards obtained from Bio-Rad Laboratories (Richmond, CA).

Amino Acid Analysis

Amino acid analysis was performed with the Pico-Tag amino acid analysis system of Waters-Millipore. The method is based on the formation of a phenylthiocarbamyl (PTC) derivative of the amino acids from acid-hydrolyzed proteins. Peptide MB-35 samples (about 1-5 μg) were hydrolyzed in 200 μl of a constant boiling HCl atmosphere containing 1% (v/v) phenol at 110°C for 24, 48, 72, and 120 h in the Pico-Tag work station. The hydrolysates were dried and the amino acids were derivatized with phenylisothiocyanate for 20 min at room temperature to yield the corresponding PTC derivatives (Bidlingmeyer et al., 1984). These derivative were analyzed with the Pico-Tag amino acid analysis system, which had been previously calibrated with a standard mixture of amino acids.

Amino Acid Sequence Analysis

Amino acid sequence analysis based on the Edman degradation of peptide was performed on Beckman 890M sequencer using Beckman standard operating program 52285. The sequencer products were identified using model 510 HPLC system (Waters) equipped with model 441 detector set at 254 nm. The peptide sequence derivative, phenylthiohydantion amino acids were reconstituted in 10 μl of acetonitrile and 2 μl was injected to the 150 x 3.9 mm Nova-Pak C_{18} column. Eluent A was 25 mM Na-acetate (pH 5) in acetonitrile (5.5:1, v/v) and eluent B was 2-propanol in water (3:2, v/v). The column temperature was held at 40°C.

Anterior Pituitary Cell Culture

Anterior pituitary cells from normal adult female Sprague-Dawley rats were dispersed as described by Spangelo et al., (1990). Normal cells were seeded into 24-well tissue culture plates (Falcon, Oxnard, CA) at a density of 0.4 x 10^6 viable cells/well in 1.5 ml of RPMI-1640 medium supplemented with 2.5% fetal calf serum, 7.5% horse serum, 7.5 μg streptomycin/ml, 15 μg gentamicin/ml, 19 μg penicillin/ml and 0.6 μg fungizone/ml (Gibco, Grand Island, NY). The cells were allowed to attach to the wells in a humidified atmosphere of 5% CO_2 -95% air at 37°C for at least 4 d before an experiment was performed. On the day of an experiment, the cells were rinsed twice (1 hour each) with serum-free RPMI-1640 medium containing antibiotics.

Prolactin and GH ASSAY

Prolactin and GH were determined by standard RIA techniques using materials and protocols supplied by the NIDDK Rat Pituitary Hormone Distribution Program. Inter - and intra-assay variations for Prolactin and GH were less than 8% and 10%, respectively. All samples were assayed in duplicate, with results expressed in terms of NIDDK standards (rat prolactin RP-3 and rat GH RP-1). Neither TF5 nor synthetic peptide MB-35 had prolactin and GH cross-reactive material in the concentrations used. The variability within a set of quadruplicate values was 5-10%. The data are expressed as the mean ± SEM of groups consisting of 4 wells. Experiments were performed independently at least, with representative results reported. Analysis of variance and the Bonferroni analysis for multiple comparisons were used for the statistical evaluation of these data; $p < 0.05$ was considered significant.

Table 1

PURIFICATION OF PEPTIDE MB-35 FROM TF5

Purification steps (Active Fractions)	Specific Activity (ng hormone released/μg protein)	
	PRL	GH
TF5	5	10
MB7	2	8
F46	6.4	21
Natural MB–35	226	98
Synthetic MB–35	212	92
Histone H2A	3	8

RESULTS

Table 1 shows the specific activity (nanogram hormone released per microgram of peptide) as a function of the different purification steps from TF5 to MB–35. Natural and synthetic peptide MB–35 appears to have similar specific activity. In contrast histone H2A has no stimulatory effect on PRL and GH release.

The preparation of natural and synthetic peptide MB–35 were identical and free of impurities as evidence by RP–HPLC, SDS–PAGE and IEF analysis. Figure 3 shows the comparison of purified synthetic and natural peptide MB–35. Isoelectric focusing on polyacrylamide gels of synthetic and natural peptide MB–35 indicates that the synthetic peptide MB–35 moves to the similar position as the natural material with pI of 9.3 (Figure 4). SDS–PAGE analysis of the synthetic and natural peptide MB–35 illustrated in Figure 5. Our results indicate that synthetic and natural peptide MB–35 contain only one protein band in the molecular weight range of 4–5 kd. Our results also indicate that purified synthetic and natural peptide MB–35 have the identical amino acid composition (Table 2).

Amino acid sequence analysis of peptide MB–35 was performed on an automated Beckman 890M microsequencer, as described in Materials and Methods. Peptide MB–35 is composed of 35 amino acid residues and has the amino acid sequence follows.

A-I-R-N-D-E-E-L-N-K-L-L-G-K-V-T-I-A-Q-G-G-V-L-P-N-I-Q-A-V-L-L-P-K-K-T

Treatment of normal anterior pituitary cells with different doses of the synthetic or natural peptide MB–35 results in a significant increase in PRL and GH release. Figures 6A and 6B show concentration-dependent influence of peptide MB–35 on PRL and GH release from normal female anterior pituitary cells. Also tested in this assay was TF5 at 1.0 and 2.0 μg/ml. Peptide MB–35 resulted in a significant (p<0.01) increase in PRL and GH release at the 0.5 μg/ml dosage which corresponds to approximately 130 nM. Peptide MB–35 is significantly more potent than partially purified TF5 in stimulating PRL and GH release.

Table 2

AMINO ACID COMPOSITION OF PEPTIDE MB-35

Amino acid composition of natural and synthetic peptide MB-35.
Amino acid analysis was performed with Pico-Tag amino acid analysis
system. 2-5 μg of peptide MB-35 were hydrolyzed with 6 M HCL,
containing 1% (v/v) phenol at 110°C for 24, 48, and 72 h. The
hydrolysates were dried and used for amino acid analysis by the Pico-Tag
standard procedure.

Amino Acid	Synthetic Peptide MB-35	Natural Peptide MB-35	# of residues from sequence
D	3.9*	4.0*	1
E	3.8*	4.0*	2
G	3.0	3.0	3
R	0.9	1.0	1
T	1.7	1.5	2
A	2.9	3.4	3
P	1.5	1.9	2
V	2.8	2.6	3
I	3.1	2.5	3
L	6.2	5.5	6
K	4.1	4.4	4
N	–	–	3
Q	–	–	2

The data are presented as numbers of residues per molecule.
* Aspartic acid and glutamic acid values are the sum of their acids and
amides.

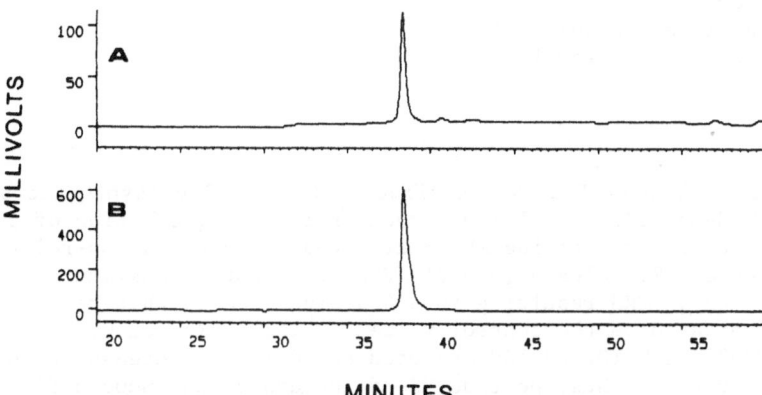

Figure 3. Comparison of natural peptide MB-35 (A) and
purified synthetic peptide MB-35 (B) on 3.0 mm x 15 cm
Delta-pak 300 Å 5 μm C_{18} column. Eluent A was 20 mM
potassium phosphate buffer (pH 6.0) and eluent B was
acetonitrile with 50% eluent A. The gradient
condition was 40 min linear gradient from 0 to 100% B
and 20 min hold at 100% B. Detection was determined at
214 nm.

IEF of Natural and
Synthetic MB-35

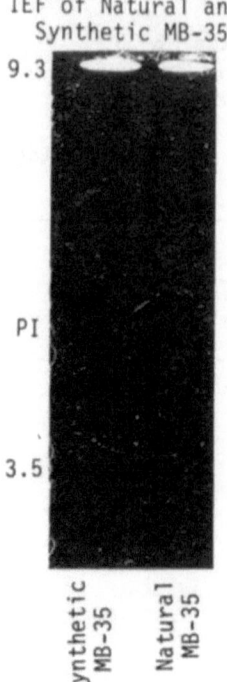

9.3

PI

3.5

Synthetic
MB-35

Natural
MB-35

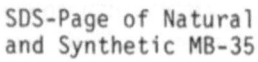

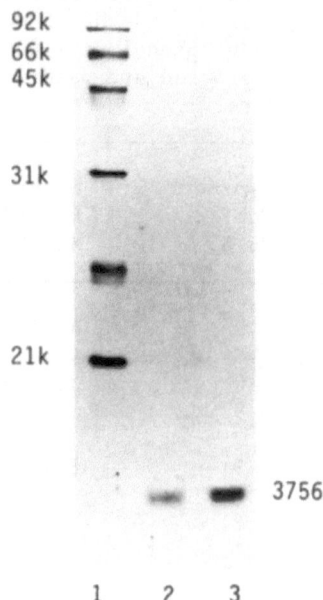

92k
66k
45k

31k

21k

3756

1   2   3

Figure 4. IEF of natural
and synthetic peptide MB-35
on Pharmacia/LKB Pagplate
(pH 3.5–9.5) was performed
by loading 50 μg of natural
and synthetic peptide MB-
35 on the gel. IEF was
carried out for 90 min on
Pharmacia/LKB multiphor
unit with cooling at 4°C.
The gel was fixed in 20%
trichloroacetic acid for 1
h.

Figure 5. SDS–PAGE of natural
and synthetic peptide MB-35. 10–
20 μg of peptide MB-35 samples
were electrophoresed on a 1.5 mm
SDS–polyacrylamide gel and
stained wtih Coomassi Blue R-250.
Lane 1: Standard proteins from
Bio-Rad. Lanes 2–3: Natural and
synthetic MB-35, respectively.

Figures 7A and 7B show the effects of natural or synthetic peptide
MB-35 on TRH–and GRF stimulated hormone release. Incubation of anterior
pituitary cells with peptide MB-35 elicited a concentration–related
stimulation of PRL release ($p<0.01$, Fig. 7A), with a maximum stimulatory
concentration of TRH resulting in a 400% increase in this release
($p<0.01$) compared to the control value. Coincubation of 0.5 or 1.0 μM
peptide MB-35 with 100 nM TRH produced an additive increase in PRL
release ($p<0.01$). Thus, peptide MB-35 increased TRH–induced PRL release
by the same increment as it increased basal PRL release. In a parallel
study treatment of anterior pituitary cells with peptide MB-35 elicited
a concentration–related increase in GH release (Fig. 7B). Similarly,
coincubation of 0.5 or 1.0 μM peptide MB-35 with a maximum
stimulatory amount of GRF (10 nM) resulted in an additive increase in GH
release ($p<0.01$).

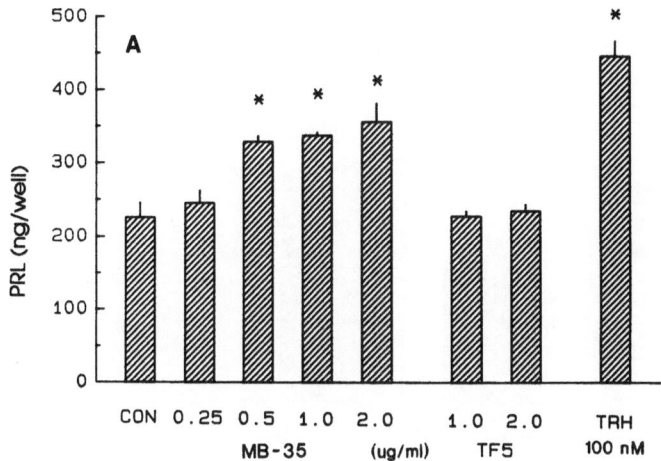

CONCENTRATION-DEPENDENT INFLUENCE OF MB-35 ON PRL
RELEASE FROM NORMAL FEMALE ANTERIOR PITUITARY CELLS

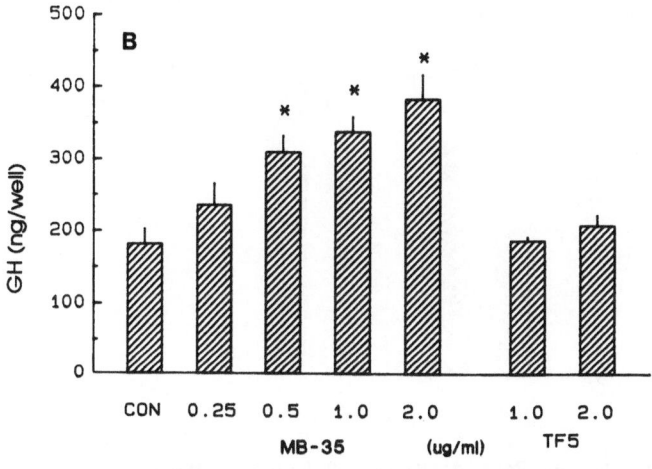

CONCENTRATION-DEPENDENT INFLUENCE OF MB-35 ON GH
RELEASE FROM NORMAL FEMALE ANTERIOR PITUITARY CELLS

Figure 6. Dose–dependent influence of peptide MB–35
and TF5 on PRL release from anterior pituitary cells.
Cells were incubated wtih RPMI–1640 medium, peptide
MB–35 (0.25–2.0 μm/ml), TF5 (1 and 2 μg/ml), or TRH
(100nM) for 30 min. Results are expressed as the mean
± SEM of four wells. Peptide MB–35 (0.5–2.0 μg/ml)
significantly stimulated PRL release from anterior
pituitary cells (P <0.01). B, Dose–dependent
influence of peptide MB–35 and TF5 on GH release from
anterior pituitary cells. The experimental conditions
are described in A.

MB-35 INCREASES TRH-STIMULATED PRL RELEASE FROM NORMAL FEMALE ANTERIOR PITUITARY CELLES

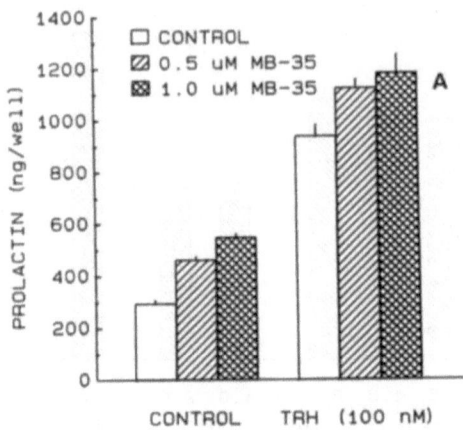

MB-35 INCREASES GRF-STIMULATED GH RELEASE FROM NORMAL FEMALE ANTERIOR PITUITARY CELLS

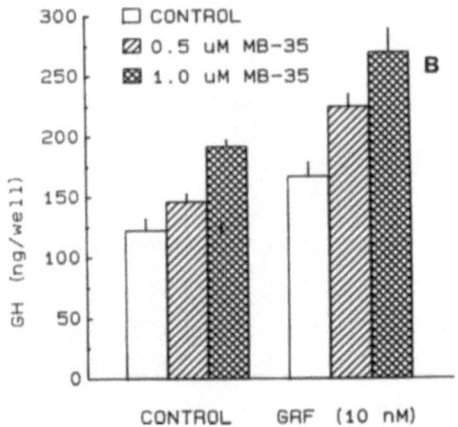

Figure 7. A, Peptide MB-35 (0.5 and 1 μM) or TRH (100 nm) treatment of normal anterior pituitary cells resulted in stimulation of PRL release (P <0.01) compared to that in vehicle-treated wells. MB-35 (0.5 and 1 μM) plus TRH (100 nM) increased PRL release compared to the effect of TRH alone (P <0.01) during a 30 min incubation. B, Normal anterior pituitary cells treated with peptide MB-35 (0.5 and 1.0 μM; P <0.01) or 10 nM GRF (P <0.05) had increased GH release compared to the control wells. MB-35 (0.5 and 1.0 μM) plus GRF (10 nM) increased GH release compared to GRF alone (P <0.01) during a 30-min incubation. Results are expressed as the mean ± SEM of four wells.

Table 3

EFFECTS OF MB-35 ON BASAL AND GRF-INDUCED
INTRA-CELLULAR cAMP ACCUMULATION

Group	Intra-cellular cAMP
Control	0.73 ± 0.05
0.5 μM MB-35	0.70 ± 0.04
1.0 μM MB-35	0.77 ± 0.05
10 nM GRF	14.3 ± 0.64
0.5 μM MB-35 + GRF	15.6 ± 0.60
1.0 μM MB-35 + GRF	14.7 ± 0.60

Values are expressed as the mean ± SEM of four determinants.

Table 3 shows effects of peptide MB-35 on basal and GRF-induced intra-cellular cAMP accumulation. The peptide MB-35 had no effect on basal or GRF-induced increases in intracellular cAMP levels in normal anterior pituitary cells.

DISCUSSION

Our current research indicates that a number of the peptide components of TF5 have novel neuroendocrine properties suggesting that the endocrine thymus may play a broader role in the physiology of the body than heretofore recognized. The question of whether the thymus which plays a specific role in the development and function of T-cell immunity may play a more general role in influencing endocrine systems has been debated for over 100 years (c.f. White and Goldstein, 1968). Our studies add support to the hypothesis that the thymus may accomplish control over immunity and perhaps other organ systems by producing peptides that both influence the functioning of T-cells and hormone producing cells of the pituitary. Our current results, showing that MB-35, a thymic-derived peptide, stimulates the release of PRL and GH from anterior pituitary cell, are consistent with the hypothesis that the thymus gland secretes soluble factors capable of regulating neuroendocrine function.

Peptide MB-35 is a very basic molecule composed of 35 amino acid residues, that has a molecular weight of 3756. The proposed structure of thymic peptide MB-35 has been confirmed by total chemical synthesis and subsequent comparison to the natural product by reverse-phase high-performance liquid chromatography, SDS-PAGE, polyacrylamide isoelectric focusing and amino acid compositional and sequence analysis. Biologically, synthetic MB-35 was determined to be as active as the natural compound in stimulating growth hormone and prolactin secretion from anterior pituitary cells.

TRH stimulation of PRL release is mediated through increased hydrolysis of polyphosphoinositide (Gershengorn, 1986). Coincubation of peptide MB-35 with an optimal amount of TRH causes an additive increase in PRL release compared to the effects of peptide MB-35 and TRH alone. These results suggest the conclusion that peptide MB-35 may have act via a mechanism(s) different from that of TRH. Similarly, GRF stimulates GH release in part through its ability to increase intracellular cAMP (Frohman and Jason, 1986). Peptide MB–35, has no effect on normal cell cAMP accumulation, and coincubation of peptide MB–35 with an optimal concentration of GRF results in greater GH release than that caused by GRF alone. The mechanism by which peptide MB–35 stimulates hormone release, therefore, does not appear to be dependent on changes in cAMP or polyphosphoinositide hydrolysis.

The primary amino acid structure of peptide MB–35 was screened for similarities with GRF and TRH polypeptides. No significant similarities were found with TRH. In contract peptide MB–35 has homology with amino acid residues of 21–23, 30, 32, and 38 of GRF polypeptide from human, porcine, and bovine.

Computer analysis of the primary sequence of peptide MB–35 using the Protein Identification Resource (PIR, National Biomedical Research Foundation, Georgetown University Medical Center, Washington, DC 20007) computer system has established that peptide MB–35 is identical to the residues 86–120 of a nuclear protein histone H2A isolated from human, chicken, rat, and bovine thymus. To the best of our knowledge, this is the first report demonstrating that a peptide fragment of nucleoprotein can stimulate PRL and GH release or for that matter be involved in the modulation of any hormonal response.

Treatment of normal anterior pituitary cells with different doses of a RP–HPLC purified commercial histone H2A (the possible–parent protein of peptide MB–35) from calf thymus did not effect PRL and GH release (Table 1).

Mammalian histone H2A is 129 residues long. Histone H2A is one of the most conserved proteins among both lower and higher eukaryotes. Such a high degree of evolutionary conservation and wide spread occurrence implies that histone H2A must play a role in one or more critical functions within the cell. Protein A24 is a dimer of histone H2A and non histone chromosomal protein (NHCP). The N–terminus portion of NHCP is termed ubiquitin. In bovine thymus A24, the two chains are linked by an isopeptide bond between histone H2A lys–119 and the carboxy–terminal Gly of NHCP. Figure 8 shows the proposed structure of nuclear protein A24 (Hunt and Dayoff, 1977; Goldknopf and Busch, 1980) and postulated relationship between histone H2A, NHCP, and the relative location of peptide MB–35. It has been proposed that the highly conserved central region (residues 12–118) of histone H2A is less exposed in the nucleosome than are the terminal, more variable regions, which may then have different functional roles (Bohm et al., 1980).

The full significance of the relationship between peptide MB–35 and histone H2A has not been fully ascertained. However, recent reports by Reichhart et al., 1985a; 1985b) suggests that some histones may exhibit hormone–like activity. Homeostatic thymus hormone (HTH) has been ascribed to have various activities, including acting as a synergist of GH. The primary amino acid structures of HTHα/H2A and HTHβ/H2B were screened for similarities between various TF5 peptides, including thymosins α_1, α_{11}, β_4, β_9, and thymopoietins. No significant similarities were found. Aten, et al., (1989) reported that the ovarian gonadotropin–releasing hormone (GnRH)–binding inhibitor is histone H2A. It inhibits the high affinity binding of GnRH to rat ovarian membrane and also evokes GnRH–like antigonadotropic responses in rat ovarian cells that do not appear to be mediated by binding to GnRH receptors. They suggest that histone H2A may have a previously unexpected role in the local regulation of ovarian function.

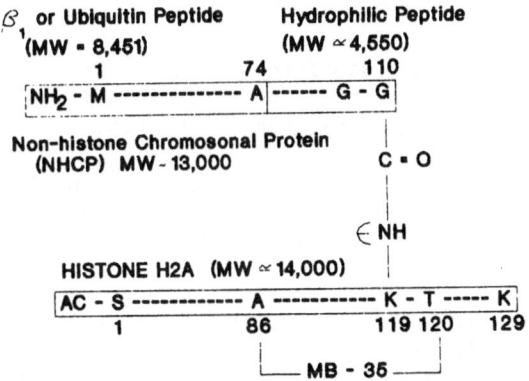

Figure 8. A proposed structure for nuclear protein A24. One of the two chains in the complex is histone H2A, with a blocked amino end. The other chain, NHCP, is composed of ubiquin plus a hydrophillic segment. The carboxyl-terminal of NHCP is linked to histone H2A through an isopeptide linkage. See Discussion for details on the possible relationship of these proteins.

The observation that some nucleoprotein components, in addition to their structural function within the cell, may have important hitherto unknown roles in regulating physiological responses is of keen interest. During cell activation it is known that histone and non-histone nucleoproteins are released by proteases and migrate to the cytoplasm (Hunt and Dayoff, 1977). Our studies suggests that some of these proteins/peptides (nucleokines) may have important extracellular paracrine and/or endocrine functions. However, at this time, the possibility that peptide MB-35 might be the degradation product of some different protein other than A24 or histone H2A cannot be excluded.

REFERENCES

Aten, R., Behrman, H., 1989. Antigonadotropic effects of the bovine ovarian gonadotropin-releasing hormone-binding inhibitor/histone H2A in rat luteal and granulosal cells. J. Biol. Chem. 264, 11072.

Badamchian, M., Wang, S.S., Spangelo, B.L., Damavandy, T., and Goldstein, A.L., 1990, Chemical and biological characterization of MB-35 a thymic-derived peptide that stimulate the release of growth hormone and prolactin from rat anterior pituitary cells, progress in NeuroEndocrinImmunology, 3(4), 258.

Badamchian, M., Spangelo, B.L., Damavandy, T., MacLeod, R.M., and Goldstein, A.L., 1991, Complete amino acid sequence analysis of a peptide isolated from the thymus that enhances release of growth hormone and prolactin, Endocrinology, 128(3):1580.

Bidlingmeyer, B.A., Cohen, S.A., and Tarvin, S.L., 1984, Rapid analysis of amino acids using pre-column derivitization. J Chromatography, 336, 93.

Bohm, L., Crane-Robinson, C., Sautiere, P., 1980, Proteolytic digestion studies of chromatin core-histone structure: Identification of a limit peptide of histone H2A. Eur. J. Biochem., 106, 525.

Farah, J.M., Jr., Hall, N.R., Bishop, J.F., Goldstein, A.L., O'Donohue, T.L., 1987. Thymosin fraction 5 stimulates secretion of immunoreactive beta-endorphin in mouse corticotropic tumor cells. J. Neurosci., Res., 18(1), 140.

Frohman, L.A., Jason, J.O., 1986. Growth hormone-releasing hormone. Endocrinol. Rev., 7, 233.

Gershengorn, M.C., 1986. Mechanism of thyrotropin releasing hormone stimulation of pituitary hormone secretion. Annu. Rec. Phys., 48, 515.

Goldknopf, I.L. and Busch, H., 1980. N-Bromosccinimide fragments of protein A_{24}(UH2A): An implication that ubiquitin is the precursor of conjugation in vivo. Biochem. Biophys. Res. Commun. 96, 1724.

Goya, R.G. Sosa, Y.E., Quigley, K.L., Gottaschall, P.E., Goldstein, A.L. and Meites, J., 1988. Differential activity of thymosin peptides (thymosin fraction 5) on plasma thyrotropin in female rats of different ages. Neuroendocrinology 47, 379.

Healy, D.L., Hodgen, G.D., Schulte, H.M., Chousos, G.P. Lorinaux, D.L., Hall, R.N., and Goldstein, A.L., 1983. The thymus-adrenal connection: thymosin has corticotropic-releasing activity in primates. Science, 222, 1353.

Hunt, L.T. and Dayoff, M.D., 1977. Amino-terminal sequence identity of ubiquitin and the nonhistone component of nuclear protein A_{24}. Biochem. Biophys. Res. Commun. 74,650.

Laemmli, U.K., 1970. Cleavage of structural proteins during the assembly of the bacteriophage T_4. Nature, 227, 680.

Rebar, R.W., Miyake, A., Low, T.L.K., and Goldstein, A.L., 1981. Thymosin stimulates secretion of luteinizing hormone-releasing factor. Science, 214, 669.

Reichart, T., Jornvall, H., Carlquist, M. and Zeppezauer, M., 1985a. The primary structure of two polypeptide chains from preparations of homeostatis thymus hormone (HTHα and HTHβ). FEBS Letters. 188, 63.

Reichhart, R., Zeppezauer, M., and Jornvall, H., 1985b. Preparations of homeostatic thymus hormone consist predominantly of histones 2A and 2B and suggest additional histone functions. Proc. Natl. Acad. Sci. 82, 4871.

Spangelo, B.L., Judd, A.M., Ross, P.C., Login, I.S., Jarvis, W.D., Badamchian, M., Goldstein, A.L., and MacLeod, R.M., 1987. Thymosin fraction 5 stimulates prolactin and growth hormone release from anterior pituitary cells in vitro. Endocrinol. 121(6), 2035.

Spangelo, B.L., MacLeod, R.M., and Isakson, P.C., 1990. Production of interleukin-6 by anterior pituitary cells in vitro. Endocrinology 126, 582.

White, A., and Goldstein, A.L., 1968. Is the thymus an endocrine gland? Old problem, new data. Perspectives in Biology and Medicine. 11(3), 475.

CYTOKINE–BASED COMBINED MODALITY APPROACHES TO THE TREATMENT OF MURINE

RENAL CANCER

Robert H. Wiltrout[1], Giovanna Damia[1], Martin MacPhee[1], Hitoyasu Futami[1], Connie R. Faltynek[2], Dan L. Longo[1], Francis W. Ruscetti[1], and Kristin L. Komschlies[3]

[1]Biological Response Modifiers Program, NCI–FCRDC, Frederick, MD, [2]Sterling Research Group, Sterling Drug, Inc., Malvern, PA, and [3]BCDP, PRI/DynCorp, Frederick, MD

INTRODUCTION

Biological response modifiers (BRM) are being developed as a potential fourth modality for cancer treatment to supplement the three currently accepted modalities, chemotherapy, radiotherapy, and surgery (1). There are several possible approaches to the use of immunoactive cytokines as part of combined modalities for cancer treatment. First, cytokines can be used in combination with one or more of the traditional modalities for cancer treatment. The rationale for such an approach is that either the mechanisms for the antitumor effects of the cytokines versus those of the other modality will differ leading to enhanced antitumor effects, or that the effects of one will enhance the activity of the other. In either case the efficacy of the combination should be greater than either modality alone. Second, different combinations of cytokines should be complementary based on their interaction as part of the cytokine cascade that regulates immune responses. We are studying different preclinical models that fall into both types of combined modality approaches. It has been reported that interleukin 1 (IL–1) can protect mice from the acute toxicity of some chemotherapeutic drugs (2–4) and that this ability to dose escalate chemotherapy translates into enhanced antitumor efficacy (4), although some late toxicity becomes evident (4). In addition, we are studying the hematoimmunological effects of various T cell–stimulating cytokines (5–7) under the hypothesis that the enhancement of the appropriate T cell functions will lead to increased antitumor efficacy.

In this report we will describe our recent results relating to the mechanism by which rhIL–1α protects mice from the acute toxicity of selected chemotherapeutic drugs, as well as our initial results on the preclinical hematoimmunological and antimetastatic effects of recombinant human interleukin 7 (rhIL–7).

MATERIALS AND METHODS

Mice. BALB/c or C57BL/6 mice were obtained from The Animal Production Area, Frederick Cancer Research and Development Center, Frederick, MD. The mice were maintained under specific pathogen–free conditions and used at 6 to 8 wk of age. After treatment with chemotherapeutic drugs, mice were maintained five per cage inside filter bonnets in an isolation room.

Agents. rhIL-1α (sp. act. $2x10^7$ U/mg protein) was generously provided by Dainippon Pharmaceutical Co. (Tokyo, Japan). Recombinant human IL-7, which was produced in E. Coli and purified by Immunex Corporation, was generously supplied by Sterling Drug, Inc., Malvern, PA. The rhIL-7 had a specific biological activity of $2-5x10^7$ U/mg of protein, as measured by proliferation of a murine pre-B cell line; endotoxin levels were <0.1 ng/mg IL-7. Recombinant human interleukin 2 (rhIL-2) was generously donated by Cetus Corporation (Emeryville, CA). The rhIL-2 had a specific activity of $18x10^6$ international (WHO) Units/mg and contained less than 0.012 ng endotoxin per mg protein. Cyclophosphamide (Cy) was purchased from Sigma Chemical Co. (St. Louis, MO), 5-fluorouracil (5FU) was purchased from LyphoMed. Inc. (Rosemont, IL), cisplatin, 1,3-bis-(2-chloroethyl)-1-nitrosourea (BCNU), and carboplatin were purchased from Bristol Laboratories, Syracuse, NY, and adriamycin was obtained from Sigma Chemical Co., St. Louis, MO.

Chemoprotection Studies. Mice were pretreated ip once per day for 7 days (0.5 μg/day) with rhIL-1α. One day after the last administration of rhIL-1α, the mice received doses of various chemotherapeutic drugs that were known to be acutely toxic for normal mice. A number of hematological parameters were monitored at various times thereafter, and a cohort of 10 mice per group was also monitored for long-term survival.

Hematoimmunological and Antimetastatic Effects of rhIL-7. Normal or tumor-bearing mice were injected with either HBSS + 0.1% normal mouse serum (NMS), IL-7 + HBSS + 0.1% NMS or IL-2 + HBSS + 0.1% NMS. At various periods of time thereafter, groups of mice were euthanized and examined for alterations in total cellularity of various lymphoid organs, changes in leukocyte subset composition in the spleen, effects on the frequency of hemopoietic progenitor cells, and antimetastatic effects.

RESULTS

Chemoprotective Effects of rhIL-1α. Previous studies from our own (4), and other laboratories (3) demonstrated that pretreatment with rhIL-1 protected mice from the acute death induced by Cy. The present study documents that this protection from acute toxicity by pretreatment with rhIL-1α also extends to a variety of other chemotherapeutic drugs that have myelosuppression as their dose-limiting toxicity. The results, summarized in Table 1, demonstrate that a 7 day pretreatment regimen with rhIL-1α protects mice against the acute toxicity (LD_{90}) of several drugs (5FU, Cy, BCNU, and carboplatin) that have myelosuppression as their primary dose-limiting toxicity. In contrast, the same pretreatment regimen of rhIL-1α administration failed to protect mice from the acute toxicity induced by an LD_{90} dose of cisplatin or adriamycin which have nephrotoxicity and cardiotoxicity as their primary dose-limiting toxicities, respectively.

The relationship of chemoprotection by rhIL-1α to myelotoxicity was further investigated by monitoring the degree of leukopenia, and the rate of recovery in mice that had been treated with 5FU or Cy alone, or with rhIL-1α in combination with 5FU or Cy. The results of these studies demonstrated that the pretreatment of mice with rhIL-1α reduced the nadir of myelosuppression slightly, but appreciably accelerated the regeneration of CFU-c and peripheral white blood cell levels. Further studies demonstrated that the performance of a bone marrow transplant

270

Table 1. Chemoprotective Effects of rhIL-1α in Mice[a]

Drug (mg/kg)	BM Recovery[b]	Chemo-protection	(% survival)[c]	Rescue by BMT[d]	Dose-limiting toxicity
5FU	Increased	Yes	(>90)	Yes	Myelosuppression
Cy	Increased	Yes	(>80)	No	Myelosuppression
BCNU	ND[e]	Yes	(>70)	ND	Myelosuppression
Carbo-platin	ND	Yes	(>70)	ND	Myelosuppression
Cisplatin	ND	No	(<20)	ND	Nephrotoxicity
Adria-mycin	ND	No	(<20)	ND	Cardiotoxicity

[a]Mice were pretreated ip with 0.5 μg of rhIL-1α daily for 7 days prior to the administration of acutely toxic doses of various chemotherapeutic drugs. Cohorts of mice were euthanized at various times thereafter for assessment of the effects of rhIL-1α on chemotherapy-induced myelosuppression and one cohort of 10 mice per group was monitored for survival.

[b]Various parameters were monitored for rate of hematopoietic recovery, including total WBC and neutrophils, as well as CFU-c levels in the bone marrow and spleen.

[c]Survival from acute toxicity was routinely assessed at day 30.

[d]Mice that had been treated with acutely toxic doses of 5FU were transplanted 4-48 hrs later with $1-3 \times 10^7$ total syngeneic bone marrow cells.

[e]ND = not determined.

(BMT) within 48 hours of the administration of a lethal dose of 5FU provided efficient rescue of these mice, suggesting that the mechanism by which pretreatment of mice with rhIL-1α protects mice from 5FU-induced toxicity is largely myeloprotective/restorative. Interestingly, BMT failed to rescue mice treated with Cy, while pretreatment with rhIL-1α was quite effective. This result suggests that pretreatment with rhIL-1α protects against both myelotoxic, as well as some non-myelotoxic, effects of Cy. Overall these results suggest that rhIL-1α may be useful for dose-intensification of a variety of chemotherapeutic drugs.

Hematoimmunological and Antimetastatic Effects of rhIL-7 in Mice. T lymphocytes are particularly potent antitumor effector cells. Therefore, cytokines that stimulate T cells should ultimately prove very useful in concert with other immunoactive cytokines and/or with chemotherapeutic drugs. Recently, rhIL-7 has been reported to affect the growth and function of both mature and immature T cells (8-11), as well as the differentiation pattern of myeloid progenitors. Based on these preliminary studies, we have undertaken a detailed analysis of the hematoimmunological effects of rhIL-7 in mice. The results of these studies are summarized in Table 2. The administration of daily doses of 5 and 10 μg rhIL-7 to mice for 4 to 7 days induces a pronounced (5-10 fold) leukocytosis in the peripheral blood and spleen, and about a 3 fold increase in lymph node cellularity. This increase occurs largely because of an increase in B220[+] B lymphocytes. In addition there is an increase in the total number of both CD4[+] and CD8[+] T cells, with the

Table 2. Hematoimmunological Effects of rhIL-7 in mice[a]

Parameter	Results
White blood cell levels	Leukocytosis in spleen and peripheral blood (5–10 fold) and lymph nodes (3–4 fold)
Subset analysis (spleen)	Increase in the % of pre–B cells. Preferential increase in the number of $CD8^+$ T cells. Reversal of the CD4/CD8 ratio. Increase in IL–2R expression.
Leukocyte Functions	No increase in NK activity. Increase in LAK activity at high doses. Increase in baseline proliferation.
Progenitor analysis	Decrease in the number of CFU–c and CFU–GEMM in the bone marrow (>90%). Increase (5–10 fold) in the number of CFU–c and CFU–GEMM in the spleen.

[a]C57BL/6 mice were treated ip twice daily with 5 or 10 μg/injection of rhIL–7. Groups of mice were euthanized on days 4 or 7 and analyzed for changes in the hematoimmunological parameters shown.

effects on $CD8^+$ T cells predominating such that the CD4/CD8 ratio goes from about 2:1 to 0.8:1. Coincident with these phenotypic changes, an increase in baseline proliferation rate was detected. Further studies revealed that rhIL–7 administration also induced a profound decrease (>90%) in the number of CFU–c and CFU–GEMM that could be cultured from bone marrow cells and a 5 to 10–fold increase in splenic CFU–c and CFU–GEMM.

Because the administration of rhIL–7 to mice caused profound perturbations in the frequency of hematopoietic progenitor cells, as well as alterations in lymphocyte subsets, studies were performed to determine whether rhIL–7 would have antimetastatic properties in mice. The data summarized in Table 3 demonstrate that the twice daily administration of rhIL–7 at doses $\geq$ 5 μg/injection for 5–10 days appreciably inhibited the number of pre–existent experimentally induced Renca metastases in the lungs of syngeneic mice. This effect is dose-dependent and has been observed in several murine tumor models. Preliminary data obtained from experiments designed to study effects of rhIL–7 on hepatic Renca metastases suggest that rhIL–7 may enhance the antimetastatic effects of rhIL–2. Overall, these results demonstrate that rhIL–7 has antimetastatic effects against at least some rodent tumors, and suggests that a further investigation of its antimetastatic potential is warranted.

DISCUSSION

The results presented herein demonstrate that rhIL–1α can be used to dose–escalate several chemotherapeutic drugs. The mechanism for these chemoprotective effects is related, but not limited to myeloprotection. The implication of these findings is that cytokines may be useful for dose–intensification of active chemotherapeutic drugs

Table 3. Antimetastatic Effects of rhIL-7 Against Murine Renal Cancer[a]

Site of Experimental Metastases	Treatment (μg/injection)	% Inhibition of the Median Number of Metastases[b]
Lung	rhIL-7 (≤ 1 μg)	<10
	rhIL-7 (≥ 5 μg)	40-75
Liver	rhIL-7 (5 μg)	<10
	rhIL-2 (10μg)	70
	rhIL-7 (5 μg) + rhIL-2 (10 μg)	90

[a]BALB/c mice were injected on day 0 with 1x10^5 Renca cells intravenously or intrasplenically for the formation of pulmonary or hepatic metastases, respectively. On days 3-8 or 3-12 cytokines were administered ip twice daily at the indicated doses. Grossly visible metastases were enumerated on days 14-16.

[b]Comparison to tumor-bearing mice treated only with HBSS.

against some tumor types. Preliminary preclinical studies have already demonstrated that this approach may lead to increased therapeutic efficacy (4). These results also re-emphasize the potential benefits of combined modality approaches to cancer treatment.

We have also begun a detailed evaluation of the effects of rhIL-7 in mice, and have reported that rhIL-7 has pronounced effects on the hematological and immunological systems as well as anti-metastatic effects. These results suggest that a more detailed investigation of the mechanism(s) for these effects will be beneficial, as will studies to relate the immunological perturbations to the antitumor effects of rhIL-7. Ultimately, rhIL-7 may prove useful as a lymphopoietic agent (12), as well as for cancer treatment. Its anticancer properties will most likely be maximized in the combined modality setting.

ACKNOWLEDGEMENTS

This project was funded in part with Federal funds from the Department of Health and Human Services, under contract number N01-CO-74102 with Program Resources, Inc./DynCorp. The contents of this publication do not necessarily reflect the views or policies of the Department of Health and Human Services, nor does mention of trade names, commercial products, or organizations imply endorsement by the U.S. Government.

REFERENCES

1. E. C. Borden, and M. J. Hawkins, Biological response modifiers as adjuncts to other therapeutic modalities. Semin. Oncol. 13:144 (1986).

2. M.A.S. Moore, and D. J. Warren, Synergy of interleukin 1 and granulocyte colony-stimulating factor: in vivo stimulation of stem-cell recovery and hematopoie.ic regeneration following 5-fluorouracil treatment of mice. <u>Proc. Natl. Acad. Sci. USA</u> 84:7134 (1987).

3. M. P. Castelli, P. L. Black, M. Schneider, R. Pennington, F. Abe, and J. E. Talmadge, Protective, restorative, and therapeutic properties of recombinant human IL-1 in rodent models. <u>J. Immunol.</u> 140:3830 (1988).

4. H. Futami, R. Jansen, M. J. MacPhee, J. Keller, K. McCormick, D. L. Longo, J. J. Oppenheim, F. W. Ruscetti, and R. H. Wiltrout, Chemoprotective effects of rhIL-1α in cyclophosphamide-treated normal and tumor-bearing mice: protection from acute toxicity, hematological effects, development of late mortality and enhanced therapeutic efficacy. <u>J. Immunol.</u> 145:4121 (1990).

5. R. R. Salup, T. A. Back, and R. H. Wiltrout, Successful treatment of advanced murine renal cell cancer by bicompartmental adoptive chemoimmunotherapy. <u>J. Immunol.</u> 138:641 (1987).

6. R. H. Wiltrout, M. R. Boyd, T. C. Back, R. R. Salup, J. A. Arthur, and R. L. Hornung, Flavone-8-acetic acid augments system natural killer cell activity and synergizes with interleukin 2 for treatment of murine renal cancer. <u>J. Immunol.</u> 140:3261 (1988).

7. T. J. Sayers, T. A. Wiltrout, K. McCormick, C. Husted, and R. H. Wiltrout, Antitumor effects of IFNα and/or IFNγ on a murine renal cancer (Renca) in vitro and in vivo. <u>Cancer Res.</u> 50:5414 (1990).

8. J. D. Watson, P. J. Morrissey, A. E. Namen, P. J. Conlon, and M. B. Widmer, Effect of IL-7 on the growth of fetal thymocytes in culture. <u>J. Immunol.</u> 143:1215 (1989).

9. P. J. Conlon, P. J. Morrissey, R. R. Nordan, K. H. Grabstein, K. S. Prickett, S. G. Reed, R. Goodwin, D. Cosman, and A. E. Namen, Murine thymocytes proliferate in direct response to interleukin 7. <u>Blood</u> 74:1368 (1989).

10. P. J. Morrissey, R. G. Goodwin, R. P. Nordan, D. Anderson, K. H. Grabstein, D. Cosman, J. Sims, S. Lupton, B. Acres, S. G. Reed, D. Mochizuki, J. Eisenman, P. J. Conlon, and A. E. Namen, Recombinant interleukin 7, pre-B cell growth factor, has costimulatory activity on purified mature T cells. <u>J. Exp. Med.</u> 169:707 (1989).

11. P. A. Welch, A. E. Namen, R. G. Goodwin, R. Armitage, and M. D. Cooper, Human IL-7: A novel T cell growth factor. <u>J. Immunol.</u> 143:3562 (1989).

12. P. J. Morrissey, P. Conlon, S. Brackly, D. E. Williams, A. E. Namen, and D. Y. Mochizuki, Administration of IL-7 to mice with cyclophosphamide-induced lymphopenia accelerates lymphocyte repopulation. <u>J. Immunol.</u> 146:1547 (1991).

RATIONALE FOR THERAPEUTIC APPROACHES WITH THYMOSIN α 1,

INTERLEUKIN 2 AND INTERFERON IN COMBINATION WITH CHEMOTHERAPY

Cartesio Favalli, Antonio Mastino, Sandro Grelli, Francesca Pica, Guido Rasi, and Enrico Garaci

Dept. of Experimental Medicine and Biochemical Sciences, University of Rome "Tor Vergata", via O. Raimondo, 00173 Rome, Italy

INTRODUCTION

Nowadays a new category of substances defined as "Biological response Modifiers" (BRMs) is currently under careful experimentation in order to ascertain its effectiveness in the stimulation of immune response. Among these various substances, the interferons (IFNs) (Bunn et al., 1986; Jaffe and Herberman, 1988), the interleukin 2 (IL-2) (Rosenberg et al., 1984; Lotze et al.,1985a; Lotze et al., 1985b), and the thymic hormones (THs) (Hooper et al., 1975; Goldstein and Schulof, 1984), are important particularly in the studies on experimental immunotherapy of cancer in animals and in humans. These substances, share the common characteristic of being physiologically involved in the regulation of the ontogenesis and of the activation of different immune cells, and are considered to exert a certain selective action on the immune response. Furthermore they are available in large quantities by biotechnological (IFNs and IL-2) or by chemical synthesis (THs) techniques. Results, however, have not always been positive and sometimes inferior to expectations and indicate that when applied alone, these BRMs display only restricted efficacy. One of the difficulties affecting these results could be that of establishing treatment dosages which must produce simultaneously both biological action and non-toxic effects. Another potential difficulty, particularly for IL-2 and IFNs, is the possibility of tumor cell resistance to cytokines, as recently described (Killion and Fidler, 1990). This resistance could be attributable either to non-responsiveness of host killer cells to the cytokines stimulating action, or to the tumor cells resistance to the cytotoxic activity by stimulated attacker cells.

Since, on the basis of the actually available results, it seems that none of the known BRMs, when utilized alone, is able to block tumoral progression in humans (Hadden ,1988), many research groups are now trying the route of combination therapies using more cytokines with or without chemotherapy. The goal of these studies is to find two or more BRMs with additive action or, more interestingly, to find combination treatments with a synergistic effect in order to obtain a powerfull antitumoral action and also to overcome the resistances to cytokines. In general a rational combination could be the use of two or more cytokines that affect, in parallel, different target cells and so stimulate

Combination Therapies, Edited by A.L. Goldstein and
E. Garaci, Plenum Press, New York, 1992

different effectors with the same target, or the use of two or more cytokines that affect , in series, the same effector at different stages of maturation in order to prepare it to be more sensitive to the effect of the following one.

With this last concept in mind, our research group has made an original contribution to the development of this new, exciting and encouraging area of research, having studied for years the combination between THs and IFN and, more recently, between THs and IL-2 (Favalli et al., 1985; Garaci et al., 1988; Favalli et al., 1989; Garaci et al., 1989; Garaci et al., 1990; Mastino et al., 1991). Here we report a review of the results of our studies in this field.

SYNERGISTIC ACTION OF THYMOSIN α 1 AND INTERFERON

During recent years it was demonstrated that treatment with thymosin was able to stimulate α and   IFN (Huang et al., 1981; Svedersky et al ., 1982). Some time after that we showed that thymosin α-1 (Tα1) (Goldstein et al., 1977) and αß IFN were able to induce a synergic action on the stimulation of NK activity in animals immunodepressed by means of cyclophosphamide (CY). In this study we found that neither Tα1 or IFN, when administered alone, were effective in restoring NK activity in CY suppressed mice; however, when both were given in combination, there was a synergistic effect and NK activity was significantly restored. Following these studies it was proved that such a synergic effect between THs and IFN, in NK activity stimulation, can also be obtained in vitro in circulating human lymphocytes (Serrate et al., 1987).

In further studies we have shown that a combined treatment with Tα1 and αß IFN powerfully stimulates NK activity in animals suppressed by tumor growth, who were not responding to IFN alone (Favalli et al., 1989).

Since it has been proved that NK activity plays an important role in host defence against tumors, we have examined the possible correlation between restored NK response and the effect on experimental tumor growth. In fact combination treatment with Tα1 and IFN caused a certain slowing-down in B16 Melanoma and in Lewis Lung carcinoma (3LL) tumor growth. It also caused an increase in animal survival time, but no long-term survival could be obtained

Table 1. Effects of in vivo administration of Tα1 and murine   interferon αß in combination with cyclophosphamide (CY) on survival time in 3LL bearing mice.

Group[a]	% mortality[b]
Untreated	100
CY	90
CY+Tα1	65
CY+IFN	90
CY+Tα1+IFN	25

a C57BL/6NcrlBR mice were challenged with 2 x 10^5 3LL viable cells s.c. Mice were then divided into experimental groups and treated as described.
b Mortality was calculated on day 90.

(Garaci et al., 1989). Since it has been demonstrated that immunotherapy could have a synergistic effect with chemotherapy, we have attempted to find out if THs and IFN treatment could prove more effective if administrated in combination with chemotherapy. As a consequence we performed experiments which demonstrated that the combination treatment with Tα1 (200 μg/Kg) for four days, followed by a single injection of murine IFN αß (3 x 10^4 IU/mouse), starting two days after CY treatment (200 mg/Kg, single injection) caused a rapid disappearance of the tumor burden in mice with 3LL. The chemo-immunotherapy protocol was effective even on the long-term survival of 75% of the animals (table 1).

Results were significantly different when compared to treatment with the single agents in conjunction with chemotherapy or to chemotherapy itself. In order to explain the mechanism of the antitumoral action, immunological studies were carried out. The results of these studies have shown that the same immunotherapy combination treatment strongly stimulated NK activity (table 2) and cytotoxicity against autologus 3LL tumor cells, in 3LL tumor bearing mice treated with CY, whereas treatments with each agent singularly did not or only slightly modified the cytotoxic activity towards both YAC-1 and 3LL target cells. The killer cells stimulated by chemoimmunotherapy combination treatment bear the phenotypic characteristics of asialo GM1 positive cells. A histological study has shown a high number of infiltrating lymphoid cells in tumors obtained from mice treated with chemoimmunotherapy combination (Garaci et al., 1990).

SYNERGISTIC ACTION OF THYMOSIN α 1 AND INTERLEUKIN 2

Previous studies have demonstrated in animals and in humans that systemic administration of IL-2, alone or in combination with IL-2 expanded lymphocyte

Table 2. Effects of in vivo administration of Tα1 and murine interferon αß on cytotoxic activity in 3LL bearing mice.

Mean LU 20/Spleen (Mean+S.D.- Mean-S.D.)	
Group[a]	TARGET: YAC-1
Normal	486.1 (527.1-448.9)
Untreated	313.7 (331.6-297.6)
CY	28.3 (32.0- 25.3)
CY+Tα1	26.6 (28.3- 25.2)
CY+IFN	29.0 (30.8- 27.3)
CY+Tα1+IFN	131.0 (147.1-116.6)

a 3LL (2x10^5 viable cells) was inoculated s.c. in the flank 14 days before testing the cytotoxicity. A group of normal, not tumor-bearing mice, was also examined.

(LAK), results in the generation of cytotoxic cells which can mediate and/or ehance tumor regression (Mulè et al., 1984; Mule'et al., 1985). Despite the wide usage of IL-2 in cancer treatment, which has sometimes had encouraging results, it is limited by marked side effects since the therapeutical blood levels of IL-2 are very toxic and poorly tolerated. As a consequence a number of attempts have been made to overcome this problem. It has been demonstrated that thymosin α 1 can upregulate the expression of high affinity IL-2 receptors in mitogen-stimulated human PBL or LGL and enhance IL-2 production (Serrate et al., 1987). Moreover, we have recently observed that in vitro or in vivo pretreatment with Tα1 potentiates IL-2 induced cytotoxic activity of spleen cells from normal mice and tumor or CY suppressed mice. Enhanced cytotoxic activity was directed against both NK sensitive YAC-1 cells and NK resistant MBL-2 cells, thus indicating a LAK-type phenomenon (Mastino et al., 1991). One possible explanation of these results could be the effect of Tα1 on the maturation of less differentiated non-cytolytic and/or IL-2-low-responsive progenitor cells. These cells may be stimulated by Tα1 to have a higher affinity for IL2 , resulting in increased cytotoxic activity after exposure to IL-2. In fact, results previously obtained by our group in bone marrow chimera experiments, suggest that Tα1 can influence the in vivo process of maturation of bone marrow progenitor cells to cytolytic effectors (Favalli et al., 1985).

We have, thus, studied the effect of the in vivo administration of an immunotherapeutic protocol with THs and IL-2, on the cytotoxic activities of 3LL tumor-bearing mice, with or without chemotherapy treatment. The results show that a combination treatment with Tα1 (200 µg/Kg) for four days, starting ten days after tumor inoculation and followed by human recombinant IL-2 (3x 50.000 U./mouse/day) for four days more, caused an evident increase in cytotoxic activity against both NK sensitive and NK resistant target cell lines. A similar

Table 3. Effects of in vivo administration of Tα1 and
human recombinant IL-2 on cytotoxic activity
in 3LL bearing mice.

Mean LU 10/Spleen (Mean+S.D.- Mean-S.D.)

Group[a]	TARGET: YAC-1	TARGET: MBL-2
Untreated	208.0 (266.5-163.8)	0.3 (18.5-<0.01)
Tα1	220.2 (266.2-183.0)	5.9 (29.6- 1.2)
IL2	340.4 (369.8-312.2)	108.5 (193.0- 61.6)
Tα1+IL2	719.6 (938.0-386.4)	532.0 (730.8-386.4)
CY	110.2 (130.0- 93.6)	1.1 (24.4- 0.4)
CY+Tα1	131.5 (139.3- 91.6)	9.5 (31.5- 2.7)
CY+IL2	187.4 (231.1-152.3)	28.6 (63.7- 13.0)
CY+Tα1+IL2	429.8 (486.6-379.3)	349.2 (522.6-233.2)

a 3LL ($2x10^5$ viable cells) was inoculated s.c. in
the flank 18 days before testing the cytotoxicity

effect was observed in CY (200 mg/Kg, single injection, on day 8 after tumor inoculation) treated mice (Table 3). Our results clearly show how a treatment with Tα1 and IL-2 <u>in vivo</u> can exert a powerful and impressive synergistic action on cytotoxic functions of immune cells.

Since IL-2 induced killer cells play a critical role in the defence against tumors, the above described results could provide an additional rationale for the novel use of Tα1 in combination with IL-2 <u>in vivo</u> in cancer treatment. Consequently we have performed experiments on the effects of Tα1 and IL-2, singularly or in combination of the two, directly on the tumorous growth of 3LL tumor. Moreover, considering the fact that it was demonstrated how chemotherapy could synergize with IL-2 and that our results demonstrate that Tα1 plus IL-2 act synergistically in CY-treated 3LL bearing mice, we have also evaluated the effect of Tα1 and IL-2 in tumor- bearing mice treated with CY.

Mice of different experiments were inoculated with 2×10^5 viable 3LL cells in 0.1 ml of HBSS subcutaneously in the right flank. Tumors were measured daily bidimensionally using caliper and survival time was controlled. Eight days after tumor inoculation, the mice were randomized, divided into different experimental groups which received or did not receive CY (200 mg/Kg in single injection on day 8 after tumor inoculation) and treated with: a) control diluent; b) Tα1 i.p. 200 μg/Kg for four days starting on day 10 after tumor inoculation: c) IL-2 150.000 I.U./day fractioned in three injections i.p. for four days starting on days 14; d) the same treatment as group b followed by treatment of group c, 24 hours after the last injection of Tα1.

The results of these experiments showed that combined immunotherapy treatment with Tα1 and IL2 can significantly slow the tumor growth and prolong survival time, with reference to non-treated controlled animals and to those which had been inoculated with the single substances. The effect is even more evident if one combines immunotherapy with CY-treatment. On the other hand,

Table 4. Effects of <u>in vivo</u> administration of Tα1 and human recombinant interleukin 2 (hrIL2) in combination with cyclophosphamide (CY) on survival time in 3LL bearing mice.

Group[a]	% mortality[b]
Untreated	100
CY	85
CY+Tα1	70
CY+hrIL2	65
CY+Tα1+hrIL2	0

a C57BL/6NcrlBR mice were challenged with 2×10^5 3LL viable cells s.c. Mice were then divided into experimental groups (20 animals each) and treated as described in the text.

b Mortality was calculated on day 90 after tumor inoculation. All surviving mice were tumor-free.

the combined immunotherapy treatment alone did not alter, in these experiments, the long-term survival of mice, while when immunotherapy was associated to CY-treatment, tumor disappearance in 100% of mice and long-term survival in all treated mice was observed (table 4)

CONCLUSIONS

Given the complexity of the immune response and the abnormalities induced in the host both by the presence of the tumor and by the therapies, it is not surprising that immunotherapy of tumors has not been very succesful. Attempts to exploit antitumoral immunotherapy will in the near future be concentrated either on phenotypic and functional study of the involved immune cells or on a deeper understanding of the complex network of intercellular messages that immunocompetent cells exchange through cytokines. This will enable us to fully exploit the potentialities of these substances, through the development of protocols of experimental and clinical models of immunotherapy. In this direction it could be reasonably be expected that combinations of different cytokines could provide better therapeutical potentialities.

The results of our studies have demonstrated that pretreatment with thymic hormones restored the IFN boosting activity in tumor, chemotherapy suppressed mice, in which none of the single agents alone was active. Furthermore, in subsequent study we proved that Thymosin α1 was able to increase the stimulating effect of IL-2 on lymphoid cells. Finally, we have now demonstrated that Tα 1, given in combination with IFN or IL-2 strikingly potentiates chemotherapy in curing 3LL tumor bearing mice. These experimental models are easily transferable to clinic practice since particular side effects are not alike to be forseen as, on the other hand, the results of a pilot study we are carrying out on man, are demonstrating.

REFERENCES

Bunn, P.A., Ihde, C.D., and Foon, K.A., 1986, The role of recombinant interferon alfa-2a., Cancer, 57: 1689.

Favalli, C., Jezzi, T., Mastino, A., Rinaldi-Garaci, C., Riccardi, C., and Garaci, E., 1985, Modulation of natural killer activity by thymosin alpha 1 and interferon., Cancer Immunol. Immunother., 20: 189.

Favalli, C., Mastino, A., Jezzi, T., Grelli, S., Goldstein, A.L., and Garaci, E., 1989, Synergic effect of thymosin alpha 1 and alpha-beta interferon on NK activity in tumor-bearing mice. Int. J. Immunopharm., 11: 443.

Garaci, E., Mastino, A., Jezzi, T., and Favalli, C., 1988, Thymic hormones and cytokines: a synergystic combination with high therapeutic potentialities, in "Recent advances in autoimmunity and tumor immunology", F. Dammacco ed., Edi-Ermes, Milano.

Garaci, E., Mastino, A., Favalli, C., 1989, Enhanced immune response and antitumor immunity with combinations of biological response modifiers., Bull. N.Y. Acad. Med., 65:111.

Garaci, E., Mastino, A., Pica, F., and Favalli, C., 1990, Combination treatment using Thymosin α 1 and interferon after cyclophosphamide is able to cure Lewis lung carcinoma in mice., Cancer Immunol. Immunother., 32: 154.

Goldstein, A.L., and Schulof, R.S., 1984, Thymosins in the treatment of cancer, in "Immunity to cancer", A.E., Reif, and M.S., Mitchell, ed., Acad.Press Inc., Orlando.

Goldstein, A.L., Low, T.L., Adoo, M., Mc Clure, J., Thurman, G.B., Rossio, G., Lay, C.Y., Chang, D., Wang, S.S., Harwey, C., Ramel, A. H., and Meienhofer, J., 1977, Thymosin alpha 1: isolation and sequence analysis of an immunologically active thymic polypeptide., Proc. Natl. Acad. Sci., 74: 725.

Hadden, J.W., 1988, New strategies of immunotherapy, in" Advances in immunomodulation", Ed. by B., Bizzini and E., Bonmassar ed., Pitagora Press, Roma.

Hooper, J.A., McDaniel, M.C., Thurman, G.B., Cohen, G.H., Schulof, R.S., and A.L., Goldstein., 1975, Purification and properties of bovine thymosin., Ann. N.Y. Acad. Sci., 249:125.

Huang, K.Y., Kind, P.D., Jagoda, E.M., and A.L., Goldstein, 1981, Thymosin treatment modulates production of interferon. J. Interferon Res., 1: 411.

Jaffe, H.S., Herberman, R.B., 1988, Rationale for recombinant human interferon-gamma adjuvant immunotherapy for cancer., J. Natl. Cancer Inst., 80: 616.

Killion, J.J., and Fidler, I.J., 1990, Evasion of host responses in metastasis: implications of cellular resistance to cytokines. Current Opinion in Immunology, 2: 693.

Lotze, M.T., Frana, L.W., Sharrow, S.O., Robb, R.J., and Rosenberg, S.A., 1985, In vivo administration of purified human interleukin-2. I. Half life and immunological effects of Jurkat cell-line derived interleukin-2., J. Immunol., 134: 157.

Lotze, M.T., Marory, Y.L., Ettinghausen, S.E., Rayner, A.A., Sharrow, S.O., Seipp, C.A.Y., Custer, M.C., and Rosenberg S.A., 1985, In vivo administration of purified human interleukin-2. II.Half life immunologic effects and expansion of peripheral lymphoid cells in vivo with recombinant IL-2., J. Immunol., 135: 2865.

Mastino, A., Favalli, C., Grelli, S., Innocenti, F., and Garaci, E., 1991, Thymosin α 1 potentiates interleukin induced cytotoxic activity in mice. Cell. Immunol., 131: 196.

Mule', J.J., Shu, S., Schwarz, S.L., and Rosenberg, S.A., 1984, Adoptive immunotherapy of established pulmonary metastases with LAK cells and recombinant interleukin-2., Science, 225: 1487.

Mule', J.J., Shu, S., and Rosenberg, S.A., 1985, The anti tumor efficacy of lymphokine-activated killer cells and recombinant interleukin-2 in vivo., J. Immunol., 135: 646.

Rosenberg, S.A., Grimm, E.A., Mcgrogan, M., Doyle, M., Kawasaki, E., and Mark, D.F., 1984, Biochemical activity of recombinant human interleukin 2 produced in Escherichia Coli., Science, 223: 1412.

Svedersky, L.P., Hui, A., May, L., McKay, P., and Stebbing, N., 1982, Induction and augmentation of mitogen-induced immune interferon production in human peripheral blood lymphocytes by α-desacetyl thymosin α1. Eur. J. Immunol., 12: 244.

MECHANISMS OF COMBINED IL-1/IL-2 AND IL-1/IFN THERAPY IN MICE INJECTED WITH METASTATIC TUMOR CELLS

F. Belardelli*, L. Gabriele*, E. Proietti*,
U. Testa**, C. Peschle** and I. Gresser***

* Dept. of Virology and ** Dept. of Hematology and
Oncology, Istituto Superiore di Sanità, 00161 Rome,
Italy; *** Lab. of Viral Oncology, I.R.S.C.,
Villejuif, France

INTRODUCTION

Several studies have recently shown that the combined treatment of tumor-bearing animals with multiple cytokines results in a more potent antitumor effect than single cytokine therapy (1-9).

In past studies we used mice transplanted with highly metastatic Friend leukemia cells (FLC) to investigate the antitumor effects of interferon (IFN)-α/β (10-12), tumor necrosis factor (TNF) α (13,14), IL-1β (15) and IL-2 (8). Peritumoral injections of IL-2, alone or in combination with LAK cells, did not inhibit the development of spleen or liver metastases, although some inhibition of the primary s.c. FLC tumor was observed (8). In contrast, injection of IFN-α/β resulted in a clear-cut inhibition of liver and spleen metastases (11,12). IL-1 β induced a marked reduction of tumor growth and an increased survival time, as compared to control mice (8,15). In particular, we have recently observed that the combined treatment of mice transplanted with FLC with both IL-1 and Il-2 resulted in an antitumor effect greater than that observed with either cytokine alone (8,9).

In this article we provide additional evidence indicating that the combined IL-1/IL-2 treatment is highly effective not only in mice injected with FLC but also in mice transplanted with a different highly metastatic tumor cell line (i.e., ESb lymphoma cells).

We describe herein that the combined IL-1/IFN-α/β treatment of mice injected with FLC also results in a synergistic antitumor effect and in a marked inhibitory effect on the development of liver and spleen metastases.

MATERIALS AND METHODS

<u>Mice.</u> Six week-old male DBA/2 mice were obtained from Charles River (Italia Calco, Italy).

Combination Therapies, Edited by A.L. Goldstein and
E. Garaci, Plenum Press, New York, 1992

Tumor cells. IFN-α/β-resistant 3Cl-8 FLC (16) were serially passaged i.p. in syngeneic DBA/2 mice (17). ESb lymphoma cells (18) were kindly provided by Dr. V. Schirrmacher (Heidelberg, FRG).

Cytokines. Mouse IFN-α/β was prepared as described elsewhere (19). Human recombinant IL-2 (Hoffmann La Roche) was obtained through the National Cancer Institute (Dr. Michael J. Hawkins, Chief of the Investigational Drug Branch). Electrophoretically pure human r-IL-1-β was provided by Sclavo (Siena and Cassina de Pecchi, Italy), through the courtesy of Dr. D. Boraschi (Centro Ricerche Sclavo, Siena).

Antibodies to asialo GM1, CD4 and CD8 antigens. Anti-asialo GM1 rabbit antibody was purchased from WAKO Chemicals GMbH (Neuss 1, West Germany). The rat hybridoma cell mAb GK1-5 producing mAb to CD4 and the rat hybridoma cell MAb 53-6.7 producing MAb to CD8 were passaged i.p. in Balb/c nude mice. Details concerning the antibody preparations and the conditions for the in vivo experiments are described elsewhere (9).

RESULTS AND DISCUSSION

1) Combined therapy with IL-1 and IL-2

Fig. 1 shows the results of a representative experiment which illustrates the synergistic antitumor effects of IL-1/IL-2 in mice injected with FLC.

DBA/2 mice were injected s.c. with FLC and, after 6 days, were treated peritumorally with IL-1β, IL-2 or a combination of both cytokines. IL-1β induced a marked inhibition of tumor growth and a clear-cut increase in survival time. In agreement with previous findings (8), s.c. treatment with IL-2 alone resulted in a slight inhibition of tumor growth (data not shown), but no increase in the mean survival time. The concomitant treatment with both IL-1 and IL-2 resulted in a synergistic antitumor effect: 60% of the IL-1/IL-2-treated tumors regressed 3-4 weeks after tumor cell injection and a few days after treatment had been discontinued.

We have studied the host mechanisms involved in the potent antitumor effects observed in FLC-injected IL-1/IL-2 treated mice (9). The antitumor action of IL-1/IL-2 treatment was abolished or markedly reduced in mice treated with antibodies to CD4 or CD8 antigens, whereas antibodies to asialo-GM1 were ineffective (9). On day 20, a clear-cut increase in the percentage of CD4+ and CD8+ cells was observed in the spleens of cytokine-treated FLC-injected mice (Fig. 2, panel A). At this time, infiltrates of host reactive cells (i.e., lymphocytes, granulocytes and monocytes) were observed in both spleen and liver from FLC-injected mice treated with IL-1/IL-2. On day 20, spleen cells from IL-1/IL-2-treated mice exerted a potent antitumor effect as determined by Winn assay experiments. This antitumor activity was abolished by preincubation of spleen cells with anti-CD8 antibody, but not significantly by treatment with antibodies to asialo-GM1 (Fig.2, panel B).

It was interest to determine whether the combined IL-1/IL-2 treatment was also effective in mice transplanted with different metastatic tumor cells. We have then investigated the antitumor effects of IL-1 and IL-2 (alone or in combination) in mice transplanted s.c. with ESb lymphoma cells, which also metastasize to the liver and to the spleen when injected s.c. in DBA/2 mice. As shown in Fig. 3, the IL-1 treatment did not result in any significant increase in the survival time of ESb cell injected mice. In contrast, in

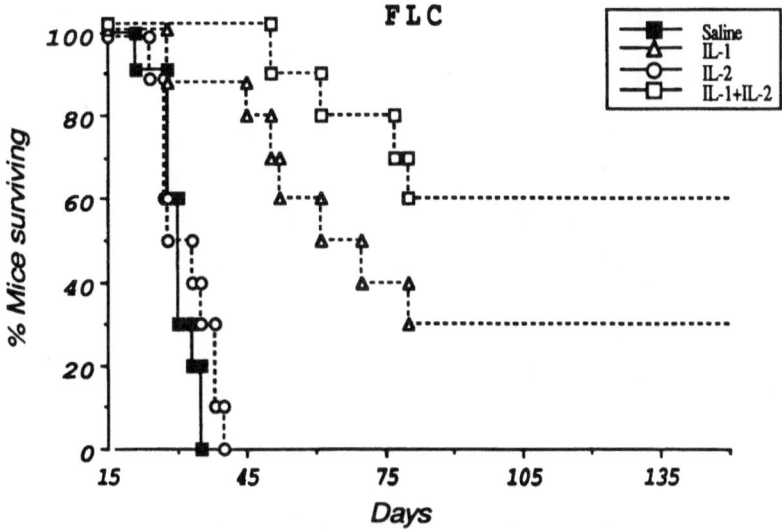

Fig. 1. <u>Antitumor effects of peritumoral injection of IL-1 β, alone or in combination with IL-2, in mice transplanted s.c. with 3Cl-8 FLC.</u>
DBA/2 mice were injected s.c. with $2x10^6$ FLC. On day 6, mice were divided into the following groups: 1) saline; 2) IL-1-β; 3) IL-2; 4) IL-1-β + IL-2.
Mice were injected peritomorally (0.2 ml per mouse, twice per day on days: 7-9;14-16;21-23. There were 10 mice for each group.
IL-1 β: 250 ng/treatment
IL-2:   20,000 U/treatment.

this tumor system, IL-2 therapy was highly effective in increasing the survival time of tumor cell injected mice and 30% of these mice were cured and did not develop liver and spleen metastases. The combined IL-1/IL-2 therapy resulted in a synergistic antitumor effect and in a complete tumor regression in 70% of the injected mice. These data emphasize that: i) the efficacy of single cytokine therapy in the same mouse host can vary with the tumor injected; ii) the combined IL-1/IL-2 therapy can result in a synergistic antitumor response not only in mice transplanted with FLC but also in mice with established metastatic ESb tumors.

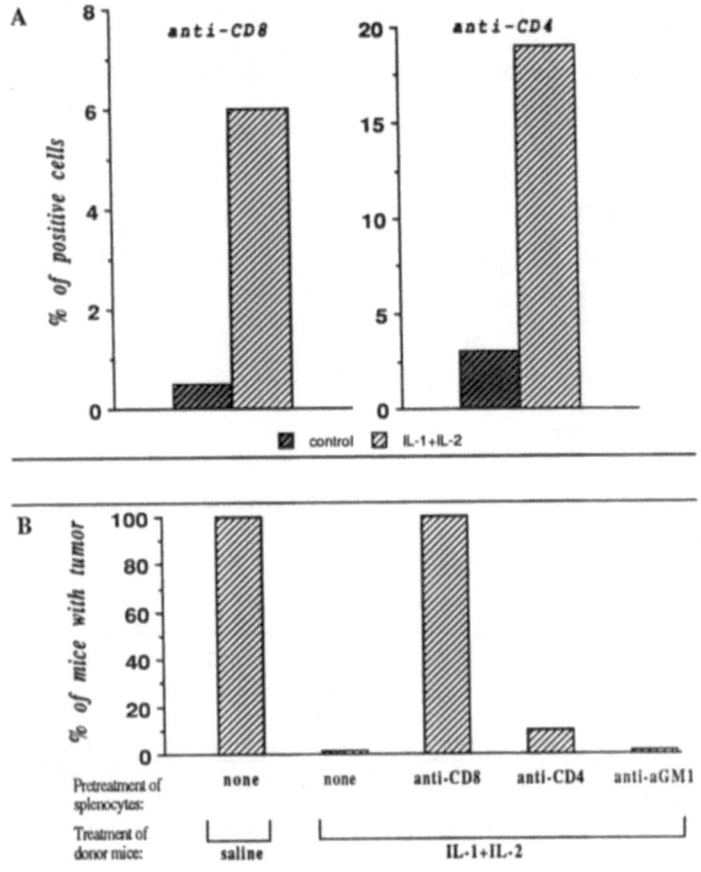

Fig. 2. Characterization of Cells endowed with antitumor activity in spleens of cytokine-treated mice.

DBA/2 mice were FLC-injected s.c. with $2x10^6$ FLC. Treatments were performed as described in the legend to Fig. 1.

Panel A: Spleen cells were recovered from FLC injected mice on day 20 and the percentage of $CD4^+$ or $CD8^+$ cells was determined by FACS analysis using fluorescein labelled monoclonal antibodies.

Panel B: On day 20, spleen cells from FLC-injected mice were preincubated for 30 min at 37°C with a suitable dilution of different antibodies. Cells were then mixed with $5x10^4$ 3Cl-8 FLC and subsequently injected s.c. in DBA/2 mice. The effector:tumor cell ratio was approximately 20:1. There were 8 mice per each group. The number of tumor-free mice in each group was determined 30 days after FLC injection.

2)   Combined therapy with IL-1 and IFN-α/β

Although repeated treatments with high doses of IFN-α/β have been shown to be highly effective in inhibiting the development of liver and spleen metastases in mice injected with FLC, it seemed of interest to determine whether the combined treatment of relatively low doses of IL-1 and IFN could result in any synergistic antitumor effect in FLC injected mice.

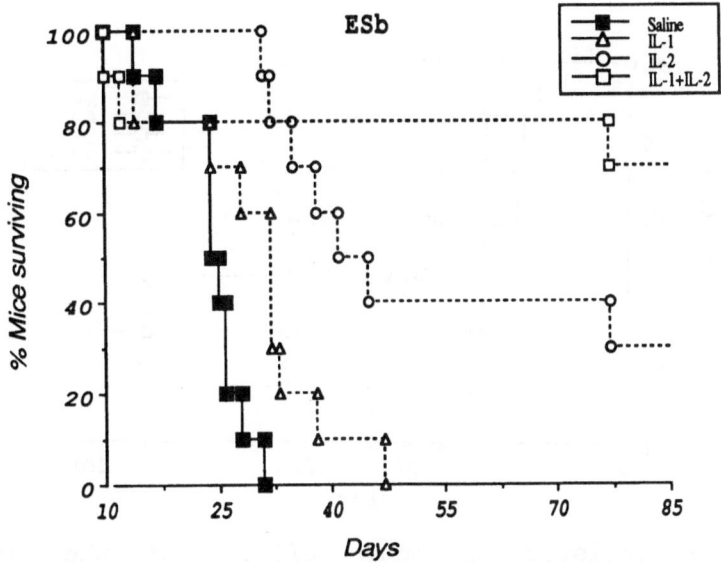

Fig. 3. <u>Antitumor effects of peritumoral injection of IL-1-β, alone or in association with IL-2, in mice injected with ESb tumor cells</u>

DBA/2 mice were injected s.c. with 10^6 ESb lymphoma cells. 5 days after tumor cell injection, mice were treated peritumorally with cytokines as described in the legend to Fig. 1 (two injections per day) on days 5-7;12-14;19 and 20. There were 10 mice/group. Dose of cytokines administered was the same as in the legend to Figure 1.

As shown in Fig. 4, a synergistic antitumor effect was observed in mice injected with both IL-1 and IFN-α/β as compared to single cytokine therapy. The antitumor action of IL-1/IFN was markedly reduced in mice treated with antibodies to CD4 antigens. This finding suggests that T cells, particularly T helper lymphocytes, are involved in the generation of the IL-1/IFN-induced antitumor response. CD4+ cells have also been shown to play a crucial role in the antitumor response in FLC injected mice treated with IL-1/IL-2 (9) or IFN-α/β (20).

NK cells also seem to participate, to some extent, to the antitumor respone in IL-1/IFN-treated FLC-injected mice, as the injection of antibody to asialo-GM1 partially inhibited the antitumor effect of the cytokine treatment; likewise, the combined IL-1/IFN treatment was less effective in NK-deficient bg/bg DBA/2 mice than in control bg/+ mice (data not shown). In this regard, it is worth mentioning that our previous studies on FLC injected mice suggested that NK cells were involved in the antitumor response in IFN-treated (20), but not in IL-1/IL-2-treated (9), animals.

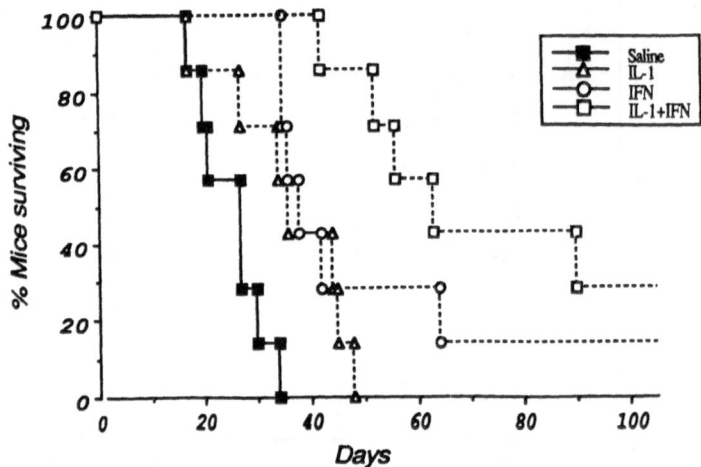

Fig. 4. <u>Synergistic antitumor effects of the combined IL-1/IFN-β treatment in mice injected s.c. with FLC.</u> DBA/2 mice were injected s.c. with 2×10^6 3Cl-8 FLC. Mice were treated peritumorally (0.2 ml per mouse, twice a day) on days: 2-4;7-9;14-16;20-22 (10 mice per group). IL-1 β: 125 ng/treatment; IFN-α/β: 20,000 U/treatment. Surviving mice were sacrificed 135 days after FLC injection and were found to be tumor-free.

Little information is available on the antitumor effects of IL-1 in mice (8,9,15,21-24). In the light of our data, it seems to us that the possible use of IL-1 as an antitumor agent, possibly in combination with other cytokines, should deserve further investigation in different experimental tumor systems.

Lastly we emphasize that the results presented in this article indicate that IFN-α/β or IL-2 can be successfully combined with suitable doses of IL-1-ß to achieve a synergistic antitumor and antimetastatic effect by activating multiple host immune mechanisms. These data suggest that similar combined cytokine therapies may represent an interesting approach to the treatment of some metastatic human cancers.

ACKNOWLEDGEMENTS

This study was supported in part by the "Progetto Italia-USA Terapia dei Tumori", the "Associazione Italiana per la Ricerca sul Cancro" and E.E.C. (SC1-0234-C).

REFERENCES

1. S. Silagi, R. Dutkowski, and A. Schaefer, Eradication of mouse melanoma by combined treatment with recombinant human interleukin 2 and recombinant murine interferon-gamma, Int. J. Cancer., 41:315 (1988).

2. J. K. McIntosh, J. J. Mulé, M. J. Merino, and S. A. Rosenberg, Synergistic antitumor effects of immunotherapy with recombinant interleukin-2 and recombinant tumor necrosis factor-alpha, Cancer Res., 48:4011 (1988).

3. M. J. Brunda, D. Bellantoni, and V. Sulich, In vivo anti-tumor activity of combinations of interferon alpha and interleukin-2 in a murine model. Correlation of efficacy with the induction of cytotoxic cells resembling natural killer cells, Int. J. Cancer., 40:365 (1987).

4. J. L. Winkelhake, S. Stampfl, and R. J. Zimmerman, Synergistic effects of combination therapy with human recombinant interleukin-2 and tumor necrosis factor in murine tumor models, Cancer Res., 47:3948 (1987).

5. J. K. McIntosh, J. J. Mulè, J. A. Krosnick, and S. A. Rosenberg, Combination cytokine immunotherapy with tumor necrosis factor alpha, interleukin 2, and alpha-interferon and its synergistic antitumor effects in mice, Cancer Res., 49:1408 (1989).

6. M. Iigo, M. Sakurai, T. Tamura, N. Saijo, and A. Hoshi, In vivo antitumor activity of multiple injections of recombinant interleukin 2, alone and in combination with three different types of recombinant interferon on various syngeneic murine tumors, Cancer Res., 48:260 (1988).

7. S. A. Rosenberg, S. L. Schwarz, and P. J. Spiess, Combination immunotherapy for cancer: synergistic antitumor interactions of interleukin-2, alpha interferon, and tumor-infiltrating lymphocytes, J. Natl. Cancer Inst., 80:1393 (1988).

8. F. Belardelli, V. Ciolli, U. Testa, E. Montesoro, D. Bulgarini, E. Proietti, P. Borghi, P. Sestili, C. Locardi, C. Peschle, and I. Gresser, Antitumor effects of interleukin-2 and interleukin-1 in mice transplanted with different syngeneic tumors, Int. J. Cancer, 44:1108 (1989).

9. V. Ciolli, L. Gabriele, P. Sestili, F. Varano, E. Proietti, I. Gresser, U. Testa, E. Montesoro, D. Bulgarini, G. Mariani, C. Peschle, F. Belardelli, Host antitumor mechanisms in the combined IL-1/IL-2 therapy in mice injected with highly metastatic Friend leukemia cells. Effects on established metastases, J. Exp. Med., 173:313 (1991).

10. F. Belardelli, I. Gresser, C. Maury, and M. T. Maunoury, Antitumor effects of interferon in mice injected with interferon-sensitive and interferon-resistant Friend leukemia cells. I, Int. J. Cancer., 30:813 (1982).

11. F. Belardelli, I. Gresser, C. Maury, P. Duvillard, M. Prade, and M. T. Maunoury, Antitumor effects of interferon in mice injected with interferon-sensitive and interferon-resistant Friend leukemia cells. III. Inhibition of growth and necrosis of tumors implanted subcutaneously, Int. J. Cancer, 31:649 (1983).

12. I. Gresser, C. Maury, D. Woodrow, J. Moss, M. G. Grutter, F. Vignaux, F. Belardelli, and M. T. Maunoury, Interferon treatment markedly inhibits the development of tumor metastases in the liver and spleen and increases survival time of mice after intravenous inoculation of Friend erythroleukemia cells, Int. J. Cancer, 41:135 (1988).

13. I. Gresser, F. Belardelli, J. Tavernier, W. Fiers, F. Podo, M. Federico, G. Carpinelli, P. Duvillard, M. Prade, C. Maury, M. T. Bandu, and M. T. Maunoury, Antitumor effects of interferon in mice injected with interferon-sensitive and interferon-resistant Friend leukemia cells. V. Comparison with the action of tumor necrosis factor, Int. J. Cancer, 38:771 (1986).

14. E. Proietti, F. Belardelli, G. Carpinelli, M. Di Vito, D. Woodrow, J. Moss, P. Sestili, W. Fiers, I. Gresser, and F. Podo, Tumor necrosis factor alpha induces early morphologic and metabolic alterations in Friend leukemia cell tumors and fibrosarcomas in mice, Int. J. Cancer, 42:582 (1988).

15. F. Belardelli, E. Proietti, V. Ciolli, P. Sestili, G. Carpinelli, M. Di Vito, A. Ferretti, D. Woodrow, D. Boraschi, and F. Podo, Interleukin-1β induces tumor necrosis and early morphologic and metabolic changes in transplantable mouse tumors. Similarities with the antitumor effects of tumor necrosis factor α or β, Int. J. Cancer, 44:116 (1989).

16. E. Affabris, C. Jemma, and G.B. Rossi, Isolation of interferon-resistant variants of Friend

erythroleukemia cells: effect of interferon and ouabain, Virology, 120:441 (1982).

17. F. Belardelli, M. Ferrantini, C. Maury, L. Santurbano, and I. Gresser, On the biologic and biochemical differences between in vitro and in vivo passaged Friend Erythroleukemia Cells I. Tumorigenicity and capacity to metastasize, Int. J. Cancer, 34:389 (1984).

18. K. Bosslet and V. Schirrmacher, High-frequency generation of new immunoresistant tumor variants during metastasis of a cloned murine tumor line (ESb), Int. J. Cancer, 29:195 (1982).

19. M. G. Tovey, J. Begon-Lours, I. Gresser, A method for the large-scale production of potent interferon preparations, Proc. Soc. Exp. Biol. Med., 146:809 (1974).

20. I. Gresser, C. Maury, C. Carnaud, E. De Maeyer, M. T. Maunoury, and F. Belardelli, Antitumor effects of Interferon in mice injected with Interferon-sensitive and Interferon-resistant Friend Erythroleukemia Cells. VIII. Role of the immune system in the inhibition of visceral metastases, Int. J. Cancer, 46:468 (1990).

21. P. G. Braunschweiger, C.S. Johnson, N. Kumar, V. Ord, and P. Furmanski, Antitumor effects of recombinant human interleukin 1β in RIF-1 and Panc02 solid tumors, Cancer Res., 48:6011 (1988).

22. S. Nakamura, K. Nakata, S. Kashimoto, H. Yoshida, and M. Yamada, Antitumor effect of recombinant human interleukin 1 alpha against murine syngeneic tumors, Jpn. J. Cancer Res. (Gann), 77:767 (1986).

23. R. J. North, R.H. Neubauer, J.J.H. Huang, R.C. Newton, and S.E. Loveless, Interleukin 1-induced, T cell-mediated regression of immunogenic murine tumors. Requirement for an adequate level of already acquired host concomitant immunity, J. Exp. Med., 168:2031 (1988).

24. M. A. Palladino, M. R. Shalaby, S. M. Kramer, B. L. Ferraiolo, R. A. Baughman, A. B. Deleo, D. Crase, B. Marafino, B. B. Aggarwal, I. S. Figari, D. Liggitt, and J. S. Patton, Characterization of the antitumor activities of human tumor necrosis factor-α and the comparison with other cytokines: induction of tumor specific immunity, J. Immunol., 138:4023 (1987).

CANCER IMMUNOTHERAPY: PRECLINICAL STUDIES WITH TRIAZENE

COMPOUNDS

L.[a],D'Tentori S.[a],Atri A.[a],Giuliani P.[b], Puccetti M.C.[b], Fioretti V.[a], Nistico' O.[c], Marelli B.[a], Bulgarini E.[a]. Bonmassar

(a) Dept.Exp.Med.Bioch.Sci., II Univ. Rome,Italy
(b) Inst. Pharm. Univ. Perugia, Italy
(c) Dept. Pharm. Univ. Milan, Italy

INTRODUCTION

A large body of evidence is now available showing that antigen-dependent immunity (ADI) and/or natural immunity (NI) can be engaged during the growth of neoplasms in their autochtonous host. However the reasons whereby the reactivity of the immune apparatus does not result in effective control of malignant growth are still largely hypotetical. Poor immunogenicity of cancer cells (1,2), suppression of antitumor responses by humoral or cellular components of the immune system (3-5), low reactivity of the host due to acquired or genetic factors, antigen modulation of tumor associated antigens (TAA), suppression of immunity by factors released from the tumor itself (6-8), and stimulation of tumor growth by immunological responses (7), have all been considered to play a role in host's unresponsiveness to a growing tumor.

One of the major goals of tumor immunology is the development of experimental procedures capable of enhancing host's control of cancer growth and progression. Several methods have been explored, including non-specific immunostimulation with a variety of biological or synthetic products (9), adoptive inmmunotherapy with specifically sensitized cytotoxic lymphocytes (10) or transfer of non-specific in vitro IL-2 activated killer lymphocytes (11).

It is conceivable that the high genetic instability of cancer cells would result in the generation of non-immunogenic and scarcely antigenic clones resistant to either ADI or NI.

Various approaches aimed at obtaining an increase of tumor-cell immunogenicity and/or conferring novel antigenic specificities have been described, e.g. as treatment with membrane-modifying enzymes (12), or haptenization with different chemicals (13). Moreover it has been suggested that antineoplastic agents could produce modifications of the antigenic profile of normal or cancer cells through various mechanisms, e.g. direct changes of the antigenic determinants, including the participation of the drug itself as a hapten, modifications of protein synthesis through direct or indirect manipulation of the genetic code (e.g. drug induced mutations or viral activation), or at transcriptional or assembling level. In other words, it could be hypothesized that, in addition to direct killing of the malignant elements, anticancer agents in non-lethal concentrations could also lead to modifications in the tumor-cell membrane composition and/or architecture resulting in modified and increased immunogenicity or antigenicity.

In 1970 we obtained the first evidence that in vivo treatment of CD2F1 mice, bearing fully histocompatible L1210 leukemia, with 5-(3-3-dimethyl-1-triazeno)-imidazole-4-carboxamide (DTIC), results in the appearance of strong and heritable transplantation antigen(s) (hereafter called drug-mediated transplantation antigen, DMTA) associated with leukemia cells following 4-6 transplant generations of treatment (14). This antitumor drug is known to be highly mutagenic, being a monomethylating agent capable of producing large amounts of O^6-methylguanine DNA adducts responsible for GC-AT transition (15) in essentially all tumor cells.

The finding that strong DMTA can be induced in vivo by drug treatment of tumor-bearing hosts appeared to open up new approaches to cancer control with immunological means. Therefore a number of investigations were carried out on DTIC-mediated induction of DMTA, a phenomenon that was called "chemical xenogenization" (CX,16). The results of these studies can be summarized as follows: a) the strenght of DTIC-induced DMTA is similar to that of alloantigens associated with H-2 incompatible tumors (17); b) DTIC-mediated CX can be obtained in a large variety of mouse lymphoma cells (18-20) and B16 melanoma (21); c) novel DMTA not detectable in the tumor of origin, are associated with DTIC-treated lymphomas, as evidenced by cell-mediated cytotoxicity (22-23), specific tolerance induction (24) and humoral antibody responses (25-26); d) tumor cell antigenicity originated from DTIC-mediated CX is not associated with drug resistance and is not the result of drug-mediated selection; e) CX induced by DTIC appears to be of somatic mutation origin. This is supported by the biochemical mechanism of action of DTIC as monomethylating agent (15), by the observation that Quinacrine, an antimutagenic compound, inhibits specifically CX (27) and by the finding that DTIC-treated tumors contain different clones expressing distinct DMTA (28); f) CX can be induced in vivo by triazenyl compounds not containing the imidazole moiety, but derived from aromatic compounds (29). Therefore CX seems to be selectively dependent on the triazenyl group; g) human tumor cells treated with a triazenyl compound in vitro undergo changes in the susceptibility to NK-mediated cytotoxicity, and presumably possess a limited amount of DMTA (30); h) DTIC is highly immunodepressant in mice (17,31,32) and abrogates host's graft responses against DTIC-induced DMTA of cancer cells. However the transfer of syngeneic mononucleated cells after DTIC treatment restores immune responsiveness in cyclophosphamide-conditioned recipients and allows CX exploitation for successful tumor immuno-chemotherapy in mice (33).

The use of mutagenic agents to increase tumor cell immunogenicity has been investigated in other laboratories, starting from 1975. In particular Boon (34) was able to isolate a large number highly immunogenic clones from mouse teratocarcinoma exposed in vitro to the mutagen N-methyl-N'-nitro-N-nitrosoguanidine (MNNG). Immunogenic sublines (i.e. "tum⁻" variants) are rejected by intact hosts unless immunodepressed with various modalities, and leave recipient mice resistant to a subsequent challenge with the scarcely immunogenic parental tumor (34). Similar results were obtained with Lewis lung carcinoma, P815 mastocytoma and various spontaneous carcinomas and leukemias in mice (34). Of particular interest appears the more recent observation of Wolfel et al.(35) who were able to transfect gene(s) coding for DMTA of "tum⁻" variants, recognized by specific cytolytic T lymphocytes.

Biochemical studies on mouse lymphoma cells exposed to MNNG, showed the appearance of new membrane proteins in immunogenic clones, not detectable in the line of origin (36). In this case the authors claim that the antigenicity was of epigenetic and not of genetic origin. However the unusually long survival times of mice challenged with the parental lymphoma render the results of difficult interpretation.

The results of studies performed in our laboratory pointed out that DMTA could be also involved in NI against DTIC-treated leukemic cells, detectable in lethally-irradiated (LI) histocompatible hosts (37).

Hemopoietic histocompatibility (Hh) factors expressed on normal blood-forming cells (38), lymphomas (39), and Friend virus-induced leukemias (40) may be regarded as tissue-specific alloantigens. These factors are controlled by a series of polymorphic genes, most of which are linked with the major histocompatibility complex (MHC) on chromosome 17 (38), and are capable of eliciting immunogenetically specific allograft reactions in vivo (rejection or reduced growth of transplanted cells). In vivo responses to Hh antigens are most unusual for they are not suppressed by acute total-body irradiation (38) or weakened by absence of the thymus (41), but are promptly abrogated upon administration of anti-macrophage agents (42). Moreover, Hh alleles are not codominant so that F_1 hybrid mice may lack parental Hh antigens and, hence, react against hemopoietic cells of parental strain donors (39).

It is possible that the expression of Hh genes on progenitor cells of the lympho-myeloid compartment, the recognition of Hh gene products by other cells, and the consequent anti-Hh response play an important physiologic role in the control of proliferation and differentiation of hemopoietic stem cells (43), surveillance over leukemogenesis (44), and genetic resistance to, and recovery from, Friend virus leukemia (45).

The present investigation was undertaken to explore whether normal bone marrow cells subjected to DTIC treatment in vivo would be susceptible to NI-mediated rejection in lethally-irradiated syngeneic recipients (i.e. through a Hh-like rejection mechanism). The preliminary results illustrated in the present report show that this was the case, at least for the H-2^d model described here.

MATERIALS AND METHODS

   Mice. Hybrid (BALB/cCr x DBA/2Cr)F1 (CD_2F_1, $H-2^d/H-2^d$) male mice, 8 weeks old, were obtained from Charles River Co (Calco, Como, Italy).

   Irradiation, transpantation and graft evaluation. Perspective recipient mice were exposed to total-body irradiation a few hours before cell injection (950 R, 4-6 hours before cell transplantation, in a ^{60}Co irradiator, Hot Spot, MKIV, Harwell, England).

   Bone marrow cells in suspension were injected into a lateral tail vein (0.5 ml/mouse), and graft cell proliferation was assessed 5 day later in spleens of irradiated recipients by a radioisotope uptake method. At the time of evaluation each mouse was injected ip with 25 ug/mouse of 5-fluoro-2'-deoxyuridine to decrease the availability of endogenous thymidine, followed by 0,5 uCi of the DNA precursor 5-iodo-2'-deoxyuridine labeled with ^{125}I (^{125}IUdR). Retention of ^{125}IUdR by donor-derived dividing cells in recipient spleens was measured in a crystal scintillation counter (Packard model 5110) and was expressed as percentage of injected radioactivity.

RESULTS AND DISCUSSION

   Donor CD2F1 mice were treated with DTIC (100 mg/Kg/day ip, day 1-5). Five days after the last DTIC injection, bone marrow (BM) cells were collected from femurs of DTIC-treated (i.e. BM/DTIC) or control untreated (i.e. BM/C) donors.

   Graded numbers of BM/C or BM/DTIC cells were injected iv into 2 groups of lethally-irradiated syngeneic hosts, non-pretreated (i.e. with intact Hh-type responses) or pretreated with cyclophosphamide [Cy, 200 mg/kg ip on day -5 before BM transplantation, depressed for Hh-type responses (46)].

   The results illustrated in the table show that : (a) marginal ^{125}UdR uptake occurred in the spleens of "radiation controls" not grafted with BM cells, non-pretreated or pretreated with Cy (i.e. groups 1 and 2); (b) BM/C proliferation was much higher than that of BM/DTIC in intact LI recipients (i.e. group 3 vs 7 and 5 vs 9); (c) no significant difference in BM cells proliferation was found in the spleens of LI recipients, intact or pretreated with Cy when inoculated with normal BM/C (i.e. groups 3 vs 4 and 5 vs 6); (d) BM/DTIC cells proliferation was much higher in the spleens of Cy-pretreated LI mice than in the spleens of non-pretreated LI controls (i.e. groups 7 vs 8 and 9 vs 10).

   Therefore it can be suggested that BM cells obtained from DTIC-treated animals can be rejected by LI syngeneic hosts. These results are consistent with the hypothesis that BM cells exposed to DTIC in vivo become somehow susceptible to Hh-type, NI-mediated suppression in LI host, since they grew better in mice with Hh reactivity impaired by Cy pretreatment. These findings could be the result of: (a) DTIC-mediated induction of novel Hh-type target structures on BM cells; (b) DTIC-mediated suppression of MHC-gene products, leading to recognition of a "missing self" on BM/DTIC by LI syngeneic recipients. Actually a recent study of Bix et al (47) pointed out that BM cells of

MHC-deficient (class I) mutant donors are rejected by wild-type LI syngeneic mice. In addition 8-10 transplant generations of treatment in vivo was found to induce a decrease in Qa-2 antigen expression in BM-derived murine lymphoma cells (Marelli O. et al., in preparation) homozygous for the H-2^d haplotype.

TABLE I

Growth of CD2F1 bone-marrow cells, untreated (BM/C) or exposed in vivo to DTIC (BM/DTIC), into lethally irradiated (LI, 950 R, total body irradiation) CD2F1 mice non pretreated (NPT) or depressed for Hh-type responses with Cyclophosphamide (Cy-PT).

Group	Bone marrow cells[a]		LI CD2F1 mice[b]	% ^{125}IUdR uptake[c]			
n.	type	number		n.obs.	Mean (SE)	P_1	P_2
1	–	None	NPT	6	0.017±0.002	–	–
2	–	None	Cy-PT	6	0.036±0.019	NS	–
3	BM/C	10^6	NPT	8	0.37 ±0.04	–	–
4	BM/C	10^6	Cy-PT	7	0.50 ±0.06	NS	–
5	BM/C	2 x 10^6	NPT	8	0.85 ±0.06	–	–
6	BM/C	2 x 10^6	Cy-PT	6	0.94 ±0.10	NS	–
7	BM/DTIC	10^6	NPT	6	0.009±0.02	–	<0.001
8	BM/DTIC	10^6	Cy-PT	6	0.17 ±0.05	<0.01	–
9	BM/DTIC	2 x 10^6	NPT	5	0.08 ±0.03	–	<0.001
10	BM/DTIC	2 x 10^6	Cy-PT	6	0.47 ±0.06	<0.001	–

a) BM/DTIC, BM cells collected from CD2F1 mice (treated with DTIC 100 mg/kg/day, day 1-5) on day 10.
b) Cy-PT, CD2F1 mice pretreated with Cy (200 mg/kg ip on day -5 before BM injection).
c) P1, probability calculated according to Student's "t" test analysis, comparing ^{125}IUdR uptake values relative to NPT vs Cy-PT groups.
   P2, probability calculated comparing ^{125}IUdR uptake values relative to NPT hosts inoculated with BM/C cells vs those injected with the same number of BM/DTIC cells (i.e. group 3 vs 7, and group 5 vs 9).

In conclusion the results of the present and previous studies suggest that Hh-type responses can be detected against DTIC-treated BM or lymphoma cells in syngeneic mice. Whether triazene compounds could alter MHC gene products leading to increased susceptibility of normal or tumor cells to NI in vivo remains to be demonstrated. Studies are in progress to elucidate the effects of triazenes on MHC antigenic make up of normal or neoplastic hematopoietic cells in the mouse.

ACKNOWLEDGEMENTS

This work has been supported by Italy-U.S.A. Program on

Therapy of Neoplasias (Legge 531, 29/12/87). The authors wish to thank Ms. Alessia De Vincenzi for her expert assistance with the preparation of this manuscript.

REFERENCES

1. Galili N., Devens B., Becker S., Klein E.: Immune responses to weakly immunogenic virally-induced tumors.I. Overcoming low responsiveness by priming mice with synergic in vitro tumor line or allogenic cross-reactive tumor.
   Eur. J. Immunol. 8:17 (1978).
2. Hewitt H.B.: The choice of animal tumors for experimental studies of cancer therapy.
   Adv. Cancer Res. 27:149 (1978).
3. Kirchner H., Chused T.M., Herbermann R.B., Lavrin D.H.: Evidence of suppressor cell activity in speel of mice bearing primary tumors induced by Moloney sarcoma virus.
   J. Exp. Med. 139:1473 (1974).
4. Hellstrom K.E., Hellstrom I.: Lymphocyte-mediated cytotoxicity and blocking serum activity to tumor antigens.
   Adv. Immunol. 18:209 (1974).
5. Fujimoto S., Greene M.I., Sbon H.B.: Regulation of immune responses to tumor antigens.I.Immuno-suppressor cells in tumor bearing hosts.
   J. Immunol. 116:791 (1976).
6. Wong A., Mankovitz R., Kennedy J.C.: Immunosuppressive and immunostimulatory factors produced by malignant cells in vitro.
   Int. J. Cancer 13:530 (1974).
7. Prehn R.T.: Do tumors grow because of the immune response of the host?
   Transplant. Rev 28:34 (1976).
8. Favalli C., Garaci E., Santoro M.G., Santucci L., Jaffe E.M.: Effect of PGA on the immune response in B16 melanoma mice.
   Prostaglandins 19:587 (1980)
9. Hersh E.M.: Current status of immunotherapy and biological therapy of cancer. In: "Advances in Immunopharmacology, 3" Chedid L., Hadden J.V., Spreafico F., Dukor P., Willoughby D. eds. pp.47. Pergamon Press (1986).
10. Greenberg P.D., Cheever M.A., Fefer A.: Therapy of established tumors by adoptive transfer of T lymphocytes. In: "Basic and Clinical Tumor Immunology" Herberman R.B. ed. pp 301. Martinus Nijhoff Publisher, Boston (1983).
11. Rosemberg S.A.: Adoptive immunotherapy of cancer using lymphokine activated killer cells and recombinant interleukin-2.
    Important Advances in Oncology 55:91 (1986).
12. Sethi K.K., Brandis H.: Neuraminidase induced loss in the transplantability of murine leukemia L1210. Induction of immunoprotection and the transfer of induced immunity to normal DBA/2 mice by serum and peritoneal cells.
    Br. J. Cancer 27:106 (1973).

13. Nagamatsu Y.: Studies on active immunization of mice with mitomycin and toyomycin-prepared Ehrlich ascites carcinoma tissue.
    Arch. Jap. Chir. 33:753 (1964).
14. Bonmassar E., Bonmassar A., Vadlumudi S. Goldin A.: Immunological alteration of leukemic cells in vivo after treatment with an antitumor drug.
    Proc. Natl. Acad. Sci. 66:1089 (1970).
15. Catapano C.V., Broggini M., Erba E., Ponti M., Mariani L., Citti L., D'Incalci M.: In vitro and in vivo methazolastone induced DNA damage and repair in L1210 leukemia sensitive and resistant to chloroethylnitrosureas.
    Cancer Res. 47: 4884 (1987).
16. Fioretti M.C., Nardelli B. Bianchi R., Nisi C., Sava G.: Antigenic changes of a murine lymphoma by in vivo treatment with triazene derivatives.
    Cancer Immunol. Immunother 11:283 (1981).
17. Bonmassar E., Bonmassar A., Vadlumudi S., Goldin A.: Antigenic changes of L1210 leukemia in mice treated with 5-(3,3-Dimethyl-1-Triazeno)-Imidazole-4-Carboxamide.
    Cancer Res. 32:1446 (1972).
18. Bonmassar E., Testorelli C., Franco P., Goldin A., Cudkowicz G.: Changes of the immunogenic properties of a radiation-induced mouse lymphoma following treatment with antitumor drugs.
    Cancer Res. 35:1957 (1975).
19. Bonmassar A., Frati L., Fioretti M.C., Romani L., Giampietri A., Goldin A.: Changes of immunogenic properties of K36 lymphoma treated in vivo with 5-(3,3-Dimethyl-1-Triazeno)-Imidazole-4-Carboxamide (DTIC).
    Europ. J. Cancer 15:933 (1979).
20. Fioretti M.C., Romani L., Bonmassar A., Taramelli D.: Appearance of strong transplantation antigens in non-immunogenic lymphoma following drug-treatment in vivo.
    J. Immunopharm. 2:189 (1980).
21. Allegrucci M.P., Romani L., Fioretti M.C.: Reduced metastatization of chemically-xenogeneized melanoma cells as a result of increased immunogenicity.
    Int. Congress Cancer Metastasis, (Bologna-Italy, 1987), p.76.
22. Nicolin A., Bini A., Franco P., Goldin A.: Cell-mediated response to a mouse leukemic sublines antigenically altered following drug treatment in vivo.
    Cancer Chemother. Rep. 58:325 (1974).
23. Romani L., Fioretti M.C., Bonmassar E.: In vitro generation of primary cytotoxic lymphocytes against L5178Y leukemia antigenically altered by 5-(3,3'-Dimethyl-1-Triazeno)-Imidazole-4-Carboxamide in vivo.
    Transplantation, 28: 218 (1979).
24. Houchens D.P., Bonmassar E., Gaston M.R., Kende M., Goldin A.: Drug-mediated immunogenic changes of virus-induced leukemia in vivo.
    Cancer Res. 36:1347 (1976).
25. Romani L., Puccetti P., Fioretti M.C., Mage M.G.: Humoral response against murine lymphoma cells xenogenized by drug treatment in vivo.
    Int. J. Cancer 36:225 (1985).

26. Testorelli C., Archetti Y.L., Aresca P., Del Vecchio L.: Monoclonal antibodies to the L1210 murine leukemia cell line and a drug-altered subline. Cancer Res. 45:5299 (1985).

27. Giampietri A., Fioretti M.C., Goldin A., Bonmassar E.: Drug mediated antigenic changesin murine leukemia cells. Antagonistic effects of Quinacrine, an antimutagenic compound. J. Natl. Cancer Inst. 64:297 (1980).

28. Fioretti M.C., Romani L., Taramelli D. Goldin A.: Antigenic properties of lymphoma sublines derived from a drug treated immunogenic L5178Y leukemia. Transplantation 26:449 (1978).

29. Nardelli B., Contessa A.R., Romani L., Sava G., Nisi C., Fioretti M.C.: Immunogenic changes of murine lymphoma cells following in vitro treatment with aryl-triazene derivatives. Cancer Immunol. Immunother 16:157 (1984).

30. Ballerini P., D'Atri S., Franchi A., Lassiani L., Ragona G., Faggioni A., Bonmassar E., Giuliani A.: Pharmacological manipulation of membrane antigens of cancer cells. In: "Advances in Immunomodulation". B. Bizzini and E. Bonmassar Eds. Pythagora Press Roma-Milan. pp. 257 (1988).

31. Giampietri A., Bonmassar E., Goldin A.: Drug-induced modulation of immune responses in mice: effects of 5-(3,3'-Dimethyl -1-Triazeno)-Imidazole-4-Carboxamide (DTIC) and Cyclophosphamide (Cy). J. Immunopharm. 1:61 (1978).

32. Puccetti P., Giampietri A., Fioretti M.C.: Long-term depression of two primary immune responses induced by a single dose of 5-(3,3'-Dimethyl-1-Triazeno)-Imidazole-4-Carboxamide (DTIC). Experientia (Basel) 34:799 (1978).

33. Giampietri A., Bonmassar A., Puccetti P., Circolo A., Goldin A., Bonmassar E.: Drug mediated increase of tumor immunogenicity in vivo for a new approach to experimental cancer immunotherapy. Cancer Res. 41:681 (1981).

34. Boon T.: Antigenic tumor cell variants obtained with mutagens. Adv. Cancer Res. 39:121 (1983).

35. Wolfel T., Van Pel A., De Plaen E., Lurquin C., Maryanski J.L., Boon T.: Immunogenic (Tum-) variants obtained by mutagenesis of mouse mastocytoma P815. 8. Detection of stable transfectants expressing a Tum-antigen with a cytolytic T cell stimulation assay. Immunogenetics 26:178 (1987).

36. Altevogt P., Von Hoegen P., Leidig S., Schirrmacher V.: Effects of mutagens on the immunogenicity of murine tumor cells: immunological and biochemical evidence for altered cell surface antigens. Cancer Res. 45:4270 (1985).

37. Riccardi C., Fioretti M.C., Giampietri A., Puccetti P., Goldin A., Bonmassar E.: Growth inhibition of normal or drug treated lymphoma cells in lethally irradiated mice. J. Natl. Cancer Inst. 60:1083 (1978).

38. Cudkowicz G.: Genetic control of resistance to allogeneic and xenogeneic bone marrow grafts in mice. Transplant Proc. 7:155 (1975).

39. Shearer G.M., Cudkowicz G.: Inducion of F_1 hybrid antiparent cytotoxic effector cells: an in vitro model for hemopoietic histoincompatibility.
Science 190:890 (1975).

40. Cudkowicz, G., Rossi G.B., Haddad J.R., Friend C.: Hybrid resistance to parental DBA/2 grafts: independence from the H-2 locus.II. Studies with Friend virus-induced leukemia cell.
J. Natl. Cancer Inst. 48:997 (1972).

41. Cudkowicz G., Bennett M.: Peculiar immunobiology of bone marrow allografts. I. Graft rejection by irradiated responder mice.
J. Exp. Med. 134:83 (1971).

42. Lotzova E., Cudkowicz G.: Abrogation of resistance to bone marrow grafts by silica aprticles. Prevention of the silica effect by the macrophage stabilizer poly-2-vinylpyridine N-oxide.
J. Immunol. 113:798 (1974).

43. McCulloch E., Gregory C.J., Till J.E.: Cellular communication early in hemopoietic differentiation. In: "Ciba Symposium on Hemopoietic Stem Cells".
Associated Scientific Publishers, Amsterdam. p.183 (1973).

44. Rossi G.B., Cudkowicz G. Friend C.: Transformation of sleen cell three hours after infection in vivo with Friend leukemia virus.
J. Natl. Cancer Inst. 50:249 (1973).

45. Kumar V., Bennett M., Eckner R.J.: Mechanisms of genetic resistance to Friend virus leukemia in mice.
J. Exp. Med. 139:1093 (1974).

46. Houchens D.P., Iorio A., Barzi A., Goldin A., Bnmassar E.: Inhibition of antilymphoma allograft response in normal and lethally irradiated mice by cyclophosphamide (NSC 26271) and isophosphamide (NSC 109724).
Cancer Chemother. Rep. 59:967 (1975).

47. Bix M., Liao N.S., Zijlstra M., Loring J., Jaemish R., Ranlet D.: Rejection of class-I MHC-deficient haematopoietic cells by irradiated MHC in matured mice.
Nature 349:329 (1991).

INDEX

AZT, *see* Azidothymidine
AZTMPDG, 124

Bacillus Calmette-Guerin (BCG), 79, 159, 185
Bacillus Calmette-Guerin (BCG) vaccine, 59
Bacterial infections, 226, *see also* specific types
B-cell lymphoma, 114
B-cell related leukemia, 13
B cells
    aspirin and, 134, 135
    cytokines / chemotherapy and, 271
    Duplan MuLV infection and, 114, 115, 120
    Fcγ receptors and, 208
    HPV and, 237
    ST 789 and, 225
BCG, *see Bacillus Calmette-Guerin*
BCNU, 67, 270
Biological response modifiers (BRMs), 59, 73–74, 269, 275, *see also* specific types
    aspirin as, 131–136
    C. albicans used in, 159–164
1,3-Bis-(2-chloroethyl)-1-nitrosourea, *see* BCNU
Blood brain barrier, 124, 128
BMT, *see* Bone marrow transplantation
Bone marrow toxicity, *see* Myelotoxicity
Bone marrow transplantation (BMT), 13, 14–15, 159, 270–271
    allogeneic, 19, 20, 25, 189–190
    autologous, 19, 20, 21, 25
    IL-2 / LAK cells and, 19–26
Bootstrap techniques, 31
Breast cancer, 15, 52, 88, 192
BRMs, *see* Biological response modifiers

cAMP, *see* Cyclic adenosine monophosphate
Cancer, *see also* specific types; Tumors
    aspirin and, 137
    in aging population, 139, 141–144
    ST 789 and, 223–227
    T-α1 and, 150
    triazene compounds and, 293–297
Candida albicans, 97, 98–100, 101
    AmpB and, 106, 108, 109, 110
    in BRMs, 159–164
    ST 789 and, 226

Candidiasis, *see Candida albicans*
Capillary leak syndrome, 142
Carboplatin, 270
Cardiotoxicity, 61, 270
Castanospermine, 124
CCNU, 80–84
CD3 cells, 21, 23, 54, 92, 151, 153, *see also* Anti-CD3 antibodies
CD4 cells
    arginine and, 224
    aspirin and, 134, 135
    cytokines and, 167, 170
    cytokines / chemotherapy and, 271–272
    HIV-1 and, 118, 123, 128, 167, 170
    IFN / T-α1 and, 7
    IL-1 / IFN-α / β and, 287
    IL-1 / IL-2 and, 284, 286
    IL-2 and, 92
    ST 789 and, 224, 225, 227
    thymosin and, 151, 153
    TILs and, 41, 44, 46, 47
CD8 cells
    aspirin and, 135
    cytokines / chemotherapy and, 271–272
    IFN / T-α1 and, 7
    IL-1 / IL-2 and, 284, 286
    IL-2 and, 92
    IL-2 / LAK cells and, 21, 23
    melanoma vaccine and, 187
    ST 789 and, 224, 225
    thymosin and, 151, 153
    TILs and, 40, 41, 44, 46, 47
CD11 cells, 151, 153
CD25 cells, 54, 91, 92
CD56 cells, 21, 23, 41, 44, 47, 200–201
CD57 cells, 200–201
cDNA clones, of Fcγ receptors, 208–209, 210
CD4-PE40, *see* CD4-pseudomonas exotoxin
CD4-pseudomonas exotoxin (CD4-PE40), 29, 32, 33, 35
Ceftazidmine, 226
Cervical carcinoma, 237–243
CFUs, *see* Colony-forming units
Chang hepatoma, 203
Checkerboard design, 29, 31
Chemical xenogenization, 294
Chemotherapy, 14, 58, 90, 100–101, 192, 245, 275–280, *see also* specific agents

Guanosine monophosphate (GMP), 161, 225

GvHD, *see* Graft-versus-host disease

GvL, *see* Graft-versus-leukemia

Hairy cell leukemia, 74

Haptenization, 293–294

HBV, *see* Hepatitis B virus

Head and neck cancer, 241–242
    IL-2 and, 90–94

Heat shock proteins, 191

Helper cells, 41, 123, 237, 287

Hematologic toxicity, 51, 71, 82, 84

Hematopoietic supportive therapy, 192

Hemodialysis, 150

Hemopoiesis, 215

Hemopoietic histocompatibility (Hh) factors, 295, 296, 297

Hepatitis B virus (HBV), 137, 149–155

Hepatitis C virus, 152

Herpes simplex virus, 127

HGP-30-KLH vaccine, 231–235

Hh factors, *see* Hemopoietic histocompatibility factors

Histocompatibility antigens, 13, *see also* HLA antigens; Majorhistocompatibility complex antigens

Histone H2A, 253–254, 258, 264, 265

HIV-1, *see* Human immunodeficiency virus-1

HLA antigens, 14–15, 19, 54, 91, 187, *see also* Major histocompatibilitycomplex antigens

Hodgkin's disease, 22

Homeostatic thymus hormone (HTH), 264

Hormone therapy, 58

HPV, *see* Human papillomavirus

HTH, *see* Homeostatic thymus hormone

Human immunodeficiency virus-1 (HIV-1), 13, 123–128
    antisense oligodeoxynucleodides and, 123, 125–127, 167, 170
    ARC and, 118
    C. albicans and, 161–162
    COMBO program on, *see* COMBO
    cytokines and, 113, 114, 120, 167–174
    immunotherapy for, 113–120
    pediatric patients with, 124
    reverse transcriptase inhibitors and, 32, 37, 123–124, 170, 173
    vaccine for, *see* AIDS vaccine

Human papillomavirus (HPV), 237–243

Hydrocortisone, 180, 181

Hypergammaglobulinemia, 114

Hypocalcemia, 52

IFN, *see* Interferon

Ig, *see* Immunoglobulin

IL, *see* Interleukin

Imexon, 114, 116–118, 120

Imidazoles, 113, 114

Immunoglobulin G (IgG), 207, 208, 209

Immunoglobulin G (IgG2a) antibodies, 201, 202, 204

Immunoglobulin M (IgM), 115

Immunotherapy, 13–15, 59–60, *see also* specific types
    active, 59
    for HIV-1, 113–120
    for tumor destruction, 189–193
    helper approach in, 88–89
    in aging population, 139–144
    passive, 59

Imuthiol, *see* Diethyldithiocarbamate

Indomethacin, 200, 203, 204

Influenza vaccine, 134–136, 139, 141, 144

Influenza viruses, 127

Inosine monophosphate methylester, 114

Interferon (IFN), 59–60, 180, 192, 275, *see also* specific types
    aging and, 139
    C. albicans and, 161–162
    CisPt and, 80–84, 237–238, 242–243
    COMBO on, 29
    HPV and, 237–238, 242–243
    T-α1 and, 1—10, 137, 149, 154, 276–277, 280

Interferon-α (IFN-α), 2, 4, 59, 67–71
    CisPt and, 237, 242
    Fcγ receptors and, 208
    5-FU and, 73–77
    HBV and, 149, 154
    HIV-1 and, 113, 114
    HPV and, 237, 242
    IFN-γ and, 60–61
    IL-1 and, 283, 284, 287–288
    IL-2 and, 49, 51–54, 61, 93
    TILs and, 62
    TNF-α and, 283

Interferon-α2a (IFN-α2a), 73–77

Interferon-α2b (IFN-α2b), 67–71

Interferon-β (IFN-β), 2, 4
    CisPt and, 80–84, 237
    Fcγ receptors and, 208

Interferon-β (IFN-β) (*cont'd*)
    HPV and, 237
    IL-1 and, 283, 284, 287–288
    TNF-α and, 283
    TS and, 80—84
Interferon-γ (IFN-γ), 103
    aging and, 139
    AM / PM treatment with, 201, 202
    aspirin and, 132, 133, 134
    C. albicans and, 98–99, 100, 162
    CisPt and, 237, 242
    Fcγ receptors and, 207, 208, 209, 210
    5-FU and, 74
    HPV and, 237, 242
    IFN-α and, 60–61
    LPS and, 198, 200
    perilymphatic injection of, 88, 89
    ST 789 and, 225, 227
    T-α1 and, 149, 154
    TNF-α and, 248
Interleukin (IL), 1, 60, *see also* specific
    types
    perilymphatic injection of, 87–94
    THs and, 177–182
Interleukin-1 (IL-1), 101, 103, 269, 270,
    272–273
    aging and, 140
    aspirin and, 132
    C. albicans and, 164
    gentamicin and, 101–102
    HIV-1 and, 120
    IFN-α / β and, 283, 284, 287–288
    IL-2 and, 283, 284–286, 288
    perilymphatic injection of, 89, 93
    ST 789 and, 225
    THs and, 177, 178, 179, 180, 181, 182
Interleukin-1α (IL-1α), 269, 270, 272–273
Interleukin-1β (IL-1β), 89, 101, 179
Interleukin-2 (IL-2), 39, 49–54, 60, 61–62,
    99, 100, 142, 270, 272, 275, 276,
    293
    aging and, 139, 140, 141–144
    arginine and, 224
    aspirin and, 131, 132, 133, 134, 135
    BMT and, 19–26
    CisPt and, 238, 242, 243
    CY and, 4, 9
    DOX and, 49, 50–51
    HIV-1 and, 114, 127, 168
    HPV and, 238, 242, 243
    IFN-α and, 49, 51–54, 61, 93
    IL-1 and, 283, 284–286, 288

Interleukin-2 (IL-2) (*cont'd*)
    in tumor control, 190, 191, 192
    LAK cells and, *see* under Lymphokine
      activated killer cells
    mAbs and, 192
    perilymphatic injection of, 88–89, 90–
      94
    PHA and, 81, 82, 83
    ST 789 and, 224, 225, 227
    T-α1 and, 149–150, 277–280
    THs and, 177, 178–179, 180, 181, 182
    TILs and, 39, 40, 41–42, 43, 44, 45,
      46, 47, 62, 92, 245–249
    TNF-α and, 245–249
Interleukin-3 (IL-3), 180
Interleukin-4 (IL-4), 99, 100
    perilymphatic injection of, 84, 93
    ST 789 and, 225
    TILs and, 39, 40, 41–42, 43, 44, 45,
      46, 47
Interleukin-6 (IL-6), 100, 177, 180, 225
Interleukin-7 (IL-7), 269, 270–272, 273
5-Iodo-2'-deoxyuridine, 296
Isoprinosine, 113, 114

Jurkat cells, 90

Kaposi's sarcoma, 13, 118
Keyhole limpet hemocyanin (KLH), 231–
    235
Klebsiella oxytoca, 226
Klebsiella pneumoniae, 226
KLH, *see* Keyhole limpet hemocyanin

LAK cells, *see* Lymphokine activated kil-
    ler cells
Lamina propria mononuclear cells
    (LPMC), 246–247, 248
L-AmpB, *see* Liposomal Amphotericin B
Langerhans cells, 243
Leishmaniasis, 106, 110
Lente viruses, 114
Leucovorin, 74, 245
Leukemia, 108, 113, 283, 284, 286, 287,
    288
    IFN-α and, 74
    IL-2 / LAK cells and, 19–26
    immune therapy and, 13–15
    traizene compounds and, 294, 295
Leukopenia, 75, 270
Leukoregulin, 237–243
Levamisole, 79, 114, 245